Acute Promyelocytic Leukemia

Oussama Abla • Francesco Lo Coco
Miguel A. Sanz
Editors

Acute Promyelocytic Leukemia

A Clinical Guide

Springer

Editors
Oussama Abla M.D.
Division of Hematology/Oncology
The Hospital for Sick Children and
University of Toronto
Toronto, Ontario, Canada

Francesco Lo Coco M.D.
Department of Hematology
University of Tor Vergata
Rome, Italy

Miguel A. Sanz M.D.
Department of Medicine, Hospital
Universitari i Politecnic La Fe,
University of Valencia
Valencia, Spain

Centro de Investigacion Biomedica en
Red de Cancer
Instituto Carlos III, Madrid, Spain

ISBN 978-3-319-64256-7 ISBN 978-3-319-64257-4 (eBook)
https://doi.org/10.1007/978-3-319-64257-4

Library of Congress Control Number: 2017962620

Printed on acid-free paper

This Springer imprint is published by the registered company Springer International Publishing AG part of Springer Nature
The registered company address is: Gewerbestrasse 11, 6330 Cham, Switzerland

Preface

Since its first identification by Leif Hillestad 60 years ago, acute promyelocytic leukemia (APL) has evolved from being the most fatal to the most curable type of acute myeloid leukemia. *Acute Promyelocytic Leukemia: A Clinical Guide* is the first book entirely dedicated to APL, a disease with a unique and fascinating biology, whose treatment has become a paradigm of modern targeted therapy.

Every chapter in this volume is written by a renowned expert in the field. The first three chapters address the historical aspects, origins, and molecular mechanisms of this leukemia. The following three chapters focus on the pathophysiology of bleeding and thrombosis, early death, and prognostic factors. The next three cover the evolution of therapy from chemotherapy-based to *all-trans* retinoic acid-chemotherapy, arsenic trioxide, and finally chemotherapy-free regimens. Subsequently, the book discusses minimal residual disease monitoring, treatment of refractory/relapsed disease, and the role of hematopoietic stem cell transplant. Special situations such as APL in children, in the elderly, and in pregnancy, therapy-related APL, and rare variants are also addressed. The final three chapters focus on therapy-related complications and management of APL in developing countries.

We would like to thank all the authors for their generous contributions to this volume.

Toronto, ON, Canada	Oussama Abla
Rome, Italy	Francesco Lo Coco
Madrid, Spain	Miguel A. Sanz

Contents

Contributors

Oussama Abla, M.D. Division of Hematology/Oncology, Department of Pediatrics, Hospital for Sick Children, Toronto, ON, Canada

Lionel Adès, M.D., Ph.D Service Hématologie Séniors, Hôpital Saint-Louis, Assistance Publique—Hôpitaux de Paris, Paris, France

Université Paris Diderot, Paris, France

Ombretta Annibali, M.D., Ph.D. UOC Hematology, Stem Cell Transplantation, University Hospital Campus Bio Medico, Rome, Italy

Luisa Corrêa de Araújo Koury, M.D. Department of Internal Medicine, Medical School of Ribeirão Preto and Centre for Cell-Based Therapy, University of São Paulo, São Paulo, SP, Brazil

Giuseppe Avvisati, M.D., Ph.D. UOC Hematology, Stem Cell Transplantation, University Hospital Campus Bio Medico, Rome, Italy

Eva Barragàn, Ph.D. Department of Medical Biopathology, Hospital Universitario La Fe, Valencia, Spain

Massimo Breccia, M.D., Ph.D. Department of Cellular Biotechnologies and Hematology, Sapienza University, Rome, Italy

Ming Chen, M.D. Department of Medicine and Pathology, Cancer Research Institute, Beth Israel Deaconess Cancer Center, Beth Israel Deaconess Medical Center, Harvard Medical School, Boston, MA, USA

Laura Cicconi, M.D. Department of Biomedicine and Prevention, University Tor Vergata, Rome, Italy

Giulia De Conti, Ph.D. Department of Experimental Oncology, European Institute of Oncology, Milan, Italy

Laurent Degos, M.D., Ph.D. Paris Diderot University—Academy of Medicine, Paris, France

Cécile Esnault, Ph.D. Université Paris Diderot, Sorbonne Paris Cité, Institut Universitaire d'Hématologie, Hôpital St. Louis, Paris, France

INSERM UMR 944, Equipe Labellisée par la Ligue Nationale contre le Cancer, Hôpital St. Louis, Paris, France

CNRS UMR 7212, Hôpital St. Louis, Paris, France

Elihu H. Estey, M.D. Department of Medicine, University of Washington, Seattle, WA, USA

Clinical Research Division, Fred Hutchinson Cancer Research Center, Seattle, WA, USA

Anna Falanga, M.D. Department of Immunohematology and Transfusion Medicine and the Hemostasis and Thrombosis Center, Hospital Papa Giovanni XXIII, Bergamo, Italy

Pierre Fenaux, M.D., Ph.D. Service Hématologie Séniors, Hôpital Saint-Louis, Assistance Publique—Hôpitaux de Paris, Paris, France

Université Paris Diderot, Paris, France

Aaron D. Goldberg, M.D., Ph.D. Leukemia Service, Memorial Sloan Kettering Cancer Center, Weill Cornell Medical College, New York, NY, USA

Gloria Iacoboni, M.D. Department of Hematology, Hospital Universitari i Politècnic La Fe, Valencia, Spain

Harry Iland, M.B.B.S., F.R.A.C.P., F.R.C.P.A. Institute of Haematology, Royal Prince Alfred Hospital, Camperdown, NSW, Australia

Matthew A. Kutny, M.D. Division of Hematology/Oncology, Department of Pediatrics, University of Alabama at Birmingham, Birmingham, AL, USA

Richard A. Larson, M.D. Department of Medicine and the Comprehensive Cancer Center, University of Chicago, Chicago, IL, USA

Sören Lehmann, M.D., Ph.D. Department of Medical Sciences, Uppsala University, Uppsala University Hospital, Uppsala, Sweden

Eva Lengfelder, M.D. Department of Hematology and Oncology, University Hospital Mannheim, Mannheim, Germany

Vikram Mathews, M.B.B.S., M.D., D.M. Department of Haematology, Christian Medical College and Hospital, Vellore, India

Lourdes Mendez, M.D., Ph.D. Department of Medicine and Pathology, Cancer Research Institute, Beth Israel Deaconess Cancer Center, Beth Israel Deaconess Medical Center, Harvard Medical School, Boston, MA, USA

Pau Montesinos, M.D., Ph.D. Department of Hematology, Hospital Universitari i Politècnic La Fe, Valencia, Spain

Centro de Investigación Biomédica en Red de Cáncer, Instituto Carlos III, Madrid, Spain

Pier Paolo Pandolfi, M.D., Ph.D. Department of Medicine and Pathology, Cancer Research Institute, Beth Israel Deaconess Cancer Center, Beth Israel Deaconess Medical Center, Harvard Medical School, Boston, MA, USA

Pier Giuseppe Pelicci, M.D., Ph.D. Department of Experimental Oncology, European Institute of Oncology, Milan, Italy

Department of Oncology and Hemathology, University of Milan, Milan, Italy

Mary-Elizabeth M. Percival, M.D. Department of Medicine, University of Washington, Seattle, WA, USA

Clinical Research Division, Fred Hutchinson Cancer Research Center, Seattle, WA, USA

Kristen Pettit, M.D. Department of Medicine and the Comprehensive Cancer Center, University of Chicago, Chicago, IL, USA

Ramy Rahmé, M.D. Service Hématologie Séniors, Hôpital Saint-Louis, Assistance Publique—Hôpitaux de Paris, Paris, France

Université Paris Diderot, Paris, France

Université Paris Diderot, Sorbonne Paris Cité, Institut Universitaire d'Hématologie, Hôpital St. Louis, Paris, France

INSERM UMR 944, Equipe Labellisée par la Ligue Nationale contre le Cancer, Hôpital St. Louis, Paris, France

CNRS UMR 7212, Hôpital St. Louis, Paris, France

Assistance Publique des Hôpitaux de Paris, Oncologie Moléculaire, Hôpital St. Louis, Paris, France

Eduardo M. Rego, M.D., Ph.D. Department of Internal Medicine, Medical School of Ribeirão Preto and Centre for Cell-Based Therapy, University of São Paulo, São Paulo, SP, Brazil

Raul Ribeiro, M.D. Division of Leukemia/Lymphoma, Department of Oncology, St. Jude Children's Research Hospital, Memphis, TN, USA

Laura Russo, Ph.D. Department of Immunohematology and Transfusion Medicine, Hospital Papa Giovanni XXIII, Bergamo, Italy

Anna Giulia Sanarico, Ph.D. Department of Experimental Oncology, European Institute of Oncology, Milan, Italy

Jaime Sanz, M.D. Department of Hematology, Hospital Universitari i Politècnic La Fe, University of Valencia, Valencia, Spain

Centro de Investigación Biomédica en Red de Cáncer, Instituto Carlos III, Madrid, Spain

Miguel A. Sanz, M.D. Department of Medicine, Hospital Universitari i Politecnic La Fe, Valencia, Spain

Centro de Investigacion Biomedica en Red de Cancer, Instituto Carlos III, Madrid, Spain

Javier de la Serna, M.D. Department of Hematology, Hospital Universitario 12 de Octubre, Madrid, Spain

Martin S. Tallman, M.D. Leukemia Service, Memorial Sloan Kettering Cancer Center, Weill Cornell Medical College, New York, NY, USA

Anna Maria Testi, M.D. Department of Cellular Biotechnologies and Hematology, Sapienza, University of Rome, Roma RM, Italy

Hugues de Thé, M.D., Ph.D. Université Paris Diderot, Sorbonne Paris Cité, Institut Universitaire d'Hématologie, Hôpital St. Louis, Paris, France

INSERM UMR 944, Equipe Labellisée par la Ligue Nationale contre le Cancer, Hôpital St. Louis, Paris, France

CNRS UMR 7212, Hôpital St. Louis, Paris, France

Assistance Publique des Hôpitaux de Paris, Oncologie Moléculaire, Hôpital St. Louis, Paris, France

Collège de France, PSL University, Paris, France

Thalia Vlachou, Ph.D. Department of Experimental Oncology, European Institute of Oncology, Milan, Italy

1 History of Acute Promyelocytic Leukemia

Laurent Degos

Introduction

Within a 60-year time span, the most severe acute leukemia—termed acute promyelocytic leukemia (APL) by the Norwegian author Leif Hillestad—was identified, characterized, and cured. The determination of a precise molecular definition of the genetic defect and the emergence of an anti-dogmatic paradigm have made the history of APL a model for the treatment of malignancies. However, the new concepts of in vivo malignant cell differentiation and cell death induced by cell modifiers were quite controversial, as illustrated by the anecdotes reported in this chapter. Furthermore, over the course of APL's history, the dialogue between onco-hematologist physicians and scientists from several worldwide hospitals and laboratories led to an impressive achievement: for the first time, a malignancy (and the most severe malignant disease of the blood, no less) was cured in standard conditions using cell modifiers without any chemotherapy, cytotoxic agents, or bone marrow grafts. Today, the prognosis for APL depends more on the timing of treatment initiation than on the treatment itself, as we shall see in this chapter.

L. Degos, M.D., Ph.D.
Paris Diderot University—Academy of Medicine, 16 rue Bonaparte, Paris, 75006, France
e-mail: laurentdegos@gmail.com

A Distinct Entity: "A Special Type of Leukemia" (1957–1987)

In the first 30 years after its identification, APL followed the conventional course of all types of leukemia: clinicians precisely described the disease and tried to manage its treatment. Long-term survival rates approached 25%, but clinicians were confronted with early bleeding diathesis. Late relapses (after 2 years) were rarely reported.

The Clinical Description

The first description of APL by Leif Hillestad, published in *Acta Medica Scandinavia* in 1957 [1], summarized the main clinical features of the disease and is still relevant today:

> "Evidence is presented for the existence of a special type of acute myelogenous leukemia. Three cases are described, characterized by:
>
> 1. A very rapid fatal course of only a few weeks' duration.
> 2. A white blood cell picture dominated by promyelocytes.
> 3. A severe bleeding tendency due to fibrinolysis and thrombocytopenia.
> 4. A normal ESR probably caused by reduced fibrinogen concentration in the plasma.
>
> It is suggested that this type is named acute promyelocytic leukemia. It seems to be the most malignant form of leukemia."

In 1959, Jean Bernard [2] reported the first series of 20 patients with APL, disclosing more

O. Abla et al. (eds.), *Acute Promyelocytic Leukemia*, https://doi.org/10.1007/978-3-319-64257-4_1

detailed criteria: numerous large granules in the cytoplasm of abnormal promyelocytes in the bone marrow, covering the nucleus and sometimes assembled in "faggots" of Auer rods, as well as a low count of blasts with a monocytoid appearance in the blood. Jacques Caen [3] more precisely defined the acquired hypofibrinogenemia. In fact, bleeding diathesis was the most impressive feature of the disease, accounting for 20–30% of deaths, which were mainly due to cerebral hemorrhages.

In 1976, the French–American–British (FAB) Nomenclature Committee assigned a specific classification of acute myelogenous leukemia (AML), the M3 type [4]. Later, the committee officially recognized a variant form of APL that combined bilobed nucleus blasts, nonvisible granules on light microscopy (microgranules), and a positive myeloperoxydase reaction, and which was often associated with high white blood cell counts and similar coagulation disorders [5]. A very rare variant form with basophilic microgranules instead of large azurophilic granules was also accepted as APL [6].

A Controversy About Treatment

The unpredictable onset of life-threatening bleeding diathesis was the major obstacle in the treatment of patients with APL. The disease seemed to be particularly sensitive to anthracycline treatment [7], showing high rates of complete remission. However, chemotherapy exacerbated bleeding diathesis and thus increased the risk of death. The central question of this era was how to manage coagulation disorders.

All hematologists agreed on platelet transfusions, so the controversies surrounded hypofibrinogenemia. Clinicians needed to determine if they were dealing with a primary or a secondary hypofibrinogenemia due to disseminated intravascular coagulopathy (DIC). These two conditions had different drug treatment options (antifibrinolytic drugs, heparin, or no coagulation drugs), platelet transfusion times, and chemotherapy initiation points (immediately or, in cases of DIC, after heparin treatment initiation). The presence of fibrinogen-fibrin degradation products in serum could not distinguish the two conditions. In France, a decrease of factors V and X led clinicians to treat patients with low-dose heparin. However, in Italy [8], normal levels of protein C and antithrombin III associated with an acquired reduction of alpha-2 plasmin inhibitor levels indicated a primary fibrinolysis.

Apart from age, the intensity of hypofibrinogenemia and high white blood cell counts were considered to be the two major prognostic factors: the first indicated an increased risk of early mortality and the second indicated a higher risk of relapse.

A Cytogenetic Signature

The abnormal cytogenetic feature that confirms the specific entity of APL was first described in 1976 as a partial deletion of chromosome 17 [9] and identified later by Janet Rowley from the same team as a balanced reciprocal translocation between the long arms of chromosome 15 and 17 [10]. The t (15;17) translocation was consistently found in APL bone marrow cells [11].

Thus, by the mid-1980s, APL could be defined not only by its morphological features and typical bleeding diathesis, but also by a specific cytogenetic abnormality.

The disease needed an adapted treatment: an aggressive and urgent initiation of anthracycline treatment, with special attention to the coagulation disorders. With this, a complete remission rate of approximately 75% was achieved, despite a high early mortality rate. Relapses still occurred in the first months after complete remission, with approximately 25% of patients surviving for more than 2 years.

A New Paradigm: The Differentiation of Malignant Cells

During the same time period, studies demonstrating the ability to transform malignant cells into terminally differentiated normal cells were received with skepticism. The dogma of the irreversible status of malignant cells was deeply anchored in the spirit of physicians and scientists.

The only accepted option to treat malignancies was to eliminate the cells by chemotherapy, radiotherapy, or surgical excision.

Abolishing the Dogma of the Irreversible Status of Malignant Cells

An Experimental Approach

In 1963, Leo Sachs (Rehovot, Israel; Fig. 1.1) developed a culture of cloned blood cells from mice [12]. From this, a number of growth factors were identified in 1970, , which he named in Hebrew; they were later renamed as granulocyte colony-stimulating factor, macrophage colony-stimulating factor, granulocyte-macrophage colony-stimulating factor, and interleukin-3. Sachs also demonstrated that cell lines from leukemic mice could be differentiated and become nondividing mature granulocytes or macrophages in cell cultures as a result of stimulation by various "differentiation factors" [13]. His presentation in 1973 at the Congress of the International Society of Genetics in Berkeley, California, was received with respect and some skepticism due to the artificial conditions of the experiments (cell lines, in vitro studies) and the absence of formal

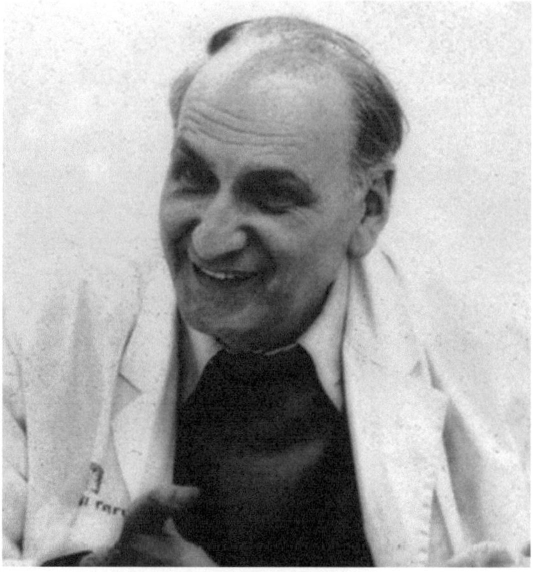

Fig. 1.1 Leo Sachs, 1924–2013

genetics. Later, in 1982, Sachs found that myeloid leukemic cells injected into embryos participated in apparent hemopoietic differentiation in the cells of adult mice [14].

A Clinical Approach

At Hospital Saint Louis in Paris, France, in June 1980, Laurent Degos proposed that his 52-year-old female patient with a resistant relapse of acute myelogenous leukemia return home for the end of life. The patient lived far away, in French Britany. Because her family was abroad, low-dose cytosine arabinoside (ARA-C; 10 mg twice a day subcutaneously) was initiated to delay the patient's death for few days. Four months later, the patient returned to the hospital in good condition with normal blood and bone marrow cell morphology. The general practitioner described a progressive improvement over several weeks. Two other patients experienced similar gradual improvements [15], with differentiation of leukemic cells in blood and bone marrow until complete remission was achieved. These clinical cases confirmed the experimental data of Leo Sachs on the reversibility of malignancies. Sachs often mentioned low-dose ARA-C as the human in vivo therapeutic achievement of his findings. The persistence of a cytogenetic signature in complete remission provided evidence in favor of the actual differentiation of malignant cells [16].

These results led to the new concept of differentiation therapy for human acute leukemia. However, in a trial using low-dose ARA-C, only 35% of patients obtained complete remission [17]. Later, alpha interferon treatment for hairy cell leukemia was also demonstrated to directly act as a cell modifier, interfering with the autocrine loop of proliferation [18].

All-Trans-Retinoic Acid as a Potential Candidate for Differentiation Therapy of APL

Although the treatment of malignancies was mainly focused on decreasing proliferation using antimitotic drugs, some scientists investigated the blockage of the differentiation of malignant cells. The arrest of maturation had been a major feature of malignancy since the first description by the pioneer Alfred Donné in 1844 [19].[1]

Murine myeloid leukemia cell lines, such as M-1 or erythroleukemia induced by the Friend virus, as well as human HL-60, KG 1, or K 562 cell lines, could be in vitro differentiated into granulocytes or monocytes using several agents, including polar plana compounds (e.g., the use of dimethyl sulfoxide for murine erythroleukemia cells by Charlotte Friend in 1971), butyric acid, hypoxanthine, ligands to nuclear receptors (vitamin D, or retinoic acid) and some antimitotic drugs (mainly ARA-C and aclacinomycin). In 1981, Theodore Breitman demonstrated the sensitivity of HL-60 cell lines to retinoids, as well as of cells from two patients with APL treated in short-term cell cultures [20]. However, an HL-60 cell line only possessing one chromosome 17 and not carrying the specific t (15-17) is not a promyelocytic cell line.

Cellular biologists and clinicians working on differentiation therapy assembled bi-annually, led by Samuel Waxman, Giovanni Battista Rossi, and Fuminaro Takaku. The first international conference on differentiation therapy in cancer was held in 1986 in Sardinia. This conference included the first generation of scientists and physicians investigating this new and antidogmatic field.

[1] *"Since I have frequently observed similar cases in the blood of individuals without purulent matter, I think that the excess of white blood cells is due to an arrest of differentiation. According to my theory about the origin and development of blood cells, that I have delivered several times, the increase of white blood cells is the consequence of an arrest of differentiation of these intermediate cells [ne sont que le résultat d'un arrêt de développement de ces particules intermédiaires]"* [19]. *John Hughes Bennett considered the presence of purulent matter in 1845 ("Two cases of disease and enlargement of the spleen in which death took place from the presence of purulent matter"). Also in 1845, Rudolph Virchow proposed that "Weisses Blut (Leukoemie)" was not purulent matter but a real new disease with splenomegaly and hemorrhage.*

The Dinner that Initiated All-Trans-Retinoic Acid Treatment for APL (1985)

Using a list of potential differentiation agents, Christine Chomienne tested more than 60 specimens of fresh bone marrow cells from various patients with leukemia (instead of cell lines) in short-term cultures. Chomienne demonstrated that the differentiating effect of retinoic acid was specific for APL. Among various vitamin A derivatives, all-trans-retinoic acid (ATRA) was potentially 10 times more effective than 13-cis or 4-oxo, whereas etretinate did not induce any differentiation [21]. At that time, etretinate (Tigazon) was the only derivative available in Europe and 13-cis (Roaccutane) was the only one available in the United States. Therefore, it was impossible to treat patients with an adequate derivative.

In 1985, a travel grant offered by Air France to Chinese professors of medicine provided an opportunity for the hematologist Wang Zhen Yi, Dean of the University of Medicine of Shanghai and French speaker by education, to visit Hospital Saint Louis. During a dinner at the home of Marie Thérèse Daniel, an FAB committee member (also attended by Chen Zhu, Wang's young student who was working in Daniel's morphology laboratory), a discussion between Laurent Degos and Wang Zhen Yi concerned a treatment designed to induce differentiation using low-dose ARA-C in patients and the specific in vitro activity of ATRA in APL (a drug not available in Western countries). The discussions resulted in the initiation of a close collaboration between the two researchers and in a decision to manufacture ATRA for APL patients in China. Several exchanges between the two institutes of hematology in Paris and Shanghai allowed for rapid progress against the disease. The two hematology institutes joined forces (Fig. 1.2) and established a formal agreement on April 25, 1987.

ATRA was first used to treat patients with APL in 1987 at Rui-Jin Hospital in Shanghai, where Laurent Degos visited to observe the remarkable effects of this treatment. Degos

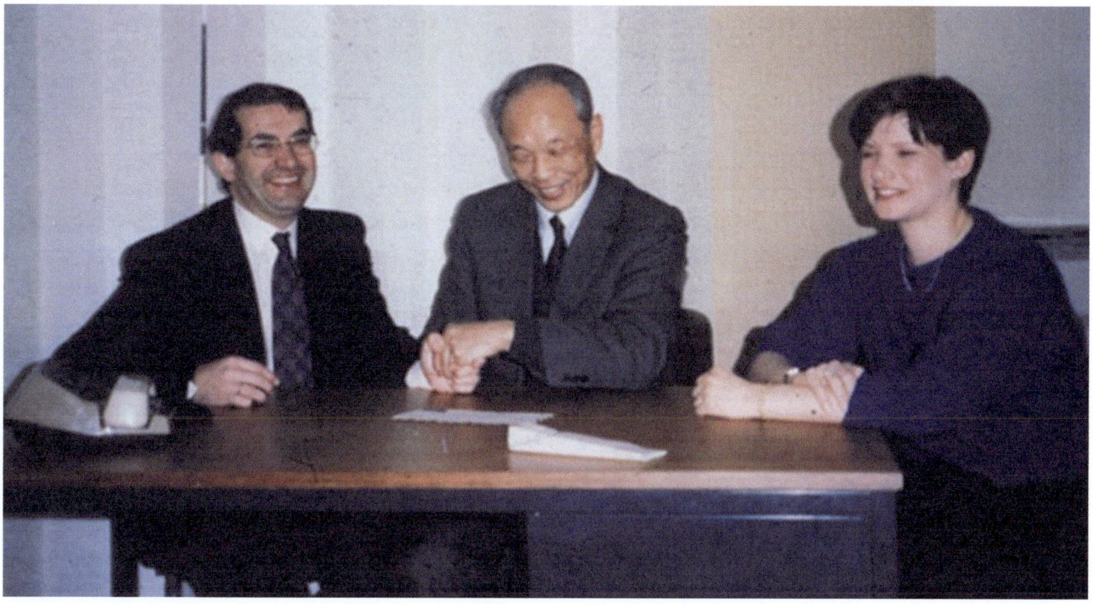

Fig. 1.2 Wang Zhen Yi with Laurent Degos and Christine Chomienne

and Wang delivered a joint presentation on differentiation therapies using low-dose ARA-C for AML and ATRA for APL at the Second Conference on Differentiation Therapy of Cancer in September 1987 in Bermuda [22]. Huang Meng Er [23] of Shanghai reported on the in vivo maturation of malignant cells until complete remission in 22 of 23 Chinese patients who were newly diagnosed with APL and treated with 45 mg/m^2 of ATRA. Sylvie Castaigne also reported on the remission of 19 of 20 patients who were treated in France after experiencing a relapse [24]. Complete remission was obtained without aplasia, alopecia, or primary resistance to the drug. Few infections were observed and coagulopathy rapidly improved within a few hours. The progressive terminal differentiation of leukemic cells in bone marrow (sometimes with the presence of Auer rods in mature granulocytes) completed the picture of unusual features for the treatment of myelogenous leukemia [24]. In response to a question from an *Impact Médecin* journalist on February 1, 1991, Wang Zhen Yi said in French: "Without the Laurent Degos team researchers and without our meeting face to face in 1985, nothing could have occurred. The Paris Saint Louis institute studies opened my eyes about the possibilities of all-trans-retinoic acid."[2]

Hoops and Hurdles

Although the availability of ATRA was no longer an obstacle, the road to a cure was not clear. Western companies still refused to manufacture the drug. ATRA was kindly provided by Shanghai producers and was transported by Chinese students when they travelled to Paris, the first of whom was Huang Meng Er.

Two anecdotes illustrate the skepticism that existed in those times on the use of ATRA as an antileukemic agent. First, when Christine Chomienne called Werner Bolag (a scientist from Roche Headquarters in Basel, Switzerland, who

[2] *"Sans les recherches de l'équipe du Pr Laurent Degos et sans notre rencontre en 1985, rien n'aurait été possible. Ce sont les travaux de Saint Louis qui m'ont ouvert les yeux quant aux possibilités de l'acide tout trans rétinoïque" Impact Médecin N°89 (1er Février 1991) p 11.*

specialized in ATRA) for some advice during the first ATRA treatment in France, he was horrified and asked her to immediately stop the treatment. Against his advice, Chomienne continued the treatment. In the second anecdote, a hematologist from New York asked the Paris team to obtain the drug for a young, relapsed patient. The package was ready to be sent with the approval of the Chinese collaborators, but the administration of the U.S. hospital refused to treat the patient with such "an experimental drug made in China and provided by French physicians." The patient subsequently died.

No More Product

Events in China in June 1989 made it difficult for Chinese students to travel. After the Tiananmen square demonstration, the French Government required all French institutions to end their collaborations with China. A shortage of ATRA occurred while several French patients were being treated. Confronted with this difficulty, Laurent Degos contacted Roche France. Victorine Carré agreed to make the drug and excluded all women from the factory during production (to prevent any teratogenous effects from retinoid contamination in the air). The board of Roche France asked Laurent Degos to restrict the administration of ATRA to French patients and to take total responsibility for any adverse events. According to the policy of Roche headquarters in Basel, vitamin A derivatives were exclusively used for patients with skin disorders.

During a 1989 spring meeting in Paris on antibodies appearing during interferon treatment for hairy cell leukemia chaired by Loretta Itri (Vice President of Roche; Nutley, NJ, USA), Laurent Degos asked her to obtain an ATRA source from Roche USA. Loretta Itri's answer was to consult her husband, Raymond Warrell, who was a hematologist at Memorial Sloan Kettering Cancer Center (MSKCC) in New York. Raymond Warrell was surprised by the differentiation effects of ATRA considering the irreversible status of malignancies. He suggested that Degos present his results in August 1989 in New York. In this presentation, Degos showed a series of bone marrow samples from several patients at various times after treatment, demonstrating the progressive terminal differentiation of malignant promyelocytes. The audience, which included the heads of MSKCC, was convinced. Raymond Warrell asked Loretta Itri to manufacture 2 million ATRA tablets—not only for patients with APL but also for extensive clinical trials involving other cancers and leukemias under the auspices of the National Cancer Institute. This happy ending opened the door to ATRA treatment for patients with APL all over the world.

Is APL a Pseudo-Leukemia?

One year later, French clinical results obtained using ATRA from China and Roche France [24] and cellular investigations [25] were published in the same issue of the journal *Blood,* which also printed images of the cells on the front cover. The journal included an editorial by Peter Wiernick, which asked whether APL was another pseudo-leukemia.[3] Is APL treated with a natural derivative of vitamin A similar to pernicious anemia treated by vitamin B12? A malignant cell could not remain malignant if its status was reversible. The concept that Leo Sachs formulated was not yet fully accepted in 1990. At that time, most thought leaders believed that if effective cell modifiers could treat a cancer, then the so-called cancer was not a malignancy.

Early Relapses with ATRA

Differentiation of malignant cells and rapid improvement of bleeding diathesis were the two breakthroughs in the treatment of APL [23, 24] confirmed in 1991 by a Chinese group [26] and by Raymond Warrell [27]. They provided evidence of the differentiation process by fluorescence in

[3]*"In 1875, William Pepper described the bone marrow of a fatal case of pernicious anemia as pseudoleukemia.... Ultimately, vitamin B12 was demonstrated to be the missing maturation and differentiation inducer, and continuous treatment with that agent uniformly cures the manifestations of the disease, but not the disease itself.... Another pseudoleukemia could be on the way out" (P.H. Wernick, Blood 1990;76:1675–1677).*

situ hybridization (FISH) and of the clonality using X chromosome-linked polymorphisms.

However, even though almost all patients experienced complete remission with ATRA (no primary resistance), all of them relapsed within 3–12 months (median: 5 months). The relapses were resistant to ATRA (secondary resistance) [24]. Considering the previous evidence that patients who were successfully treated with high-dose daunorubicin chemotherapy [28] had few relapses after 2 years, Laurent Degos decided to initiate a combination of ATRA and chemotherapy in 1990. Patients first received ATRA until they achieved complete remission. ATRA was then followed by intensive chemotherapy (induction and two courses of consolidation) to combine the positive effects of the two treatments—that is, complete remission with rapid disappearance of bleeding diathesis by ATRA and a relapse-free survival by intensive chemotherapy.

Hope for a Curable Disease

The first nonrandomized trial treated 26 patients using ATRA until complete remission, followed by three courses of daunorubicin and ARA-C. These results were compared to historical control groups of patients who received the same chemotherapy without ATRA [29]. The addition of ATRA greatly reduced early mortality and the number of early relapses. These favorable results prompted French investigators to launch the first randomized trial in 1991 using a similar study design but comparing the results to a control group instead of a historical group of patients. The trial ended prematurely after 18 months at the end of 1992 because event-free survival was significantly higher with ATRA [30]. This was the starting point for a big jump in long-term survival for patients with APL, from 25 to 75%.

Worldwide Enthusiasm

The second pivotal randomized trial was launched in 1993 by the same European Cooperative Group. The trial compared patients who were receiving ATRA followed by chemotherapy (the reference treatment) with patients who were receiving ATRA and concomitant chemotherapy followed by two courses of consolidation [31]. This trial demonstrated the superiority of the simultaneous regimen and the advantages of a maintenance therapy.

At that time, nonrandomized trials conducted by Wang Zhen Yi in China, Raymond Warrell in New York, and Akihisa Kamaru in Japan confirmed the beneficial effects of ATRA. Meanwhile, in 1993, an Italian group (Gruppo Italiano Malattie Ematologiche Maligne dell' Adulto, or GIMEMA) launched by Giuseppe Avvisati investigated a combinatorial approach of ATRA plus idarubicin (AIDA) for induction followed by three courses of consolidation [32]. This approach was further refined by a Spanish group (Programa Español de Tratamientos en Hematología, or PETHEMA) led by Miguel Sanz, which explored the benefits of treatment deintensification (especially in the consolidation phase). Japanese investigators led by Luizo Ohno made efforts to organize a controlled multicenter trial (the Japan Adult Leukemia Study Group, or JALSG). Furthermore, a U.S. intergroup also met several times to find a consensus for a study including ATRA. They started a randomized trial comparing ATRA plus two courses of chemotherapy to three courses of chemotherapy. In 1997, Martin Tallman reported better results when ATRA was administered, but an unexplained lower complete remission rate than the other cooperative groups (68% vs. ~90%) [33].

By the end of 1993, a high rate of complete remission, a reduced risk of early mortality, an absence of primary resistance, and a low relapse rate generated hope for curing at least 75% of patients with APL [34]. The first meeting on APL entitled "APL, A Curable Disease" was organized in Rome and chaired by Franco Mandelli, the founder of the GIMEMA group (Fig. 1.3). This positive outlook on a new original treatment for malignancies encouraged national and international collaborations, which led to larger studies: the European Cooperative group, which including French, Belgian, and Swiss researchers; the U.S. intergroup; a Japanese cooperative group; Chinese cooperative trials; PETHEMA in Spain enrolling

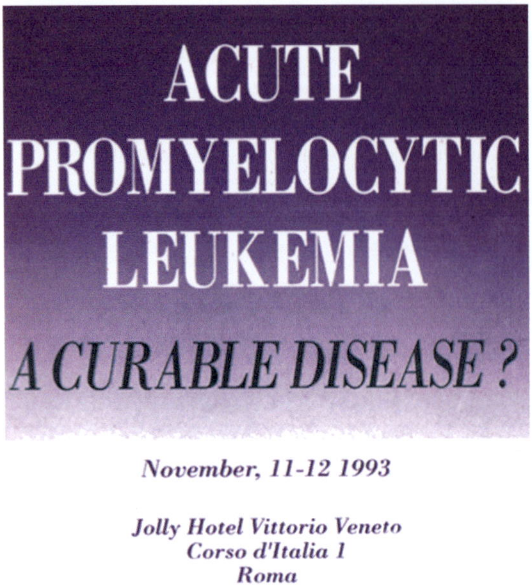

Fig. 1.3 First meeting on APL in Rome

patients from South America and Hovon in the Netherlands; a France-India cooperation; several meta-analyses jointly conducted by GIMEMA-PETHEMA and the French-Belgian-Swiss group in collaboration with PETHEMA; and finally, as we shall see later, the Italian-German GINEMAZ-SAL-AMSLG group.

New Clinical Horizons, Unknown Conditions

Hematopathologists were captivated by the features of progressive differentiation of malignant cells with distinctive Auer rods in mature polymorphonuclear cells. The nuclear bodies disrupted into multiple spots in leukemic cells but were reconstructed within 5 days of ATRA treatment [35]. The cell abnormalities of APL seemed to be restored by ATRA treatment—a treatment approach that was previously totally unknown for other malignancies. However, ATRA treatment led to three major unpredicted adverse effects: leukocyte activation, secondary resistance to ATRA, and thrombosis.

During the early days of treatment with ATRA, physicians were surprised by a potentially lethal syndrome, particularly in hyperleukocytic and microgranular forms of the disease. These patients experienced fever, weight gain, dyspnea due to pleural and pericardial effusions, pulmonary infiltrates, and sometimes renal failure [24]. The “ATRA syndrome” affected a third of patients in Western countries and Japan (but not in China). It was often preceded by an increase of white blood cells, but it was treated by early chemotherapy (European group) and high doses of corticosteroids (New York group). The syndrome was considered to be leukocyte activation related to cytokine release by the differentiating cells [36].

Using ATRA alone, very rare primary resistance to ATRA (in part attributed to rare mutations of the retinoic receptor pocket) contrasted with a short-lived complete remission (3–12 months) and a permanent secondary resistance when relapses occurred. Additional genetic defects of the retinoic receptor could not be involved because all patients acquired resistance to ATRA; the resistance was sometimes reversible after 12 months. Consequently, catabolic mechanisms were suspected and confirmed by a decrease in ATRA plasma concentrations; this was due to an increase of cytochrome P450 induced by ATRA itself, together with upregulation of the expression of cytoplasmic protein binding protein (CRABP II) depriving the nucleus of ATRA. Optimal intranuclear ATRA concentrations correlated with the range of differentiation of APL cells.

Bleeding diathesis rapidly disappeared after few days of ATRA treatment, with a concomitant decrease of primary fibrinolysis (and of extended proteolysis due to endocellular cathepsin G, elastase, and myeloblastin) [37]. The prothrombotic trend (DIC) was not counteracted by ATRA treatment, which explained why severe thrombosis occurred in some patients (particularly those receiving ATRA alone) and indicated the need for low-dose heparin in such cases.

Nonstandard Regimens

Patients with high white blood cell counts (>10 G/L) are often associated with a microgranular variant, which has a higher risk of early death due to hemorrhages or ATRA syndrome and a higher risk of relapse. Massive platelet transfusion, early chemotherapy, and high-dose corticosteroids can greatly improve the prognosis of these patients. The questions in the 1995s were the role of ARA-C in induction and consolidation (PETHEMA-GIMEMA), risk stratification, and the advantages and disadvantages of maintenance therapy. After long discussions among cooperative groups, the results of a French-Spanish collaborative meta-analysis and other studies suggested that ARA-C did not appear to be mandatory in induction therapy (mainly when idarubicin was proposed) but could be beneficial for high-risk patients, who were also most likely to need consolidation. The modalities of maintenance therapy (intermittent treatment with 6-mercaptopurine, methotrexate, and ATRA) were also a matter of controversy. Positive findings were observed by European (France, Belgium, Switzerland) and American groups but not by Italian and Japanese groups (see Chap. 8, p. 106). This could be a posteriori explained by the intensity of front line treatment: two courses of chemotherapy by the American group, three courses of chemotherapy by the European group, and four courses of chemotherapy by the Italian group.

APL is rare in children (10% of APL cases), with a higher incidence before the age of 4 years. Pediatricians were surprised by children's particular sensitivity to ATRA at the standard adult dose, with the occurrence of pseudotumor cerebri syndrome in 3–4% of cases. In response, ATRA was administered to pediatric patients at a half dose (25 mg/m^2), which was demonstrated to be as effective as the standard adult dose (45 mg/m^2).

Furthermore, ATRA seemed to abrogate any unfavorable conditions. For instance, compared to other secondary acute leukemias, patients with therapy-related APL experienced similar outcomes as patients with de novo APL when ATRA was included in the treatment scheme. Approximately 10–15% of APL cases occurred after chemotherapy or radiotherapy, mainly when they included anthracycline and/or mitoxantrone for breast cancer or multiple sclerosis. Another striking effect of ATRA was the similar survival of patients with or without other cytogenetic abnormalities that are usually considered to be poor prognostic factors for leukemia.

Molecular Defects

The specific sensitivity of APL to ATRA treatment and the genetic signature t (15;17) were intriguing. Clinicians contacted molecular biologists to answer the question.

First Attempts at Molecular Approaches

In 1988, Marie Geneviève Mattei in Montpelier [38] located the retinoic acid receptor alpha (RARA) on band q21 of the long arm of chromosome 17. One year prior, Martin Petkovitch (Pierre Chambon laboratory, Strasbourg) had cloned the RARA gene [39]. These two findings, in conjunction with the demonstration of ATRA sensitivity, prompted Laurent Degos and Christine Chomienne to go to Strasbourg and obtain the RARA probe to investigate the possible location of the RARA site translocation.

After initial attempts with Huang Meng Er (who recently moved from Shanghai) to explore RARA mRNA products in the blasts of patients with APL, the researchers contacted Hughes de Thé from Anne Dejean's laboratory at Pasteur Institute, who had previously cloned the RAR beta, and proposed a collaboration. Together, they found abnormalities of mRNA in the RARA of patients with APL but not of patients with other types of leukemia.

Early in 1989, they submitted an article describing these mRNA results to the *New England Journal of Medicine*. The manuscript was rejected. The reviewers believed that the observations were due to artefacts and polymorphisms at restriction sites, and they quoted a previous article from an American team that showed no particular expression pattern of RARA mRNA in APL. In fact, the blots from the quoted article depicted the RARA abnormalities, but the figures were printed upside down.

Meanwhile, the French group cloned and sequenced the breakpoint on the RARA gene [40] using the NB4 cell line established by Michel Lanotte [41] from a patient followed by Sylvie Castaigne. The partner gene of RARA was first named myl. Two other teams conducted concomitant investigations following different pathways and reached the same conclusions: one headed by Helen Solomon [42] on chromosome 17, and the second headed by Pier Giuseppe Pelicci [43] on several potential partner genes. One year later, the partner gene of RARA in the t (15;17) was sequenced by the French group [44] and Ron Evans's team [45]. Both groups published their results in the same issue of the journal *Cell*. The gene was renamed PML for promyelocytic leukemia, avoiding any confusion of myl with the myosin light chain gene. The PML-RARA fusion gene was definitively considered to be the precise signature of APL.

Clinical Consequences: Diagnostic and Follow-Up Tools

Reverse-transcription polymerase chain reaction (RT-PCR) was rapidly established in France and Italy. A European Biomed Program led by Christine Chomienne organized a series of technical workshops to standardize the tests. The GIMEMA studies demonstrated that the RT-PCR reaction after the end of consolidation therapy was negative in 95% of the patients. A conversion from a negative reaction to a positive reaction predicted a relapse, which led to an anticipated early salvage and thus improved the outcome [46]. This strategy of RT-PCR follow-up was further developed and adopted by several other investigators, including David Grimwade in the United Kingdom.

Hughes de Thé in France, Jacqueline Dick in the United States, and Brunangelo Falini [47] in Italy produced antibodies against the PML protein, allowing for a better description of nuclear bodies [35], the location of the PML protein on the outer shell of the bodies in any cell of the body, and the association of PML with several other molecules. A PML molecule involved in the structure of a nuclear body could be responsible for the oncogenesis by itself (truncated PML) and/or for the effect of disruption of the body on companion products in the clone of leukemic cells. Brunangelo Falini proposed that the disruption and rapid reconstruction of nuclear bodies be used as a diagnostic tool and as a determinant of ATRA sensitivity, respectively. The novel PML gene and protein were scrutinized. The two major breaking points leading to long and short PMLs and seven groups of protein isoforms were compared to clinical status. Some correlations but no clear stratification with the prognosis were reported (see Chap. 2, p. 18 and Chap. 11, p. 153).

Several other very rare leukemias (sometimes represented by just one single case report) were found to harbor a translocation involving the RARA gene and partner genes other than PML. Some of them were sensitive to ATRA (NPM, NuMA partners) but others were not (PLZF, Stat 5 partners). These findings helped biologists to better understand the oncogenesis and specific effects of ATRA.

Toward a Biological Explanation of Oncogenesis and Restoration

Among retinoic acid receptors, RARA was recognized by Hughes de Thé [48] as the most involved in myelopoiesis. PML-RARA transfections impaired the normal function of the RARA receptor of Cos cells, halting the differentiation of HL-60 cells usually obtained by ATRA, whereas RARA-deficient mice had normal (and increased) hematopoiesis. The paradox between the leukemia induced by PML-RARA and the normal granulopoiesis observed in RARA-deficient mice was intriguing. RARA treatment seemed to alleviate the blockage of differentiation, allowing for the effects of coactivators.

PML-RARA suppression was extensively studied by Suk Hyun Hong, Hugues de Thé, Pier Giuseppe Pelicci, Anne Dejean, Ron Evans, and other teams. RARA, a nuclear receptor (transcription factor) acts as a dimer with the retinoic X receptor (RXR) and binds co-repressors (SMRT, N-COR, and histone deacetylase) in the absence of a ligand (retinoic acid). In the presence of retinoic acid, it becomes an activator linked to histone acetylase. It was suggested that the PML-RARA product blocked the nuclear receptor at a suppressor status, but pharmacological doses of ATRA overcame the suppression (see Chap. 2, p. 19 and Chap. 4, p. 44 and p. 48). APL became a model for the study of the link between gene expressions and chromatine reshaping through deacetylation of histones and methylation of promotors. Histone deacetylation inhibitors such as trichostatin A, valproate, and demethylating agents were investigated as tools for experiments and potential anticancer drugs.

Later, Chen Zhu (who had returned to Shanghai) found more than 150 retinoic acid–induced genes (RIG) using differential display techniques on the NB4 cell line before and after ATRA treatment [49]. Pier Giuseppe Pelicci investigated interferences on other genes, such as the p53 product. Several avenues with few clear explanations were presented at the second APL meeting in November 1997. Only simple conclusions could be reached: RARA is involved in granulopoiesis, PML-RARA blocks the differentiation, and ATRA restores the normal differentiation. Furthermore, PML is involved in leukemogenesis through a structural disruption of nuclear bodies and ATRA restores the normal structure.

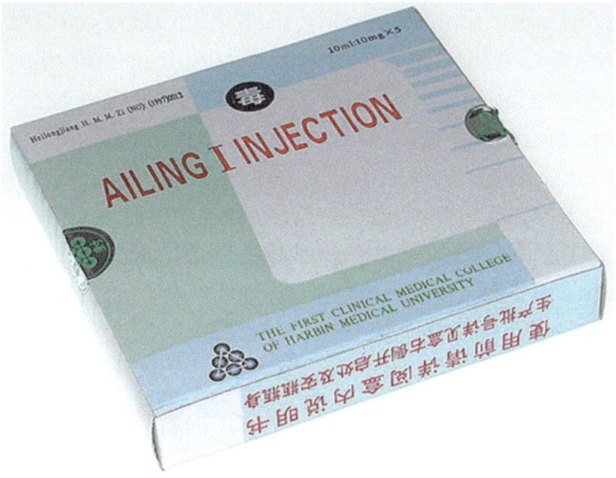

Fig. 1.4 Original Chinese ATO drug

Arsenic, a Manchurian Traditional Medicine (1995)

During the congress of the Chinese Society of Hematology at Da Lian (1995), to which Laurent Degos and Luizo Ohno were invited, two separate groups from Harbin in Manchuria reported that complete remission of APL was obtained with 10 mg/day of purified arsenic trioxide (ATO) given intravenously. The first trial was started in 1971 and included 60 patients—30 with de novo and 30 with relapsed disease; of these, 73% and 53% experienced complete remission, respectively. The second trial enrolled 72 patients; in this trial, 73% of the 30 patients with de novo and 52% of the 32 patients with relapsed disease obtained complete remission. A previous article from one of the groups, published in a relatively unknown Chinese journal [50], reported that 31 of the 42 patients treated with the AL-1 Harbin drug since 1971 achieved complete remission.

A Second Era for Clinicians

Chen Zhu's team in Shanghai used ATO with the so-called AILING I injection, manufactured by the "First Clinical Medical College of Harbin Medical University" (Fig. 1.4), to treat 10 patients with APL who relapsed after ATRA and chemotherapy. Of these patients, nine obtained complete remission. The only nonresponder lost the t(15;17) in malignant cells at relapse. They demonstrated differentiation and apoptotic effects at low and high concentrations, respectively [51].

Arsenic (Fowler liquor) had been designated since 1890 as an antileukemic drug in medical textbooks in Europe, with some rare but good outcomes. The spectacular effect of ATO in APL was first confirmed at MSKCC and then by several groups in Europe and Japan. Similarly to ATRA therapy, bleeding diathesis disappeared rapidly with ATO, eliminating not only the primary fibrinolysis but also the DIC. Like ATRA, ATO induced an "ATRA syndrome" consisting of leukocyte activation. Also like ATRA but with faster kinetics, the PML-RARA transcript was cleared.

ATO was rapidly manufactured (at a high price) in the United States and was used by many groups for relapsed patients to induce a second complete remission. The question at that time was whether to introduce ATO in first-line regimens. Some teams combined ATO with ATRA and chemotherapy during consolidation treatment and later during induction treatment to reduce the amount of chemotherapy needed; their results were at least similar to those obtained with classical ATRA–chemotherapy regimens. In other countries (mainly China, India, and Iran, who were manufacturing their own drugs at low prices), ATO was used alone, yielding complete remission rates of approximately 90% and long-term survival rates of approximately 70%. Thus, a second effective drug was available for patients with APL. However, Chinese researchers, who had acquired great experience with ATO, found that it was highly toxic for the liver in de novo patients when given in association with ATRA.

A Better Biological Understanding

Chen Zhu, in collaboration with Arthur Zelent, identified the first translocation that included the RARA gene with a different partner, namely PLZF [52]. The resistance of this rare disease to ATRA treatment was investigated by several groups. It was determined to be a result of a second binding to histone deacetylase through PLZF. For an unknown reason, the disease was sensitive to the association of ATRA plus a granulocyte colony-stimulating factor.

Animal models were used to gain a better understanding of the effect of the two drugs, ATRA and ATO (see Chap. 4). RARA knockout mice were viable, with no obvious defect in myelopoiesis. This was explained by the natural gene repression of RARA in the absence of a ligand. The absence of the receptor not only allowed for but also accelerated myelopoiesis. Italian scientists also aimed to reproduce APL disease in mouse models. PML-RARA transgenic mice were generated by Pier Giuseppe Pelicci and other groups using regulatory elements of the gene in promyelocytes, mainly cathepsin G or hMRP8. The mice developed ATRA-sensitive leukemia after a a long preleukemic state. Pier Paolo Pandolfi produced several transgenic mice (including transgenic, double transgenic, and knockout mice) by inserting not only PML-RARA or RARA-PML but also PLZF-RARA and other X-RARA fusion genes. Whatever the partner of RARA was, the mice developed a form of leukemia.

Using an APL model by transplanting spleen cells from APL transgenic mice, Valérie Lallemand and Hughes de Thé [53] demonstrated that ATRA and ATO had beneficial effects on induced APL in mice, but also that the combination of ATRA and ATO eradicated the disease. These findings gave hope for a definitive cure of the disease, encouraging clinicians to overcome the threats of the toxicity of ATRA-ATO combination previously described by Chinese investigators. A meeting jointly organized in October 2001 by Francesco Lo Coco and Samuel Waxman for the third symposium on "APL, a Curable Disease" chaired by Franco Mandelli and the 9th international conference on differentiation therapy led by Samuel Waxman envisaged new avenues for treatments, not only for patients with APL but also for patients with other malignancies using cell modifier agents.

ATRA-ATO Combination in Patients: From Curable to Cured APL

The next achievements are described in each chapter of this book. To summarize, in the 1991–2001 decade, international cooperative groups improved the outcomes of patients with APL using a combination of ATRA and chemotherapy by refining therapy though the addition or omission of maintenance treatment, grading the disease in high- and low/intermediate-risk groups of patients, adapting treatment to these criteria, modulating the chemotherapy for elderly patients, and decreasing the ATRA dose for children. Trials for relapsed patients also prompted to the implementation of worldwide cooperative groups due to the rarity of this event.

The synergic action of ATRA and ATO was further demonstrated by collaborative research between Shanghai and Paris, which showed that arsenic targeted PML moiety, whereas ATRA acted on the RARA moiety of the PML-RARA fusion gene. Several complementary (or controversial) studies led to the conclusion that the PML-RARA oncogenic product is degraded (and eliminated) through an ubiquitination at the RARA end by ATRA and through a sumoylation at the PML end by ATO.

The simultaneous use of ATRA and ATO in the first-line treatment of patients with APL in nonrandomized trials was previously approached by Chen Zhu (China) and Elihu Estey (United States), who demonstrated a synergistic effect in inducing prolonged complete remissions. Elihu Estey first proposed this combination as an alternative to chemotherapy for newly diagnosed patients and published excellent outcomes using a protocol that completely omitted chemotherapy.

The GIMEMA group, led by Francesco Lo Coco, conducted a randomized trial in 2006 in collaboration with German cooperative groups AMLSG and SAL [54], which challenged the conventional use of ATRA and idarubicin (AIDA) against the ATRA-ATO scheme designed by Estey [55]. The results demonstrated the superiority of the latter approach and ultimately the extraordinary achievement of the ATO-ATRA venture: APL is a malignant disease cured by cell-modifying agents without any chemotherapy. The GIMEMA-SAL-AMLSG study published in July 2013 in the *New England Journal of Medicine* and another independent randomized study conducted by the Medical Research Council led by Alan Burnett and presented at the 6th APL Symposium in Rome (October 2013) clearly showed that, at least in patients with low- to intermediate-risk APL, ATRA-ATO was better than ATRA-anthracycline-based chemotherapy. Nearly 100% of patients were event free at 2 years, without notable toxicity [56].

However, despite these compelling data, ATO was still not available for first-line treatment in Western countries. Regulatory bodies (mainly the European Medicines Agency, or EMA) did not provide market approval because the trials were conducted by academic groups and not by the industrial companies manufacturing the drug. In February 2015, a common letter signed by all European thought leaders and chairs of large cooperative groups on APL treatment was sent to the EMA, requesting a solution to this unfavorable situation. Hematologists needed drug approval for first-line therapy of APL without having to conduct further randomized trials, which would be unethical given the compelling results published in randomized studies. The EMA reacted with an open-minded attitude and proposed a meeting to discuss the issue with all involved partners and stakeholders (regulatory experts, manufacturing companies, thought leaders, and patient advocacy representatives) in London in July 2015. Solutions were explored and the way was paved toward a solution.

And Beyond: Lessons and Questions

History has demonstrated that a cure for APL using cell modifiers was not obtained by chance. Rather, it resulted from a long-term aim to modify malignant cells. Collaboration between several institutes of hematology around the world counteracted the obstacles. Clinical and biological findings were achieved by academic collaborations, often against the strategies of companies. The APL story is a model for international academic collaboration, both in clinical and laboratory investigations.

ATRA and ATO, the two cell-modifying agents, were neither promoted nor defended by companies. They were not actually recognized as innovative drugs, or even considered as nonconventional drugs. They were often the subject of controversies and discussions that delayed their use in patients. Conversely, when Gleevec, another target therapy, appeared 10 years later in the market, the support of the company facilitated the approval.

Today, the outcomes of patients with APL around the world are partly attributable to treatment choices and the availability of clinical facilities, but mostly attributable to rapid diagnosis and the delivery of appropriate treatment. In fact, the risk of early mortality before the initiation of ATRA treatment still persists and is the main obstacle to an APL cure. Some countries are educating physicians (including general practitioners and residents) and laboratories to shorten the time between the first symptom and hemogram, between the hemogram and myelogram, and between the myelogram and treatment. APL outcomes are related to the healthcare facility, so the differences in developed countries (early mortality rates before treatment ranging from 5% to 20%) should be further investigated and improved.

The purpose of ATRA and ATO targeted treatment is unique compared with the other targeted drugs used for cancer therapy (e.g., the series of antikinases). ATRA and ATO modify and restore normal transcription activities, whereas antikinases are generally antienzyme agents that inhibit hypersignals of transduction. The pathway to transcription normalization is still unclear: Is it the degradation of the oncogenic PML-RARA product, histone reshaping, or a mix of both mechanisms? Concerning the PML protein, what are the respective roles of PML and its partners on the nuclear body? Which metabolic pathway is modified (P53, others) and restored? Do the effects of ATO mainly consist of differentiation, restoration of apoptosis, normal self-renewal, or normal senescence? What is the role of the proteasome? Would a proteasome inhibitor block the effects of ATRA and/or ATO? What is the pathway between sumoylation and degradation of the product, and is it a degradation or an autophagy? So many question remain without definitive answers.

It is also unclear why one series of ATRA plus ATO is enough to definitively cure patients, whereas Gleevec (and other target antikinase drugs) are often administered for the rest of a patient's life. Does it eradicate the clone and the stem cell upstream to which the clone is derived? Why does the change from co-repressor to co-activator remain for life? How could degradation of the PML-RARA product erase a clone? Is it due to an immunological effect, like a vaccine (which was investigated by Rose Ann Padua)? What is the immunogenic product? Could a relapse occur in cases of immune deficiency?

More intriguing facts are as yet unexplained. When ATRA or ATO are administered, additional cytogenetic abnormalities do not affect prognosis, as commonly occurs in other leukemias. Is the differentiation of malignant cells the major defect to be treated, whatever the other events may be? If so, should we abandon the other avenues to cure patients that target, for instance, proliferation? Except for Gleevec in chronic myeloid leukemia, where cells are already well differentiated, any targeted antiproliferative treatment (i.e., antikinases) has delayed the progression of disease and patients were not cured. Although few studies have focused on the restoration of normal transcription and normal differentiation (probably due to the difficulty of manipulating transcription factors), the APL story should encourage researchers to move in this direction.

Conflict of Interest Laurent Degos has no conflict of interest to disclose.

References

1. Hillestad LK. Acute promyelocytic leukemia. Acta Med Scand. 1957;159:189–4.
2. Bernard J, Mathé G, Boulay J, Ceoard B, Chome J. Acute promyelocytic leukemia: a study made on 20 cases. Schweiz Med Wochenschr. 1959;89:604–8.
3. Caen J, Larrieu MH, Bernard J. Afibrinemies acquises. Rev French Clin Biol. 1959;4:363–6.
4. Bennett JM, Catowsky D, Daniel MT, Flandrin G, Galton D, Gralnick M, Sultan C. Proposals for the classification of acute leukemias. Br J Haematol. 1976;33:451–8.
5. Bennett JM, Catowsky D, Daniel MT, Flandrin G, Galton D, Gralnick M, Sultan C. A variant form of hypergranular promyelocytic leukemia. Br J Haematol. 1980;44:169–70.
6. McKenna RW, Parkin J, Bloomfield CD, Sunberg RD, Brunning RD. Acute promyelocytic leukaemia: a study of 39 cases with identification of a hyperbasophilic microgranular variant. Br J Haematol. 1982;50:201–14.
7. Bernard J, Weil M, Boiron M, Jacquillat C, Flandrin G, Gemon MF. Acute promyelocytic leukemia. Results of treatment with daunorubicin. Blood. 1973;41:489–96.
8. Avvisati G, ten Cate JW, Sturk A, Lamping R, Petti MC, Mandelli F. Acquired alpha2 antiplasmin deficiency in acute promyelocytic leukaemia. Br J Haematol. 1988;70:43–8.
9. Golomb HM, Rowley J, Vardiman J, Baron J, Locker G, Krasnow S. Partial deletion of long arm of chromosome 17: a specific abnormality in acute promyelocytic leukemia? Arch Intern Med. 1976;136:293–6.
10. Rowley J, Golomb HM, Dougherty C. The 15/17 translocation: a consistent chromosomal change in acute promyelocytic leukemia. Lancet. 1977;1:549–50.
11. Larson RA, Kondo K, Vardiman JW, Butler AE, Golomb HM, Rowley J. Evidence for a 15;17 translocation in every patient with acute promyelocytic leukemia. Am J Med. 1984;76:827–41.
12. Ginsburg H, Sachs L. Formation of pure suspensions of mast cells in tissue culture by differentiation of lymphoid cells from the mouse thymus. J Natl Cancer Inst. 1963;31:1–40.
13. Paran M, Sachs L, Barak Y, Resnitzky P. In vitro induction of granulocyte differentiation in hematopoietic cells from leukemic and non-leukemic patients. Proc Natl Acad Sci. 1970;67:1542–9.

14. Gootwine E, Webb CG, Sachs L. Participation of myeloid leukemic cells injected into embryos in haematopoietic differentiation in adult mice. Nature. 1982;299:63–5.
15. Housset M, Daniel MT, Degos L. Small doses of ARA-C in the treatment of acute myeloid leukemia: differentiation of leukemic cells? Br J Haematol. 1982;51:125–9.
16. Tilly H, Bastard C, Bizet M, Piguet H, Castaigne S, Degos L. Low-dose cytarabine: persistence of a clonal abnormality during complete remission of acute nonlymphocytic leukemia. N Engl J Med. 1986;314(4):246–7.
17. Tilly H, Castaigne S, Bordessoule D, Sigaux F, Daniel MT, Monconduit M, Degos L. Low-dose cytosine arabinoside treatment for acute nonlymphocytic leukemia in elderly patients. Cancer. 1985;55(8):1633–6.
18. Génot E, Bismuth G, Degos L, Sigaux F, Wietzerbin J. Interferon-alpha downregulates the abnormal intracytoplasmic free calcium concentration of tumor cells in hairy cell leukemia. Blood. 1992;80(8):2060–5.
19. Degos L. Alfred Donné. Hematol J. 2001;2 (1).
20. Breitman TR, Collin SJ, Keene BR. Terminal differentiation of human promyelocytic leukemic cells in primary culture in response to retinoic acid. Blood. 1981;57:1000–4.
21. Chomienne C, Balitrand N, Abita JP. Inefficacy of the synthetic aromatic retinoid etretinate and its free acid on the in vitro differenciation of leukemic cells. Leuk Res. 1986;10:1079–81.
22. Degos L, Castaigne S, Chomienne C, Huang ME, Tilly H, Bordessoule D, et al. Therapeutic trials of acute myeloid leukemias and myelodysplastic syndromes by LD ARA-C and treatment of acute promyelocytic leukemia by retinoic acid. In: Waxman S, Rossi GB, Takaku F, editors. The status of differentiation therapy of cancer. Vol. 45. Serono Symposium Publications, Raven Press; 1988. p. 361–73.
23. Huang ME, Yu-Chen Y, Shu-Rong C, Jin-Ren C, Lu JX, Zhoa L, Gu LJ, Wang ZY. Use of all trans retinoic acid inthe treatment of acute promyelocytic leukemia. Blood. 1988;72:567–72.
24. Castaigne S, Chomienne C, Daniel MT, Ballerini P, Berger R, Fenaux P, Degos L. All-trans retinoic acid as a differentiation therapy for acute promyelocytic leukemia. I. Clinical results. Blood. 1990;76:1704–9.
25. Chomienne C, Ballerini P, Balitrand N, Daniel MT, Fenaux P, Castaigne S, Degos L. All-trans retinoic acid in acute promyelocytic leukemias. II. In vitro studies: structure-function relationship. Blood. 1990;76:1710–7.
26. Chen XJ, Xue YQ, Zhang R, Tao RF, Xia XM, Li C, Wang W, et al. A clinical and experimental study on all trans retinoic acid treated acute promyelocytic leukemia patients. Blood. 1991;78:1413–9.
27. Warrell RP, Frankel SR, Miller WH, Scheinberg DA, Itri L, Hittelman WN, Vyas R, et al. Differentiation therapy of acute promyelocytic leukemia with tretinoin (all trans retinoic acid). N Engl J Med. 1991;324:1385–93.
28. Marty M, Ganem G, Fisher J, Flandrin G, Berger R, Schaison G, Degos L, Boiron M. Leucémie aigue promylocytaire: étude retrospective de 119 malades traités par daunorubicine. Nouv Rev Fr Hematol. 1984;26:371–8.
29. Fenaux P, Castaigne S, Dombret H, Archimbaud E, Duarte M, Morel P, Lamy T, et al. All trans retinoic acid followed by intensive chemotherapy gives a high complete remission rate and may prolong remissions in newly diagnosed acute promyelocytic leukemia: a pilot study on 26 cases. Blood. 1992;80:2176–81.
30. Fenaux P, Le Deley MC, Castaigne S, Archimbaud E, Chomienne C, Link H, Guerci A, et al. Effect of all trans retinoic acidin newly diagnosed acute promyelocytic leulemia. Result of a multicenter randomized trial. European APL 91 Group. Blood. 1993;82:3241–9.
31. Degos L, Dombret H, Chomienne C, Daniel MT, Miclea JM, Chastang C, Castaigne S, Fenaux P. All trans retinoic acid as a differentiating agent in acute promyelocytic leukemia. Blood. 1995;85:2643–53.
32. Avvisati G, Lo Coco F, Diveiro D, Falda M, Ferrara F, Lazzarino M, Russo D. AIDA (all-trans retinoic acid + idarubicin) in newly diagnosed acute promyelocytic leukemia: a Gruppo Italiano Malattie Ematologiche Maligne dell'Adulto (GIMEMA) pilot study. Blood. 1996;88:1390–8.
33. Tallman MS, Andersen JW, Schiffer CA, Appelbaum FR, Feusner JH, Ogden A, Shepherd L, et al. All trans retinoic acid in acute promyelocytic leukemia. New Engl J Med. 1997;337:1021–8.
34. Degos L. Is acute promyelocytic leukemia a curable disease? Treatment strategy for long term survival. Leukemia. 1994;8:56s–8s.
35. Daniel MT, Koken M, Romagne O, Barbey S, Bazarbachi A, Stadler M, Guillemin MC, Degos L, et al. PML expression in hematopoietic and APL cells. Blood. 1993;82:1858–67.
36. Dubois C, Schlateger MH, de Gentile A, Balitrand N, Toubert ME, Krawice I, Fenaux P, et al. Hematopoietic growth factor expression and ATRA sensitivity in acute promyelocytic leukemia. Leukemia. 1994;8:1750–7.
37. Dombret H, Scrobohaci ML, Daniel M, Miclea JM, Castaigne S, Chomienne C, Fenaux P, Degos L. In vivo thrombin and plasmin activities in patients with acute promyelocytic leukemia (APL): effect of all trans retinoic acid (ATRA) therapy. Leukemia. 1995;9:19–24.
38. Mattei MG, Petkovitch M, Mattei JF, Brand N, Chambon P. Mapping of the human retinoic acid receptor to the q21 band of chromosome 17. Hum Genet. 1988;80:186–8.
39. Petkovitch M, Brand NJ, Krust A, Chambon P. A human retinoic acid receptor which belong to the family of nuclear receptors. Nature. 1987;330:444–50.
40. de Thé H, Chomienne C, Lanotte M, Degos L, Dejean A. The t(15;17) translocation of acute promyelocytic leukaemia fuses the retinoic acid receptor alpha gene to a novel transcribed locus. Nature. 1990;347:558–61.

41. Lanotte M, Martin-Thouvenin V, Najman S, Ballerini P, Valensi F, Berger R. NB4 a maturation inducible cell line with t(15;17) marker isolated from a Human acute promyelocytic leukemia (M3). Blood. 1991;77:1080–6.
42. Borrow J, Goddard A, Sheer D, Solomon E. Molecular analysis of acute promyelocytic leukemia breakpoint cluster region on chromosome 17. Science. 1990;249:1577–80.
43. Longo L, Diviero D, Pandolfi PP, Biondi A, Rambaldi A, Mencarelli A, Lo Coco F, et al. Rearrangement and aberrant expression of the retinoic acid receptor alpha gene in acute promyelocytic leukemia. J Exp Med. 1990;172:1571–5.
44. de Thé H, Lavau C, Marchio A, Chomienne C, Degos L, Dejean A. The PML-RAR alpha fusion mRNA generated by the t(15;17) translocation in acute promyelocytic leukemia encodes a functionally altered RAR. Cell. 1991;66:675–84.
45. Kakizuka A, Miller WH Jr, Umesono K, Warrell RP, Frankel SR, Murty VS, Dimitrovsky E, Evans R. Chromosomal translocation t(15;17) in human acute promyelocytic leukemia fuses RAR alpha with a novel putative transcription factor PML. Cell. 1991;66:663–74.
46. Lo Coco F, Diviero D, Pandolfi PP, Biondi A, Rossi V, Avvisati G, Rambaldi A, Arcese W, et al. Molecular evaluation of residual disease as a predictor of relapse in acute promyelocytic leukemia. Lancet. 1992;340:1437–8.
47. Falini B, Flenghi L, Fagioli M, Lo Coco F, Cordone I, Diverio D, Pasqualucci L, et al. Immunocytochemical diagnosis of acute promyelocytic leukemia (M3) with the monoclonal antibody PG-M3 (anti-PML). Blood. 1997;90:4046–53.
48. De Thé H, Marchio A, Tiollais P, Dejean A. Differential expression and ligand regulation of the retinoic acid alpha and beta genes. EMBO J. 1989;8:429–33.
49. Mao M, Yu M, Tong JH, Ye J, Zhu H, Huang QH, Fu G, Yu L, et al. RIG-E, a human homolog of the murine Ly-6 family is induced by retinoic acid during the differentiation of acute promyelocytic leukemia cell. Proc Natl Acad Sci. 1996;93:5910–4.
50. Sun HD, Ma L, Hu XC, Zhang TD. Treatment of acute promyelocytic leukemic by AL-1 therapy. Chin J Integrat Tradit West Med. 1992;12:170–2.
51. Chen GQ, Zhu J, Shi XG, Hi JH, Zhong HJ, Si GY, Jin XL, et al. In vitro studies on cellular and molecular mechanisms of arsenic trioxide (As2O3) in the treatment of acute promyelocytic leukemia. Blood. 1996;78:1052–61.
52. Chen ZC, Brand NJ, Chen A, Chen SJ, Tong SH, Wang ZY, Waxman S, Zelent A. Fusion between a novel Krüppel-like zinc finger gene and the retinoic acid receptor alpha locus due to a variant(11;17)translocation associated with acute promyelocytic leukemia. EMBO J. 1993;12:1161–7.
53. Lallemand-Breitenbach V, Guillemin MC, Janin A, Daniel MT, Degos L, Kogan SC, Bishop JM, de Thé H. Retinoic acid and arsenic synergize to eradicate leukemic cells in a mouse model of acute promyelocytic leukemia. J Exp Med. 1999;189:1043–52.
54. Lo-Coco F, Avvisati G, Vignetti M, Thiede C, Orlando SM, Iacobelli S, Ferrara F, Fazi P. Gruppo Italiano Malattie Ematologiche dell'Adulto; German-Austrian Acute Myeloid Leukemia Study Group; Study Alliance Leukemia. Retinoic acid and arsenic trioxide for acute promyelocytic leukemia. N Engl J Med. 2013;369:111–21.
55. Estey E, Garcia-Manero G, Ferrajoli A, Faderl S, Verstovsek S, Jones D, et al. Use of all-trans retinoic acid plus arsenic trioxide as an alternative to chemotherapy in untreated acute promyelocytic leukemia. Blood. 2006;107:3469–73.
56. Burnett A, Russell NH, Hills RK, et al. Arsenic trioxide and all-trans retinoic acid treatment for acute promyelocytic leukemia in all risk groups (AML17): results of a randomised, controlled, phase 3 trial. Lancet Oncol. 2015;16:1295–305.

Molecular Targets of Treatment in Acute Promyelocytic Leukemia

2

Ramy Rahmé, Cécile Esnault, and Hugues de Thé

Introduction

Acute promyelocytic leukemia (APL) is the M3 subtype of acute myeloid leukemia (AML), characterized at the cellular level by a differentiation block of the granulocytic lineage at the promyelocytic stage. On the molecular level, more than 98% of APL cases are caused by the chromosomal translocation t(15;17) which implicates the two genes promyelocytic leukemia (PML) and retinoic acid receptor alpha (RARA), leading to the expression of the *PML/RARA* fusion oncoprotein [1]. In the RARA gene, the breakdown always occurs in the intron 2, whereas three breakdown regions were described occurring in the PML gene and resulting in the expression of two long isoforms (bcr1 and bcr2 transcripts) and one short isoform (bcr3 transcript) (Fig. 2.1) [1–3]. Other translocations were reported in APL always involving the RARA gene with various gene partners, of which PLZF is the most common [4]. This chapter will discuss the role of *PML/RARA* in the development of APL while focusing on the importance of treatment-triggered *PML/RARA* degradation and PML/P53-driven senescence in the pathophysiology of cure.

R. Rahmé, M.D.
Service Hématologie Séniors, Hôpital Saint-Louis, Assistance Publique—Hôpitaux de Paris, Paris, France

Université Paris Diderot, Paris, France

Université Paris Diderot, Sorbonne Paris Cité, Institut Universitaire d'Hématologie, Hôpital St. Louis, Paris, France

INSERM UMR 944, Equipe Labellisée par la Ligue Nationale contre le Cancer, Hôpital St. Louis, Paris, France

CNRS UMR 7212, Hôpital St. Louis, Paris, France

Assistance Publique des Hôpitaux de Paris, Oncologie Moléculaire, Hôpital St. Louis, Paris, France
e-mail: ramy.rahme@gmail.com

C. Esnault, Ph.D.
Université Paris Diderot, Sorbonne Paris Cité, Institut Universitaire d'Hématologie, Hôpital St. Louis, Paris, France

INSERM UMR 944, Equipe Labellisée par la Ligue Nationale contre le Cancer, Hôpital St. Louis, Paris, France

CNRS UMR 7212, Hôpital St. Louis, Paris, France

H. de Thé, M.D., Ph.D. (✉)
Université Paris Diderot, Sorbonne Paris Cité, Institut Universitaire d'Hématologie, Hôpital St. Louis, Paris, France

INSERM UMR 944, Equipe Labellisée par la Ligue Nationale contre le Cancer, Hôpital St. Louis, Paris, France

CNRS UMR 7212, Hôpital St. Louis, Paris, France

Assistance Publique des Hôpitaux de Paris, Oncologie Moléculaire, Hôpital St. Louis, Paris, France

Collège de France, PSL University, Paris, France
e-mail: hugues.dethe@inserm.fr

O. Abla et al. (eds.), *Acute Promyelocytic Leukemia*, https://doi.org/10.1007/978-3-319-64257-4_2

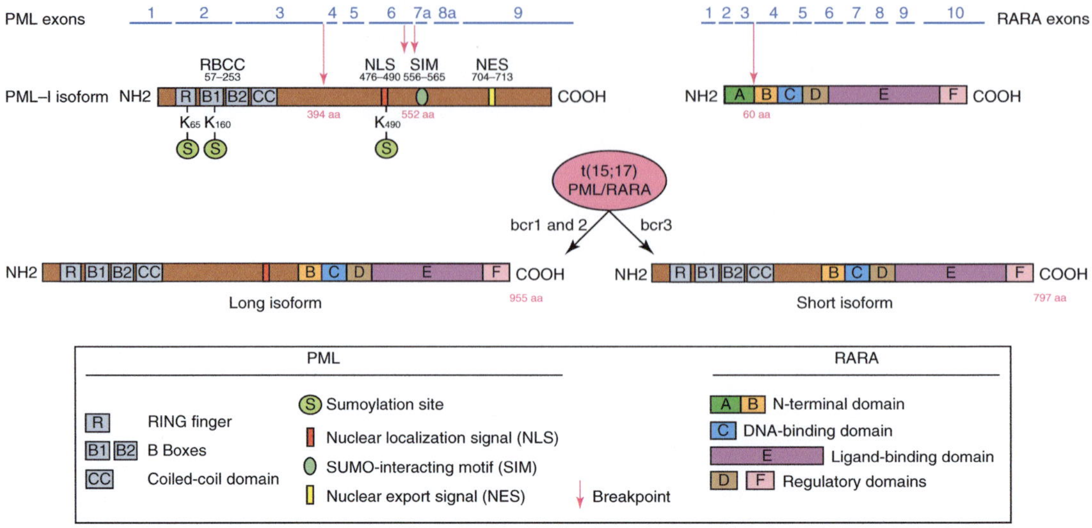

Fig. 2.1 The t(15;17) translocation partners. The t(15;17) translocation involves two genes, PML and RARA, leading to the expression of the PML/RARA fusion protein. The breakpoints always occur in the intron 2 of the RARA gene, whereas three breakdown regions were described in the PML gene: in the intron and exon 6 for bcr1 and bcr2 transcripts, respectively, and in the intron 3 for bcr3 transcript. This results in the expression of two long PML/RARA isoforms (bcr1 and 2) and one short (bcr3). PML/RARA retains all the functional domains of RARA (notably the DNA- and ligand-binding domains) and PML (in particular the RING finger and coiled-coil domains). *bcr* breakpoint cluster region

The Translocation Partners: RARA and PML

RARA, the retinoic acid (RA) receptor alpha, is a nuclear transcription factor activated by retinoids—such as all-trans retinoic acid (ATRA). Upon heterodimerization with its cofactor the retinoic X receptor (RXR) [5], the RARA/RXR complex binds to specific DNA RA response elements (RARE) composed typically of two direct repeats of a core hexameric motif, PuG [G/T] TCA; the classical RARE is a 5 bp-spaced direct repeat [6]. In the absence of the ligand, RARA/RXR interacts with nuclear receptor corepressors such as N-CoR (nuclear receptor corepressor) and SMRT (silencing mediator of retinoid and thyroid hormone receptor). This interaction leads to the recruitment of Sin3A and histone deacetylase (HDAC) complexes which maintain chromatin in a compacted and repressed state [7, 8]. The binding of retinoids induces conformational changes in the ligand-binding domain (LBD) of RARA, the most striking one being the repositioning of helix 12. This structural modification causes corepressor release and recruitment of coregulator complexes, some members of which exhibit enzymatic activities such as CBP/p300, then allowing transcription of target genes [9, 10]. Some of these target genes accelerate myeloid differentiation toward granulopoiesis. Accordingly, in vivo granulopoiesis is delayed in the presence of RARA, reflecting the basal repressive activity of unliganded RARA, while it is accelerated by RA solely in the presence of RARA [11].

The PML gene was originally identified in APL [3, 12] and is encoded by nine exons. Seven isoforms are generated by alternative splicing: six are nuclear isoforms designated PML-I to PML-VI, and one is cytoplasmic, PML-VII. PML belongs to the TRIM family, many of which are ubiquitin ligases [13, 14]. Several members of this family are oncogenes: few of them were shown to promote malignant transformation as partners of fusion genes [15]. PML protein contains several regions: a RBCC/TRIM motif (amino acids 57–253 in exons 1–3) which harbors a C_3HC_4 RING finger, two B boxes (B1 and B2), and an α-helical coiled-coil homodimerization domain [14, 16, 17], a nuclear localization signal (NLS) (amino acids 476–490 in exon 6), a SUMO-interacting motif (SIM) (amino acids 556–565 in exon 7a) present only in PML-I to PML-V, and a nuclear export signal (NES) (amino acids 704–713 in exon 9) found only in PML-I and consistent with its nuclear and cytoplasmic distribution [17]. Some domains were described in isoform-specific sequences, like the interaction domain between PML-IV and ARF, a positive regulator of p53 [18], and the exonuclease-like domain in PML-I [19].

PML proteins aggregate in the nucleus and form speckles known as PML nuclear bodies (NBs). These domains are tightly associated with senescence and control of p53 activation, as recently reviewed [20]. Indeed, PML is required for senescence induction, as demonstrated upon stress, DNA damage, oncogene activation, or simply during replicative senescence [21]. At least, some of these functions are mediated through PML NBs which have been implicated in partner sequestration and/or posttranslational modifications, notably phosphorylation, sumoylation, and ubiquitinylation [22, 23]. PML NBs are dynamic structures which harbor a few constitutive, and numerous transiently, client proteins depending on different conditions (i.e., stress, interferon (IFN) treatment, viral infections) like the death domain-associated protein Daxx [22], p53, and many of its regulators [24–26]. Indeed, PML NBs regulate the subcellular localization of Daxx, thereby controlling its proapoptotic activity, and appear to be important for activation of p53-mediated senescence, most likely through posttranslational modifications [27, 28]. In addition, PML-controlled senescence can be initiated and furthermore reinforced at the transcriptional level: PML promoter contains IFN and p53 response elements, creating a positive feedback loop during senescence induction [27, 29].

The Oncoprotein PML/RARA

The expression of *PML/RARA* is sufficient to drive leukemogenesis by deregulating RA-dependent cell differentiation pathways and enhancing the self-renewal of myeloid progenitors [30]. In murine transgenic models, *PML/RARA* expression yields typical APL, although at variable penetrance [31]. From a structural point of view, the *PML/RARA* fusion protein retains all the functional domains of RARA (notably the DNA- and the ligand-binding domains) and PML (in particular the RING finger and coiled-coil domains). On one hand, PML/RARA binds DNA via its RARA domain and acts in a dominant-negative manner to repress the transcription of RARA target genes by strengthening the recruitment of corepressors (N-CoR and SMRT) and HDACs, enforcing DNA methylation and gene silencing. PML/RARA oligomers are complexed to RXR which greatly enhances PML/RARA ability to bind DNA and recognize highly degenerate sites [32, 33]. As RARA signaling regulates myeloid differentiation, its inhibition could explain the block in differentiation that is observed in APL cells. On the other hand, PML/RARA also heterodimerizes with PML via its coiled-coil domain leading to the disruption of NBs: in APL cells, PML is redistributed in a microspeckled pattern (Fig. 2.2). This could abrogate the PML-controlled senescence pathways and contribute to APL pathogenesis. Accordingly, PML/RARA expression was conclusively linked to defective p53 activation [26, 28], thus leading to senescence deregulation, as well as increased self-renewal.

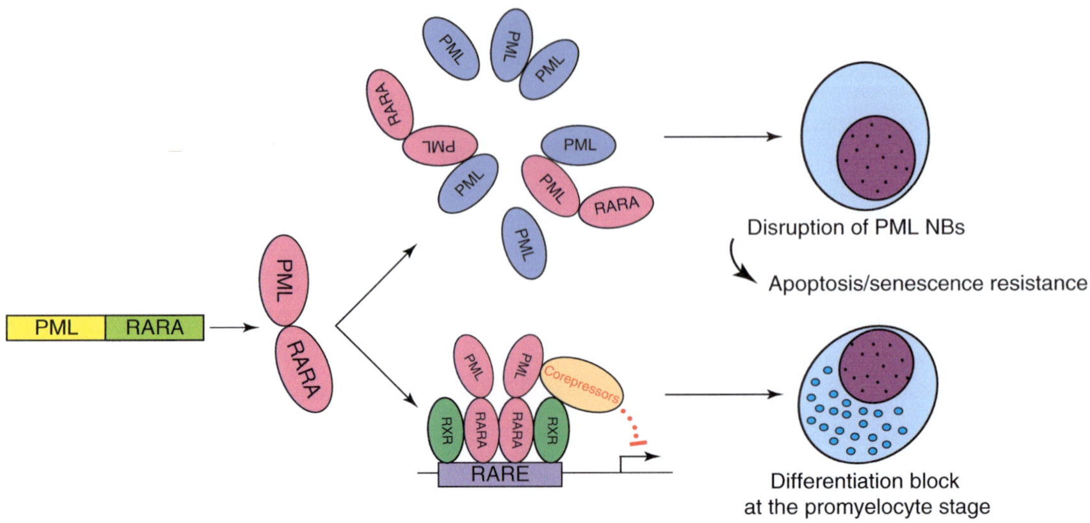

Fig. 2.2 Dual action of PML/RARA oncoproteins. The PML/RARA fusion protein interacts with PML via the coiled-coil domain of its PML moiety, resulting in the disruption of PML NBs. PML/RARA forms a heterodimer with RXR via its RARA moiety and binds DNA with poor selectivity to repress transcription of many genes, including RARA targets, by recruiting corepressors. This collectively causes the characteristic differentiation block of APL cells at the promyelocytic stage

Therapeutic Effects of Retinoic Acid in APL

In the 1980s, APL patients were treated with chemotherapy alone and had poor prognosis despite a complete remission rate of 50–90%. This was explained by a high rate of relapse. The addition of RA to anthracycline-based chemotherapy marked a major advance in the treatment of APL by increasing rates of clinical remission and cure. With these optimized historical regimens, the 5-year overall relapse-free survival is up to 75% [34]:

Uncoupling Differentiation and Loss of Clonogenicity Under RA Treatment

RA treatment of APL constitutes the first example of differentiation therapy in patients [35–38]. RA binds to the ligand-binding domain on the RARA moiety of PML/RARA, triggering a conformational change that releases corepressors and recruits transcriptional coactivators. This allows the activation of RARA target gene transcription and differentiation of leukemic cells (Fig. 2.3). It was first believed that the therapeutic effect of RA stems solely from its ability to reverse repression of myeloid differentiation. Nevertheless, experiments from APL transgenic mice have demonstrated that blast differentiation can be uncoupled from loss of leukemia-initiating cells (LIC) [39]. As reviewed below, multiple settings were described in which full differentiation was not accompanied by significant APL regression or prolongation of survival [40]. For example, in PML/RARA mice, treatment with various RA doses (low, intermediate, and high) or synthetic retinoids similarly yielded terminal granulocytic differentiation; however, survival of treated mice sharply differed by dose and retinoid type. In fact, loss of LIC was dose dependent with only intermediate and high all-trans RA was able to impede clonogenicity in secondary recipients [39–41]. In PLZF-RARA transgenic mice (PLZF-RARA APL is RA resistant in patients), cell differentiation levels upon RA treatment

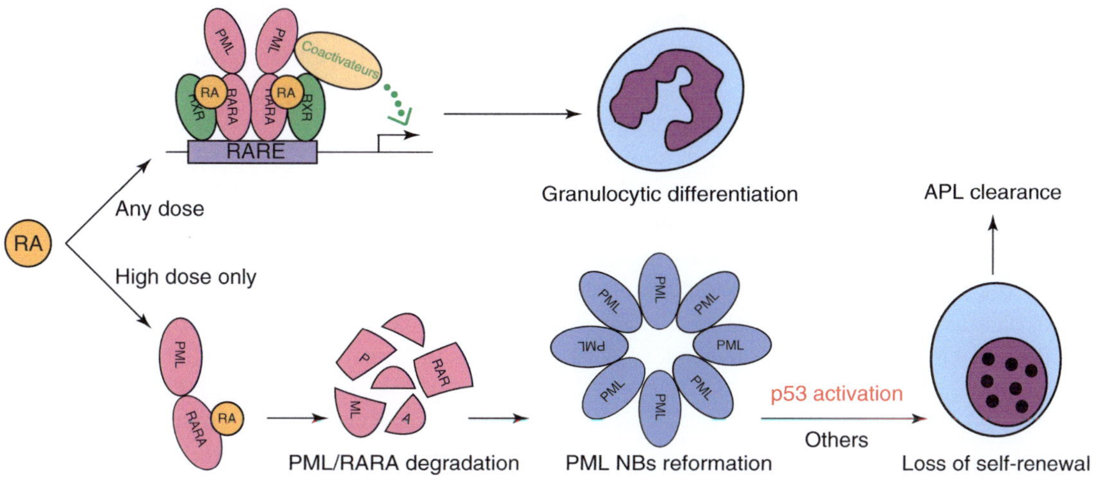

Fig. 2.3 Model of APL eradication with RA treatment. RA binds to RARA LBD of PML/RARA and elicits a conformational change releasing transcription corepressors and leading to the recruitment of coactivators. This allows transcription of RARA target genes and the terminal granulocytic differentiation of the blast. Moreover, RA treatment leads to PML/RARA proteasomal degradation that is followed by PML NB reformation and activation of p53. This latter effect results in loss of LIC

were comparable to that observed in PML/RARA mice but with a strong difference in survival of primary- and secondary-treated recipients [41]. Moreover, RA-resistant APL cells are highly sensitive to cAMP-induced differentiation, particularly in the presence of RA but fail to regress [39, 42]. Similarly, treatment of PML/RARA leukemic mice with histone deacetylase inhibitors (HDACi) led to tumor regression as well as a release in the differentiation block; however, HDACi failed to induce disease clearance [43]. Collectively, those results clearly establish the uncoupling of blast differentiation and tumor eradication in APL: significant transcriptional activation can indeed be obtained with small doses of RA, whereas clearance of LIC necessitates exposure to higher RA levels, an observation that was not yet fully transferred to clinical protocols. Indeed, a unique study has reported the use of single-agent liposomal RA in the treatment of APL patients and has found that some patients—mainly low-risk APL—can be cured without any additional chemotherapy [44], supporting the existence of dose-response in patients upon treatment with RA.

RA-Induced PML/RARA Degradation

Several studies have shown that RA triggers PML/RARA proteasomal degradation [40, 45, 46, 47]. Indeed, RA binding to PML/RARA allows direct recruitment of the proteasome to the ligand-activated transcriptional activation domain AF2 of RARA moiety, leading to PML/RARA degradation (Fig. 2.3) [46, 47]. This proteasome-mediated degradation is additionally modulated by a cAMP-triggered PML/RARA phosphorylation at serine 873 [39, 48]. A caspase-dependent cleavage was also reported [49]. Resistance to RA of some APL cell lines was associated with failure to degrade the fusion protein [46, 50]. In fact, most of these cell lines were mutated for PML/RARA [51, 52]. Thus, PML/RARA proteolysis seems to be linked to clearance of leukemic cells under RA treatment. Phosphorylation at serine 873 sharply enhances RA-induced LIC clearance [39], and the use of theophylline, an inhibitor of cAMP degradation, was beneficial in the treatment of a RA-resistant APL patient [42]. Ablain et al. further showed that treating

APL mice with retinoids other than RA did not affect PML/RARA degradation, although cell differentiation was induced. In secondary recipient experiments, loss of clonogenicity was only observed with RA [40] demonstrating that PML/RARA degradation by RA is followed by reformation of PML NBs [53]. Collectively, these data pharmacologically prove the uncoupling of differentiation and blast clearance and underscore the key role of PML/RARA in vivo degradation in APL eradication.

Role of PML and p53 in the Cure of APL Under RA Treatment

Loss of RA-treated PML/RARA leukemic cells was linked to cell cycle arrest and P53 activation. Examination of bone marrow transcriptome revealed that genes strongly associated with cell cycle arrest were activated only when APL mice were treated with high RA doses that also significantly affect LIC survival. Among the 30 most upregulated genes in this context, 10 were drivers of cell senescence directly linked to p53. For example, a massive induction of the master senescence gene Serpine1, also known as plasminogen activator inhibitor-1 (PAI-1), was observed. PML/RARA degradation was followed by PML NB reformation and triggered p53 stabilization, possibly through posttranslational modifications occurring on NBs (Fig. 2.3). This leads to a cell cycle arrest with senescence-like features resulting in elimination of leukemia-propagating cells [41]. The role of p53 in RA-induced APL elimination was demonstrated by in vivo survival experiments in $p53^{+/+}$ and $p53^{-/-}$ PML/RARA-driven APLs [41]. In addition, the importance of PML in inducing p53 activation and APL clearance was further established by mice survival experiments showing a much shorter survival of $Pml^{-/-}$ APL compared to that of $Pml^{+/+}$ APL. Definitely, these data demonstrate that functional PML NB reorganization upon RA treatment leading to p53 activation is a determining step in the cure of APL.

Therapeutic Effects of Arsenic Trioxide in APL

Arsenic trioxide (ATO) was first utilized in APL patients in the early 1990s and led to cure in 70% of patients [54, 55]. Thereby, APL is exquisitely sensitive to ATO which, in contrast to RA, may cure APL as a single agent. Moreover, the combination of RA and ATO in clinical trials appeared to be much superior to the conventional treatment with RA and chemotherapy [56]:

ATO-Induced PML NB Reformation and PML/RARA Degradation

Although RA and ATO are two unrelated therapeutic agents in APL, they share the biochemical property of inducing PML/RARA degradation. As described above, PML/RARA loss was directly linked to loss of self-renewal in leukemic cells and cure of APL [39]. Furthermore, ATO-induced PML/RARA loss could explain the differentiation observed in vivo in APL cells upon ATO exposure by a promoter clearance mechanism [57]. At the molecular level, while RA targets the RARA moiety of the fusion oncoprotein, ATO targets its PML moiety [50, 58] and induces its oxidation [59]. The same effect is observed on normal PML, and a specific ATO binding site was identified in the second B box. Arsenic sharply enhances the reformation of PML NBs by multimerization of PML and PML/RARA proteins. Then, through recruitment of UBC9 SUMO-E2 ligase, it favors the sumoylation of PML [23, 60]. Sumoylation of PML is followed by recruitment of the

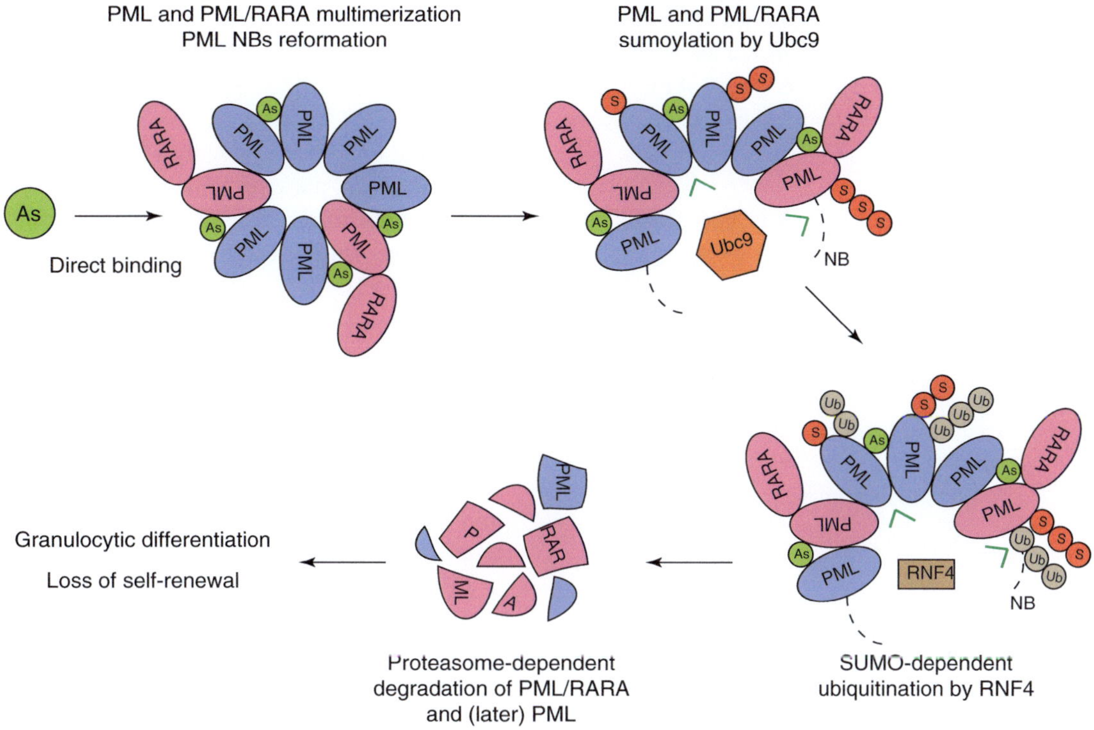

Fig. 2.4 ATO-induced degradation of PML/RARA. ATO prompts PML and PML/RARA multimerization that triggers PML NB reorganization. This is followed by recruitment of SUMO E2 ligase Ubc9 which sumoylates PML and PML/RARA on its PML part. Then, the sumoylated proteins are polyubiquitinated by the SUMO-dependent ubiquitin E3 ligase RNF4 resulting in their degradation. This likely explains the great efficacy of ATO in APL treatment. As is ATO

SUMO-dependent ubiquitin E3 ligase RNF4, which catalyzes polyubiquitination and subsequent proteasome-mediated proteolysis of PML and PML/RARA (Fig. 2.4) [61, 62]. In conclusion, degradation of PML/RARA and enhanced NB biogenesis are the two main effects of ATO which results in p53 activation and clearance of APL LICs. Note that the dual targeting of PML/RARA and PML likely explains the clinical superiority of this drug.

RA and ATO Synergy in APL Cure

In several mice models, combined RA and ATO treatment causes a rapid disappearance of APL cells and cures leukemia. Yet, those two therapeutic agents do not synergize (even antagonize) to induce cell differentiation [63–65], but they do cooperate to induce PML/RARA degradation by non-overlapping biochemical pathways [39, 50, 58]. Actually, NB reformation with RA-ATO treatment was much more complete in APL blasts than with RA alone, which can be explained both by the synergistic effect of both drugs on PML/RARA degradation but also by the direct PML targeting by ATO [41]. Accordingly, this treatment elicited enhanced activation of p53 target genes [41]. Hence, ATO cooperates with RA to cure APL by increasing RA-induced PML/RARA degradation and also by potentiating PML NB reorganization yielding enhanced NB formation, p53 activation, and senescence (Fig. 2.5).

This model for PML NB-based APL eradication was strongly supported by the discovery of a mutation in normal PML gene in a therapy-resistant patient [66–68]. Strikingly, this mutation (A216V), located immediately next to the ATO binding site on PML, is the predominant one observed within PML/RARA in ATO-resistant patients (Fig. 2.6) [69–72]. Finally, mutations in the p53 gene have been reported in rare, fully therapy-resistant patients [51, 52].

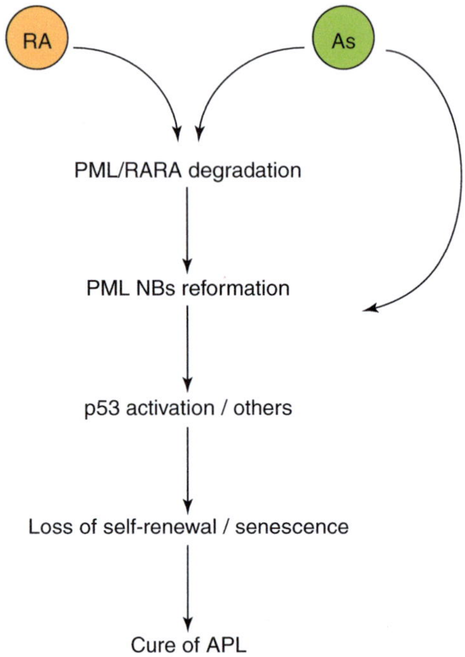

Fig. 2.5 Molecular effects of treatment combination in APL cure. PML/RARA degradation is strongly enhanced by the two therapeutic agents as well as PML NB reformation. This effect drives a greater NB reformation and p53 activation than with RA alone. Hence, ATO cooperates with RA to cure APL

Conclusions

PML/RARA degradation by RA and/or ATO appears to be the driving force underlying the cure of APL patients. Triggering the degradation of oncoproteins in other leukemias and sarcomas caused by fusion proteins could be a promising therapeutic approach as in APL. Downstream of PML/RARA degradation and PML NB reformation drives P53 activation and is required for loss of self-renewal by a senescence-like program. Importantly, targeting PML by ATO could drive cancer cell senescence in other diseases. Indeed, there are some indications that PML may be important in other hematological malignancies, like adult T-cell leukemia/lymphoma (ATL). Thus, this model of APL cure not only constitutes a success story of molecularly targeted therapy but may actually open new therapeutic avenues in other malignancies.

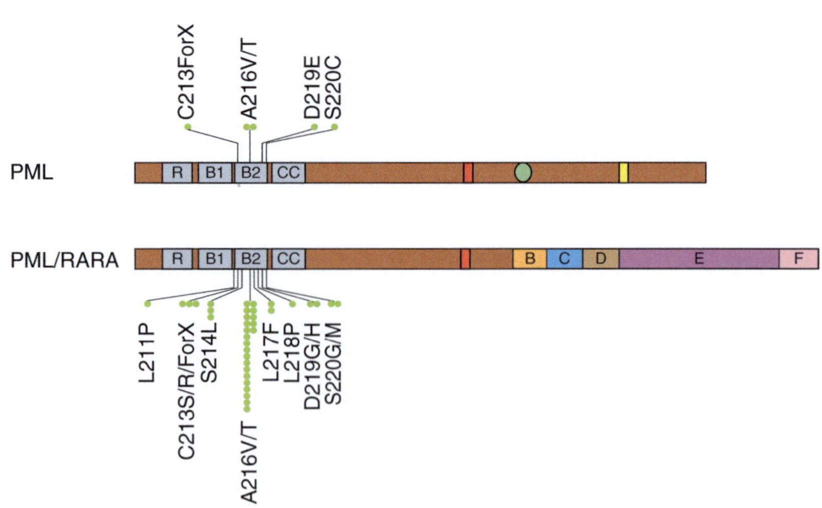

Fig. 2.6 Spectrum of mutations in PML and PML/RARA in ATO-resistant patients. Schematic representation of PML and PML/RARA proteins with observed mutations. *Circles* depict individual mutations

References

1. de The H, Chomienne C, Lanotte M, Degos L, Dejean A. The t(15;17) translocation of acute promyelocytic leukaemia fuses the retinoic acid receptor alpha gene to a novel transcribed locus. Nature. 1990;347(6293):558–61.
2. Borrow J, Goddard AD, Sheer D, Solomon E. Molecular analysis of acute promyelocytic leukemia breakpoint cluster region on chromosome 17. Science. 1990;249(4976):1577–80.
3. de The H, Lavau C, Marchio A, Chomienne C, Degos L, Dejean A. The PML-RAR alpha fusion mRNA generated by the t(15;17) translocation in acute promyelocytic leukemia encodes a functionally altered RAR. Cell. 1991;66(4):675–84.
4. Chen Z, Brand NJ, Chen A, Chen SJ, Tong JH, Wang ZY, et al. Fusion between a novel Kruppel-like zinc finger gene and the retinoic acid receptor-alpha locus due to a variant t(11;17) translocation associated with acute promyelocytic leukaemia. EMBO J. 1993;12(3):1161–7.
5. Mangelsdorf DJ, Thummel C, Beato M, Herrlich P, Schutz G, Umesono K, et al. The nuclear receptor superfamily: the second decade. Cell. 1995;83(6):835–9.
6. Chambon P. A decade of molecular biology of retinoic acid receptors. FASEB J. 1996;10(9):940–54.
7. Nagy L, Kao HY, Chakravarti D, Lin RJ, Hassig CA, Ayer DE, et al. Nuclear receptor repression mediated by a complex containing SMRT, mSin3A, and histone deacetylase. Cell. 1997;89(3):373–80.
8. Farboud B, Hauksdottir H, Wu Y, Privalsky ML. Isotype-restricted corepressor recruitment: a constitutively closed helix 12 conformation in retinoic acid receptors beta and gamma interferes with corepressor recruitment and prevents transcriptional repression. Mol Cell Biol. 2003;23(8):2844–58.
9. Onate SA, Tsai SY, Tsai MJ, O'Malley BW. Sequence and characterization of a coactivator for the steroid hormone receptor superfamily. Science. 1995;270(5240):1354–7.
10. Yao TP, Ku G, Zhou N, Scully R, Livingston DM. The nuclear hormone receptor coactivator SRC-1 is a specific target of p300. Proc Natl Acad Sci U S A. 1996;93(20):10626–31.
11. Kastner P, Lawrence HJ, Waltzinger C, Ghyselinck NB, Chambon P, Chan S. Positive and negative regulation of granulopoiesis by endogenous RARalpha. Blood. 2001;97(5):1314–20.
12. Kakizuka A, Miller WH Jr, Umesono K, Warrell RP Jr, Frankel SR, Murty VV, et al. Chromosomal translocation t(15;17) in human acute promyelocytic leukemia fuses RAR alpha with a novel putative transcription factor, PML. Cell. 1991;66(4):663–74.
13. Meroni G, Diez-Roux G. TRIM/RBCC, a novel class of 'single protein RING finger' E3 ubiquitin ligases. Bioessays. 2005;27(11):1147–57.
14. Reymond A, Meroni G, Fantozzi A, Merla G, Cairo S, Luzi L, et al. The tripartite motif family identifies cell compartments. EMBO J. 2001;20(9):2140–51.
15. Hatakeyama S. TRIM proteins and cancer. Nat Rev Cancer. 2011;11(11):792–804.
16. Kastner P, Perez A, Lutz Y, Rochette-Egly C, Gaub MP, Durand B, et al. Structure, localization and transcriptional properties of two classes of retinoic acid receptor alpha fusion proteins in acute promyelocytic leukemia (APL): structural similarities with a new family of oncoproteins. EMBO J. 1992;11(2):629–42.
17. Nisole S, Maroui MA, Mascle XH, Aubry M, Chelbi-Alix MK. Differential roles of PML isoforms. Front Oncol. 2013;3:125.
18. Ivanschitz L, Takahashi Y, Jollivet F, Ayrault O, Le Bras M, de The H. PML IV/ARF interaction enhances p53 SUMO-1 conjugation, activation, and senescence. Proc Natl Acad Sci U S A. 2015;112(46):14278–83.
19. Condemine W, Takahashi Y, Le Bras M, de The H. A nucleolar targeting signal in PML-I addresses PML to nucleolar caps in stressed or senescent cells. J Cell Sci. 2007;120(Pt 18):3219–27.
20. Lallemand-Breitenbach V, de The H. PML nuclear bodies. Cold Spring Harb Perspect Biol. 2010;2(5):a000661.
21. Ivanschitz L, De The H, Le Bras M. PML, SUMOylation, and senescence. Front Oncol. 2013; 3:171.
22. Ishov AM, Sotnikov AG, Negorev D, Vladimirova OV, Neff N, Kamitani T, et al. PML is critical for ND10 formation and recruits the PML-interacting protein daxx to this nuclear structure when modified by SUMO-1. J Cell Biol. 1999;147(2):221–34.
23. Lallemand-Breitenbach V, Zhu J, Puvion F, Koken M, Honore N, Doubeikovsky A, et al. Role of promyelocytic leukemia (PML) sumoylation in nuclear body formation, 11S proteasome recruitment, and As2O3-induced PML or PML/retinoic acid receptor alpha degradation. J Exp Med. 2001;193(12):1361–71.
24. Fogal V, Gostissa M, Sandy P, Zacchi P, Sternsdorf T, Jensen K, et al. Regulation of p53 activity in nuclear bodies by a specific PML isoform. EMBO J. 2000;19(22):6185–95.
25. Guo A, Salomoni P, Luo J, Shih A, Zhong S, Gu W, et al. The function of PML in p53-dependent apoptosis. Nat Cell Biol. 2000;2(10):730–6.
26. Pearson M, Carbone R, Sebastiani C, Cioce M, Fagioli M, Saito S, et al. PML regulates p53 acetylation and premature senescence induced by oncogenic Ras. Nature. 2000;406(6792):207–10.
27. de Stanchina E, Querido E, Narita M, Davuluri RV, Pandolfi PP, Ferbeyre G, et al. PML is a direct p53 target that modulates p53 effector functions. Mol Cell. 2004;13(4):523–35.
28. Insinga A, Monestiroli S, Ronzoni S, Carbone R, Pearson M, Pruneri G, et al. Impairment of p53 acetylation, stability and function by an oncogenic transcription factor. EMBO J. 2004;23(5):1144–54.
29. Hubackova S, Novakova Z, Krejcikova K, Kosar M, Dobrovolna J, Duskova P, et al. Regulation of the PML tumor suppressor in drug-induced senescence

of human normal and cancer cells by JAK/STAT-mediated signaling. Cell Cycle. 2010;9(15):3085–99.
30. Du C, Redner RL, Cooke MP, Lavau C. Overexpression of wild-type retinoic acid receptor alpha (RARalpha) recapitulates retinoic acid-sensitive transformation of primary myeloid progenitors by acute promyelocytic leukemia RARalpha-fusion genes. Blood. 1999;94(2):793–802.
31. de The H, Chen Z. Acute promyelocytic leukaemia: novel insights into the mechanisms of cure. Nat Rev Cancer. 2010;10(11):775–83.
32. Kamashev D, Vitoux D, De The H. PML-RARA-RXR oligomers mediate retinoid and rexinoid/cAMP cross-talk in acute promyelocytic leukemia cell differentiation. J Exp Med. 2004;199(8):1163–74.
33. Martens JH, Brinkman AB, Simmer F, Francoijs KJ, Nebbioso A, Ferrara F, et al. PML-RARalpha/RXR alters the epigenetic landscape in acute promyelocytic leukemia. Cancer Cell. 2010;17(2):173–85.
34. Ades L, Guerci A, Raffoux E, Sanz M, Chevallier P, Lapusan S, et al. Very long-term outcome of acute promyelocytic leukemia after treatment with all-trans retinoic acid and chemotherapy: the European APL Group experience. Blood. 2010;115(9):1690–6.
35. Breitman TR, Collins SJ, Keene BR. Terminal differentiation of human promyelocytic leukemic cells in primary culture in response to retinoic acid. Blood. 1981;57(6):1000–4.
36. Castaigne S, Chomienne C, Daniel MT, Ballerini P, Berger R, Fenaux P, et al. All-trans retinoic acid as a differentiation therapy for acute promyelocytic leukemia. I. Clinical results. Blood. 1990;76(9):1704–9.
37. Fenaux P, Chastang C, Chomienne C, Degos L. Tretinoin with chemotherapy in newly diagnosed acute promyelocytic leukaemia. European APL Group. Lancet. 1994;343(8904):1033.
38. Huang ME, Ye YC, Chen SR, Chai JR, Lu JX, Zhoa L, et al. Use of all-trans retinoic acid in the treatment of acute promyelocytic leukemia. Blood. 1988;72(2):567–72.
39. Nasr R, Guillemin MC, Ferhi O, Soilihi H, Peres L, Berthier C, et al. Eradication of acute promyelocytic leukemia-initiating cells through PML-RARA degradation. Nat Med. 2008;14(12):1333–42.
40. Ablain J, Leiva M, Peres L, Fonsart J, Anthony E, de The H. Uncoupling RARA transcriptional activation and degradation clarifies the bases for APL response to therapies. J Exp Med. 2013;210(4):647–53.
41. Ablain J, Rice K, Soilihi H, de Reynies A, Minucci S, de The H. Activation of a promyelocytic leukemia-tumor protein 53 axis underlies acute promyelocytic leukemia cure. Nat Med. 2014;20(2):167–74.
42. Guillemin MC, Raffoux E, Vitoux D, Kogan S, Soilihi H, Lallemand-Breitenbach V, et al. In vivo activation of cAMP signaling induces growth arrest and differentiation in acute promyelocytic leukemia. J Exp Med. 2002;196(10):1373–80.
43. Leiva M, Moretti S, Soilihi H, Pallavicini I, Peres L, Mercurio C, et al. Valproic acid induces differentiation and transient tumor regression, but spares leukemia-initiating activity in mouse models of APL. Leukemia. 2012;26(7):1630–7.
44. Tsimberidou AM, Tirado-Gomez M, Andreeff M, O'Brien S, Kantarjian H, Keating M, et al. Single-agent liposomal all-trans retinoic acid can cure some patients with untreated acute promyelocytic leukemia: an update of The University of Texas M. D. Anderson Cancer Center Series. Leuk Lymphoma. 2006;47(6):1062–8.
45. Yoshida H, Kitamura K, Tanaka K, Omura S, Miyazaki T, Hachiya T, et al. Accelerated degradation of PML-retinoic acid receptor alpha (PML-RARA) oncoprotein by all-trans-retinoic acid in acute promyelocytic leukemia: possible role of the proteasome pathway. Cancer Res. 1996;56(13):2945–8.
46. Zhu J, Gianni M, Kopf E, Honore N, Chelbi-Alix M, Koken M, et al. Retinoic acid induces proteasome-dependent degradation of retinoic acid receptor alpha (RARalpha) and oncogenic RARalpha fusion proteins. Proc Natl Acad Sci U S A. 1999;96(26):14807–12.
47. Kopf E, Plassat JL, Vivat V, de The H, Chambon P, Rochette-Egly C. Dimerization with retinoid X receptors and phosphorylation modulate the retinoic acid-induced degradation of retinoic acid receptors alpha and gamma through the ubiquitin-proteasome pathway. J Biol Chem. 2000;275(43):33280–8.
48. Parrella E, Gianni M, Cecconi V, Nigro E, Barzago MM, Rambaldi A, et al. Phosphodiesterase IV inhibition by piclamilast potentiates the cytodifferentiating action of retinoids in myeloid leukemia cells. Cross-talk between the cAMP and the retinoic acid signaling pathways. J Biol Chem. 2004;279(40):42026–40.
49. Nervi C, Ferrara FF, Fanelli M, Rippo MR, Tomassini B, Ferrucci PF, et al. Caspases mediate retinoic acid-induced degradation of the acute promyelocytic leukemia PML/RARalpha fusion protein. Blood. 1998;92(7):2244–51.
50. Zhu J, Lallemand-Breitenbach V, de The H. Pathways of retinoic acid- or arsenic trioxide-induced PML/RARalpha catabolism, role of oncogene degradation in disease remission. Oncogene. 2001;20(49):7257–65.
51. Akagi T, Shih LY, Kato M, Kawamata N, Yamamoto G, Sanada M, et al. Hidden abnormalities and novel classification of t(15;17) acute promyelocytic leukemia (APL) based on genomic alterations. Blood. 2009;113(8):1741–8.
52. Karnan S, Tsuzuki S, Kiyoi H, Tagawa H, Ueda R, Seto M, et al. Genomewide array-based comparative genomic hybridization analysis of acute promyelocytic leukemia. Genes Chromosomes Cancer. 2006;45(4):420–5.
53. Koken MH, Linares-Cruz G, Quignon F, Viron A, Chelbi-Alix MK, Sobczak-Thepot J, et al. The PML growth-suppressor has an altered expression in human oncogenesis. Oncogene. 1995;10(7):1315–24.
54. Ghavamzadeh A, Alimoghaddam K, Rostami S, Ghaffari SH, Jahani M, Iravani M, et al. Phase II study of single-agent arsenic trioxide for the front-line therapy of acute promyelocytic leukemia. J Clin Oncol. 2011;29(20):2753–7.

55. Mathews V, George B, Chendamarai E, Lakshmi KM, Desire S, Balasubramanian P, et al. Single-agent arsenic trioxide in the treatment of newly diagnosed acute promyelocytic leukemia: long-term follow-up data. J Clin Oncol. 2010;28(24):3866–71.
56. Platzbecker U, Avvisati G, Cicconi L, Thiede C, Paoloni F, Vignetti M, et al. Improved outcomes with retinoic acid and arsenic trioxide compared with retinoic acid and chemotherapy in non-high-risk acute promyelocytic leukemia: final results of the randomized Italian-German APL0406 Trial. J Clin Oncol. 2017;35(6):605–12.
57. Vitaliano-Prunier A, Halftermeyer J, Ablain J, de Reynies A, Peres L, Le Bras M, et al. Clearance of PML/RARA-bound promoters suffice to initiate APL differentiation. Blood. 2014;124(25):3772–80.
58. Quignon F, Chen Z, de The H. Retinoic acid and arsenic: towards oncogene-targeted treatments of acute promyelocytic leukaemia. Biochim Biophys Acta. 1997;1333(3):M53–61.
59. Jeanne M, Lallemand-Breitenbach V, Ferhi O, Koken M, Le Bras M, Duffort S, et al. PML/RARA oxidation and arsenic binding initiate the antileukemia response of As2O3. Cancer Cell. 2010;18(1):88–98.
60. Sahin U, Ferhi O, Jeanne M, Benhenda S, Berthier C, Jollivet F, et al. Oxidative stress-induced assembly of PML nuclear bodies controls sumoylation of partner proteins. J Cell Biol. 2014;204(6):931–45.
61. Lallemand-Breitenbach V, Jeanne M, Benhenda S, Nasr R, Lei M, Peres L, et al. Arsenic degrades PML or PML-RARalpha through a SUMO-triggered RNF4/ubiquitin-mediated pathway. Nat Cell Biol. 2008;10(5):547–55.
62. Tatham MH, Geoffroy MC, Shen L, Plechanovova A, Hattersley N, Jaffray EG, et al. RNF4 is a poly-SUMO-specific E3 ubiquitin ligase required for arsenic-induced PML degradation. Nat Cell Biol. 2008;10(5):538–46.
63. Chen GQ, Shi XG, Tang W, Xiong SM, Zhu J, Cai X, et al. Use of arsenic trioxide (As2O3) in the treatment of acute promyelocytic leukemia (APL): I. As2O3 exerts dose-dependent dual effects on APL cells. Blood. 1997;89(9):3345–53.
64. Chen GQ, Zhu J, Shi XG, Ni JH, Zhong HJ, Si GY, et al. In vitro studies on cellular and molecular mechanisms of arsenic trioxide (As2O3) in the treatment of acute promyelocytic leukemia: As2O3 induces NB4 cell apoptosis with downregulation of Bcl-2 expression and modulation of PML-RAR alpha/PML proteins. Blood. 1996;88(3):1052–61.
65. Shao W, Fanelli M, Ferrara FF, Riccioni R, Rosenauer A, Davison K, et al. Arsenic trioxide as an inducer of apoptosis and loss of PML/RAR alpha protein in acute promyelocytic leukemia cells. J Natl Cancer Inst. 1998;90(2):124–33.
66. Iaccarino L, Ottone T, Divona M, Cicconi L, Cairoli R, Voso MT, et al. Mutations affecting both the rearranged and the unrearranged PML alleles in refractory acute promyelocytic leukaemia. Br J Haematol. 2016;172(6):909–13.
67. Lehmann-Che J, Bally C, de The H. Resistance to therapy in acute promyelocytic leukemia. N Engl J Med. 2014;371(12):1170–2.
68. Madan V, Shyamsunder P, Han L, Mayakonda A, Nagata Y, Sundaresan J, et al. Comprehensive mutational analysis of primary and relapse acute promyelocytic leukemia. Leukemia. 2016;30(8):1672–81.
69. Chendamarai E, Ganesan S, Alex AA, Kamath V, Nair SC, Nellickal AJ, et al. Comparison of newly diagnosed and relapsed patients with acute promyelocytic leukemia treated with arsenic trioxide: insight into mechanisms of resistance. PLoS One. 2015;10(3):e0121912.
70. Goto E, Tomita A, Hayakawa F, Atsumi A, Kiyoi H, Naoe T. Missense mutations in PML-RARA are critical for the lack of responsiveness to arsenic trioxide treatment. Blood. 2011;118(6):1600–9.
71. Lou Y, Ma Y, Sun J, Ye X, Pan H, Wang Y, et al. Evaluating frequency of PML-RARA mutations and conferring resistance to arsenic trioxide-based therapy in relapsed acute promyelocytic leukemia patients. Ann Hematol. 2015;94(11):1829–37.
72. Zhu HH, Qin YZ, Huang XJ. Resistance to arsenic therapy in acute promyelocytic leukemia. N Engl J Med. 2014;370(19):1864–6.

The Leukemic Stem Cell

3

Thalia Vlachou[†], Giulia De Conti[†],
Anna Giulia Sanarico, and Pier Giuseppe Pelicci

Abbreviations

AML	Acute myeloid leukemia
APL	Acute promyelocytic leukemia
ATO	Arsenic trioxide
ATRA	All-trans retinoic acid
BM	Bone marrow
CSC	Cancer stem cell
FAB	French-American-British classification
FACS	Fluorescence-activated cell sorting
FISH	Fluorescent in situ hybridization
GO	Gemtuzumab ozogamicin
HSC	Hematopoietic stem cell
LIC	Leukemia-initiating cell
LSC	Leukemia stem cell
MSC	Mesenchymal stromal cell
NOD/SCID	Nonobese diabetic SCID
NSG	NOD/SCID IL2Rg null
RA	Retinoic acid
ROS	Reactive oxygen species
SC	Stem cell
SCID	Severe combined immunodeficiency
TIC	Tumor-initiating cell

[†] Thalia Vlachou and Giulia De Conti contributed equally to this work.

T. Vlachou, Ph.D. • G. De Conti, Ph.D • A.G. Sanarico
Department of Experimental Oncology, European Institute of Oncology,
Via Adamello 16, 20139 Milan, Italy

P.G. Pelicci, M.D., Ph.D. (✉)
Department of Experimental Oncology, European Institute of Oncology, Via Adamello 16,
20139 Milan, Italy

Department of Oncology and Hemathology, University of Milan, Milan, Italy
e-mail: piergiuseppe.pelicci@ieo.it

The Cancer Stem Cell Theory

Tumors can be envisioned as aberrant organs harboring a complex and hierarchical cellular organization, similar to that of their normal tissue counterparts, with cancer stem cells (CSCs) placed at the apex of this hierarchy [1]. As their name indicates, CSCs are cancer cells endowed with stem cell (SC) properties, namely, the ability to self-renew and to generate more differentiated progeny forming the bulk of the tumor [2]. According to the CSC theory, which was formulated between years 1990 and 2000, CSCs constitute a minor cell fraction of the tumor, which serves as the functional reservoir of cancer cells. In this view, CSCs are thought to be indispensable for tumor initiation, maintenance, and propagation and can be, therefore, considered the only responsible for the appearance of distant metastases and disease relapse after initial remission [1].

Although the CSC concept has gained increasingly attention and acceptance within the

O. Abla et al. (eds.), *Acute Promyelocytic Leukemia*, https://doi.org/10.1007/978-3-319-64257-4_3

scientific community, most currently used therapeutic approaches target highly proliferating cells and find their rationale on a different model of tumorigenesis. In the so-called "classical" or "stochastic" model of tumor growth (Fig. 3.1a), all cancer cells have equal self-renewal ability and tumorigenic potential, while stem-like behavior is randomly expressed by different cells in the heterogeneous cancer population. In this case, intratumoral phenotypic heterogeneity is usually attributed to the acquisition of distinct mutations that establish subclonal populations within the tumor. In contrast, in the CSC or "hierarchical" model (Fig. 3.1b), tumorigenicity and self-renewal are considered properties of rare cells, the CSCs. Furthermore, CSCs are thought to be responsible for the generation of intratumoral cell heterogeneity, due to their intrinsic ability to perform asymmetric cell divisions, by which they simultaneously self-renew and produce non-CSCs [1, 3]. Understanding the nature of intratumoral heterogeneity is vital for the development of efficient therapeutic approaches: if the hierarchical model is correct, elimination of CSCs is necessary and sufficient for tumor eradication [1].

Both models of tumorigenesis can be employed to explain certain aspects of intratumoral cell heterogeneity. For instance, only a small fraction of cancer cells possess the property to produce a colony of cells *in vitro* [4]. Indeed, *in vitro* clonogenicity can be seen either as a property shared by all cancer cells but expressed in a stochastic manner at any given time or as a specific property of the rare CSC or progenitor subpopulations. However, the stochastic model fails to provide a coherent explanation regarding other phenotypic traits, such as the ability to form tumors at distant sites (metastases). If all cancer cells were endowed with metastatic potential, any disseminated cell should eventually lead to the development of a metastasis. Instead, it has been long reported that cancer cells are frequently shed from tumors and released in the blood and lymphatic circulation without necessarily giving rise to metastatic lesions [5, 6]. As an interpretation of this phenomenon, it has been suggested that low numbers of cancer cells might be indeed efficiently targeted and eliminated by the patient's immune system before tumor initiation at a distant location occurs [1]. Although depicting a plausible scenario, this interpretation is inconsistent with the frequency of disease recurrence after seemingly successful treatments. In these cases, resistance should be restricted to a small—clinically undetectable—population of cancer cells,

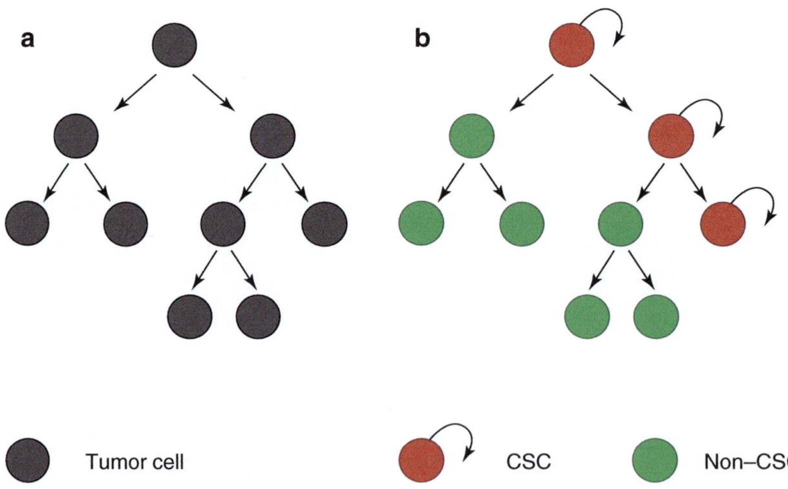

Fig. 3.1 Stochastic versus hierarchical model of tumor growth. The stochastic model of tumor growth (**a**) foresees that all tumor cells have equal self-renewal potential. In the hierarchical model (**b**), instead, only a small fraction of the tumor cells (viz., the CSCs) retains the ability of long-term self-renewal (indicated by the *curved arrow*) and differentiation (depicted by the generation of non-CSCs)

and, therefore, the probability of evading immune surveillance at such numbers and stochastically reinitiating tumor formation would be expected to be very low. On the contrary, the existence of a rare population of tumorigenic cells within tumors can account for both phenomena, as the dissemination or survival of these cells—and these cells only—would inevitably seed a metastasis or lead to tumor relapse.

Although the CSC theory was formally established quite recently, the concept that tumor growth could be driven and sustained by cells with stem-like properties is much older. The earliest reports go back to the nineteenth century and to the "embryonic rest theory", which postulated that either delocalized or overabundant embryonic cells could persist in adulthood and lead to tumor formation [7, 8]. Studies on teratocarcinomas in the twentieth century led to the identification of pluripotent SCs within tumoral populations (embryonal carcinoma cells) and provided the first evidence for the hierarchical organization of tumors [9]. Finally, the development of functional assays with the use of xenotransplantation models in the 1990s allowed for the isolation and characterization of human leukemic populations with increased *in vivo* self-renewal and differentiation capacity, which were later termed leukemia stem cells (LSCs) or leukemia-initiating cells (LICs).

Defining Stemness in Leukemia

In vitro clonogenic and *in vivo* transplantation assays paved the way for the identification of tumoral cell populations with variable tumorigenic potential and the designation of CSCs as the only cells able to sustain tumor initiation and progression in vivo. Pioneering studies in John Dick's lab demonstrated the existence of such a population in acute myeloid leukemias (AMLs), by the prospective isolation and xenotransplantation into immunocompromised murine hosts of leukemic populations with different combinations of CD34 and CD38 antigen expression. These studies documented that only the $CD34^{+}CD38^{-}$ compartment retains tumorigenic ability *in vivo* [10, 11]. There is great heterogeneity in the expression profile of the CD34/CD38 surface markers among different patient samples, and LSCs have been subsequently identified with varying frequencies and in different cellular subpopulations in many AML samples [12, 13]. For instance, LSC activity is commonly found in the $CD34^{-}$ compartment in *NPM*-mutated AMLs, which are generally characterized by low CD34 expression [13]. In $CD34^{+}$ leukemias, instead, the $CD34^{+}CD38^{-}$ subset has been associated with higher tumorigenic capacity, using limiting dilution xenotransplantation assays [14, 15]. The existence of CSCs, or more precisely of tumor-initiating cell (TIC) populations, has been then demonstrated also in numerous solid tumors, including breast cancer [16], glioblastoma [17], and colorectal cancer [18]. However, there are also tumors that do not seem to follow strictly the CSC model or that suggest a higher plasticity within this intrinsic hierarchy. In melanoma, nearly each tumor cell seems to possess tumorigenic potential, as single-cell transplantations in immunocompromised murine hosts have proven their high *in vivo* tumor reconstitution capacity [19]. Nevertheless, also melanomas show some extent of intratumoral phenotypic [20] and functional heterogeneity [21].

The concomitant development of lineage-specific monoclonal antibodies and fluorescence-activated cell sorting (FACS) enabled the characterization and prospective isolation of phenotypically distinct tumor subpopulations and to operationally define CSCs as TICs, meaning the cells that retain the ability to seed a tumor in murine hosts [2]. It should be noted that the two terms are not synonymous even though they are often used interchangeably in the literature to denote cells bestowed with *in vivo* tumor initiation capacity. The discrepancy between them is obvious in the case of melanoma, where the high frequency of TICs scored in transplantation assays is the reason for which melanoma is considered a non-hierarchically organized tumor [22].

Although *in vivo* transplantation experiments provided the first evidence for the existence of LSCs, there are several limitations inherent to these assays. One of the main caveats is that stemness (or tumorigenicity) is assessed at a population and not at a single-cell level. As a result, this approach does not allow for the isolation of "pure" populations but rather for the detection of SC activity and the segregation of tumorigenic from non-tumorigenic subpopulations. In fact, limiting dilution transplantation assays are used to measure the frequency of LICs in the isolated tumorigenic populations and, thus, to define their purity. Nevertheless, it is not given that the cells that initiate tumor growth in the murine host are indeed the same cells that initiate or sustain the tumor in the patient. To some extent, xenotransplantation measures the ability of cells to successfully engraft and repopulate an "alien" and potentially hostile microenvironment. Indeed, the transition from athymic (nude) mice which lacked T lymphocytes to the various SCID (severely combined immunodeficient) strains allowed the engraftment of liquid cancers in the first place, while the introduction of more immunodeficient models led to significantly higher sensitivity in xenotransplantation assays [19, 23]. Finally, the use of monoclonal antibodies for the purpose of cell isolation might introduce experimental bias by itself [12].

All cells within a normal tissue are the progeny of somatic SCs, which possess increased self-renewal potential and the capacity of multilineage differentiation. Therefore, normal SCs are both defined by their intrinsic properties (self-renewal and differentiation) and as the cells from which all other cells originate. In tumors, however, CSCs (i.e., the cells that sustain tumor growth and disease progression) do not necessarily originate from the malignant transformation of normal SCs [22, 24]. Despite the high similarity between CSCs and their normal counterparts, which would indicate normal SCs as the cell target of transformation (cell of origin), studies on murine models of spontaneous leukemogenesis have shown that oncogenic mutations can also confer self-renewal properties to hematopoietic cells with limited regenerative potential [25, 26]. It is worth thinking that the biological properties of LSCs, then, may vary with regard to the immunophenotype, transcriptome, genetics, cell cycle status, and multilineage potential of the cell of origin [27]. Indeed, several marker combinations have been used to isolate nearly pure HSC populations, both human and murine. Human HSCs are enriched in Lin^-, $Thy1^+$, $CD34^+$, and $CD38^{neg/low}$ cell populations [28], while murine HSCs are enriched in Lin^-, $Thy1^{low}$, $Sca1^+$, Kit^+, $CD34^-$, and $Flk2^-$ populations [29] (Table 3.1). As previously mentioned, initially, many studies observed that for most AMLs, the only cells capable of transplanting leukemia in nonobese diabetic SCID (NOD/SCID) mice have a $CD34^+CD38^-$ phenotype, similar to that of normal human HSCs, whereas the $CD34^+CD38^+$ leukemic blast cells cannot transfer the disease to mice [30]. However, xenograft experiments in later studies led to the detection of LICs in AML populations with variable phenotypes downstream of the $CD34^+CD38^-$ profile. This is consistent with the observation that in individual patients, LSCs of variable immunophenotypes coexist together and has important implications for the development of targeted therapies (see section "Implications for Therapy").

Table 3.1 Immunophenotype of human and murine hematopoietic stem and progenitor cells

	Human	Mouse
HSCs	Lin^- $CD34^+$ $CD38^-$ Thy^+	Lin^- $Sca1^+$ Kit^+ $CD34^-$ $Flk2^-$
Early progenitors	Lin^- $CD34^+$ $CD38^+$ Thy^-	Lin^- $Sca1^+$ Kit^+ $CD34^+$
Myeloid progenitors	Lin^- $CD34^+$ $CD38^+$	Lin^- $Sca1^-$ Kit^+ $CD34^+$ $CD33^+$
Committed myeloid cells (promyelocytes)	Lin^+ $CD34^-$ $CD33^+$	Lin^+

The Case of APL

The study of LSCs in APL has been historically difficult due to the low efficiency of human APL engraftment into immunodeficient mice [10]. Indeed, only in 2012, Patel and colleagues were able to obtain engraftment of CD3-depleted APL samples into irradiated NOD/SCID IL2Rg^{null} (NSG) mice, formally demonstrating the presence of LICs in human APL [31]. On the other hand, several mouse models of APL have been developed, in which the expression of PML-RARα in different hematopoietic progenitors shed light on the issue of the cell of origin of the disease. There are two main types of APL mouse models: (1) transgenic mice, harboring the human PML-RARα cDNA derived from at (15;17) translocation and (2) mice transplanted with hematopoietic cells previously transduced with viral constructs coding for the PML-RARα fusion protein.

The most widely diffuse transgenic APL mouse models harbor PML-RARα cDNA under the control of human MRP8 (migration inhibitory factor-related protein-8) [32] or the human CG (cathepsin G) promoters [33]. Both of these promoters become active relatively early during the process of myeloid differentiation. Instead, PML-RARα expression under the control of CD11b promoter, which is active in more differentiated myeloid cells (myelocytes), does not lead to APL development [34]. A common feature of APL transgenic mice is the long latency and low penetrance of disease development, suggesting that PML-RARα expression is not sufficient alone to cause leukemia and that the acquisition of other mutations is required in the APL leukemogenic process. Indeed, mouse models harboring other mutations like the reciprocal translocation RARα-PML [35], FLT3-ITD mutation [36], or BCL-2 overexpression [37] develop leukemia with a shorter latency or higher penetrance. Finally, Westervelt and colleagues targeted PML-RARα cDNA into the murine CG locus obtaining a knock-in mouse model which develops APL with high penetrance (90%) but still after a prolonged latency. In this model, PML-RARα expression levels are much lower than in the previously mentioned transgenic mice suggesting that very low levels of PML-RARα expression in early myeloid cells are sufficient for the development of APL in mice [38].

Analyses of transgenic mouse models further allow studies on the preleukemic phase preceding overt APL. During preleukemia, PML-RARα expression does not modify the proportion of stem and progenitor populations in the bone marrow, but it is able to confer, *in vitro*, self-renewal properties to early myeloid progenitors and promyelocytes. Preleukemic promyelocytes are endowed with the ability to engraft in lethally irradiated recipient mice, demonstrating that PML-RARα confers self-renewal potential to committed cells prior to APL development [39]. When mice develop APL, their bone marrow shows a marked reduction of the normal stem and progenitor compartments in favor of more committed myeloid progenitors and promyelocytes, which are the only population able to propagate the disease in recipient mice. These findings suggest that APL LICs reside in the promyelocytic population [39, 40]. The possibility of APL originating from myeloid-committed cells like promyelocytes implies that the fusion oncoprotein should be able to extend their limited self-renewal by itself or with specific additional mutations.

Viral transduction of purified cell populations and subsequent transplantation in recipient mice provided further information regarding the cell susceptible of PML-RARα-induced transformation. Minucci and colleagues obtained an APL mouse model by transplanting murine Lin$^-$ progenitors transduced with a PML-RARα-coding retroviral vector. Mice receiving PML-RARα-expressing Lin$^-$ cells develop leukemia with a short latency (4 months) and high penetrance (80%) suggesting that the expression of PML-RARα was enforced in a compartment enriched in the oncogene target cells [41]. In addition, this model confirms the existence of a preleukemic phase in APL, during which mice display only minor impairment in myeloid maturation, hinting to the requirement of a second hit to develop overt leukemia.

PML-RARα transduction of human early progenitors (Lin$^-$CD34$^+$CD71$^-$) results in a rapid induction of myeloid differentiation to the promyelocytic stage (CD34$^-$) and subsequent retinoic acid (RA)-sensitive maturation block, *in vitro*. Moreover, hematopoietic progenitors show a strong bias toward the granulocytic lineage, regardless of cytokine stimuli, and become resistant to apoptosis induced by *in vitro* cytokine withdrawal. These findings suggested that the PML-RARα target cell could be an early progenitor [42].

More recently, Matsushita and colleagues established a humanized APL model via retroviral transduction of PML-RARα into CD34$^+$ human cord blood cells and transplantation into immunodeficient mice. PML-RARα expression in human CD34$^+$ cells induces myeloid differentiation and maturation block at the promyelocytic stage until, eventually, mice develop a disease similar to human APL and characterized by CD34$^-$ blasts. In particular, among the CD34$^+$ cells, CD34$^+$CD38$^+$ progenitors induce APL with higher efficiency in NSG mice. APL cells have a low transplantation potential into secondary recipients, but CD34$^-$ blasts exhibit the ability to function as LICs *in vivo* [43]. These findings suggest that, in APL, the tumor initiation and maintenance potential could reside in different cell populations.

The first studies on APL SCs go back to the 1990s when different groups investigated the presence of PML-RARα translocation in the CD34$^+$CD38$^-$ population (HSCs) rather than in the CD34$^+$CD38$^+$ compartment (multipotent progenitor cells) by Southern blot or fluorescent in situ hybridization (FISH) analyses, obtaining contradictory results [44, 45]. An interesting attempt to reconcile the conflicting findings in the field was proposed by Grimwade and Enver. The authors introduced the possibility that different subtypes of APL could arise from different target cells, where more committed progenitors may give rise to the classical and less aggressive hypergranular APL, while earlier progenitors may give rise to the hypogranular form of APL, which is characterized by the presence of lymphoid markers and the expression of the fusion gene in the stem compartment (CD34$^+$CD48$^-$) [46].

In 2016, a humanized ossicle xenograft mouse model was reported to allow efficient engraftment of CD3-depleted APL with a high level of bone marrow chimerism. These mice have been subcutaneously injected with human bone marrow mesenchymal stromal cells (BM-MSCs) resulting in the formation of a functional humanized bone marrow niche. Injection of human APL into the humanized niche allows complete engraftment of the ossicle and, thus, analyses of the APL SC identity. Injection of CD34$^+$CD38$^-$ fraction from APL samples gives rise to normal lymphoid and myeloid progeny, which do not express PML-RARα. On the contrary, injection of APL bulk gives rise only transiently to normal hematopoiesis, before its abrogation by the expansion of myeloid blasts harboring the oncogenic translocation. Moreover, FISH analysis of subpopulations isolated from human APL samples demonstrated that PML-RARα is absent in stem and early progenitor cells, while it is present in CD34$^-$ myeloid-committed progenitors (promyelocytes) which are also able to engraft in humanized ossicle xenograft mice [47]. Up to now, this is the best demonstration that human APL LSCs reside in a myeloid-committed progenitor.

Implications for Therapy

CSCs are clinically relevant, as they appear to be intrinsically resistant to different drugs and can therefore persist during treatment and lead to the emergence of a relapse. The significance of this observation is further highlighted by the increased frequency of CSCs [48, 49] and the prevalence of CSC transcriptional signatures [14, 50] in the most aggressive tumors. Several studies have reported a correlation between LSCs and clinical outcome, specifically in AML. For instance, high LSC content (CD34$^+$CD38$^-$ cells) in AML samples at diagnosis has been associated with better engraftment in NOD/SCID mice [49], and, in turn, successful engraftment of patient leukemic blasts in NOD/SCID mice has been linked to poor prognosis [49, 51]. Different biological features among LSC-specific properties may underlie the inability of certain AML samples to engraft in immunodeficient mice and at the same time to exhibit higher responsiveness to current therapies, as happens in the case of APL. It has been further shown that poor clinical outcome correlates with the degree of overlap between the gene expression profile of functionally validated LSCs and normal HSCs [14]. In addition, integrated LSC gene expression and DNA methylation analysis led to the identification of an epigenetic signature that is able to segregate AMLs according to their FAB classification and, potentially, according to the cell of origin of the disease [52]. More recently, Ng and colleagues developed a core biomarker list of 17 genes related to stemness (the LSC17 score), which are differentially expressed between the LSC and non-LSC fractions from 78 AML patients, and were functionally validated by xenotransplantation. The LSC17 score was highly prognostic in five independent patient cohorts belonging to different AML subtypes and predicted therapy resistance. Patients with high LSC17 scores had poor outcomes with current treatments, while APL patient samples significantly segregated with low LSC17 scores [53].

The ability of SCs and CSCs to evade chemotherapy and radiotherapy has been associated with various functional properties and molecular mechanisms such as quiescence [54–56], apoptosis evasion [57–59], enhanced DNA damage response [60, 61], and lower concentration of reactive oxygen species (ROS) [58, 62]. Even though the relationship between these properties and stemness, per se, has not been fully delineated, accumulating evidence stresses the need for efficient therapeutic interventions that target specifically the CSC population for complete tumor eradication. For instance, glioblastoma cells positive for the CSC marker prominin-1 (CD133+) have been found enriched after ionizing radiation both *in vitro*, after short-term cultures, and *in vivo*, in the brains of immunocompromised mice, as well as in tumor samples obtained from patients. Importantly, the higher frequency of CD133+ cells after radiation was linked to the development of more aggressive tumors upon transplantation in secondary recipient mice, suggesting that glioblastoma CSCs might survive radiotherapy and lead to the relapse of the disease [60]. Similarly, breast CSCs identified by aldehyde dehydrogenase 1 expression (ALDH1) in the samples of patients who failed to achieve remission after treatment have been associated with resistance to chemotherapy [63].

Indeed, indirect evidence points to LSC quiescence as the source of resistance and eventual relapse. Quiescence has been linked to therapy resistance [55, 56], while cell cycle-restricted LSCs are crucial for the development of leukemia [61]. Longitudinal single-cell analyses in two AML patients, from diagnosis to relapse, allowed lineage reconstruction depicting the genomic distance based on microsatellite mutations. In contrast to studies on driver mutations, this approach enables the approximation of cell depth at relapse or, in other words, the number of cell replication events prior to the emergence of the relapse clone. Although lacking direct evidence, this study indicated that mutations carried in minor slowly expanding subclones were maintained after treatment, suggesting that cells with shorter replicative histories may be more apt to survive chemotherapy [64]. Quiescent cells are also characterized by lower levels of oxidative phosphorylation, and LSCs have been shown to have lower ROS levels and oxygen consumption rates. At the same time, LSCs are highly dependent on oxidative phosphorylation, which can be targeted by Bcl-2 inhibitors leading to eradication of LSCs [57, 58]. As normal HSCs, LSCs are mostly quiescent [65], and *in vivo* tracking of individual LSCs in serially transplanted NOD/SCID mice showed that, like in the normal HSC compartment, distinct hierarchically organized LSCs are present. The diverse LSC behavior derives from heterogeneous self-renewal and proliferation potential [66]. Nevertheless, quiescent LSCs can be recruited into the cell cycle becoming sensitive to chemotherapeutic agents [56]. Despite shared features between LSCs and

HSCs, it may be possible to target gene networks that are indispensable for the survival of malignant stem cells only. This is the case of miR-126, which was found to promote quiescence and increase self-renewal in primary LSCs, while it plays opposite role in HSCs [67].

The design of novel therapeutic strategies in AML should include the specific targeting of LSCs while sparing normal HSCs. For instance, CD47 is a protein highly expressed on the surface of cancer cells, and its role is linked to cancer evasion from innate immune surveillance [68]. LSCs overexpress CD47, as compared to normal HSCs, thus fulfilling the above criteria [69]. Since markers commonly used to study LSCs in human AML are based on the immunophenotype of normal hematopoietic cells, a lot of effort has been invested into identifying specific molecules able to efficiently discriminate LSCs both from normal HSCs and the bulk of leukemic blasts. This is also necessary for APL, where series of evidence suggest that LSCs reside in a myeloid-committed progenitor population. Many surface markers have been proposed to be specific for LSC identification in different AML subtypes, with the exception of APL, also due to the low engraftment efficiency in xenograft models which makes the characterization of APL LSCs difficult. However, the proposed markers allowed identification and only partial elimination of LSCs. Among other markers, the CD33 antigen is highly expressed in APL/AML blasts and in normal human myeloid-committed progenitors, while it is not expressed on normal HSCs [70]. Therefore, CD33 is a potential target for new therapies, and specific antibodies are in clinical trials. In particular, GO (gemtuzumab ozogamicin) is an anti-CD33 monoclonal antibody conjugated to the toxin calicheamicin, which gave significantly increased remission rates in advanced and relapsed APL [71, 72]. GO is highly active against APL, as compared to other AMLs, suggesting that APL stem cells reside in the $CD33^+$ compartment and have a mature phenotype [73]. However, in 2010 Pfizer voluntarily withdrew GO due to safety concerns, and the drug is currently available only for palliative use [74]. SGN-CD33A, a novel anti-CD33 antibody conjugated to two molecules of a pyrrolobenzodiazepine dimer drug, is currently in clinical trials for AML, including APL. It has demonstrated antileukemic activity with 47% of complete remission and rapid blast clearance with relatively modest toxicity [75].

Even though the CSC theory has been fairly established, the nature of CSCs has raised an ongoing debate. If stemness is not a fixed property of a specific cancer cell population but rather a cell state controlled or influenced by microenvironmental cues and cell-cell interactions, then, any cancer cell could potentially gain stem properties and reestablish a tumor. This “dynamic CSC model” [76] poses both clinical and conceptual challenges. If CSCs are a moving target, how could they be identified and efficiently targeted? It has been indeed proposed that cancer cells might be endowed with higher plasticity, and therefore dedifferentiation events might be more frequent in tumors than in normal tissues [77]. If this is the case, CSC-specific therapies would fail in curing patients. Nevertheless, differentiation therapies should be successful, regardless of the identity of CSCs and potential cancer cell plasticity. APL is a paradigm for targeted differentiation therapies in cancer as, in the last decades, treatments have evolved from all-trans retinoic acid (ATRA) and chemotherapy, for all newly diagnosed patients, to ATRA and arsenic trioxide (ATO). The ATRA and ATO combination has been demonstrated to eradicate APL-initiating cells via PML-RARα degradation [78]. The effective LSC eradication in APL is demonstrated by the high rate of complete remission and the low incidence of relapses, especially for low-risk patients [79]. APL transgenic mouse models have been used to elucidate the molecular mechanisms underlying PML-RARα-targeted therapy with ATRA and ATO. Mice transplanted with murine APL and treated with ATRA show a rapid differentiation of APL blasts in the bone marrow. Subsequent transplantation of ATRA treated bone marrow cells into secondary recipients leads to the development of APL, indicating the persistence of LSCs after ATRA treatment. Therefore, while ATRA is effective in inducing blast terminal differentiation, it is insufficient in

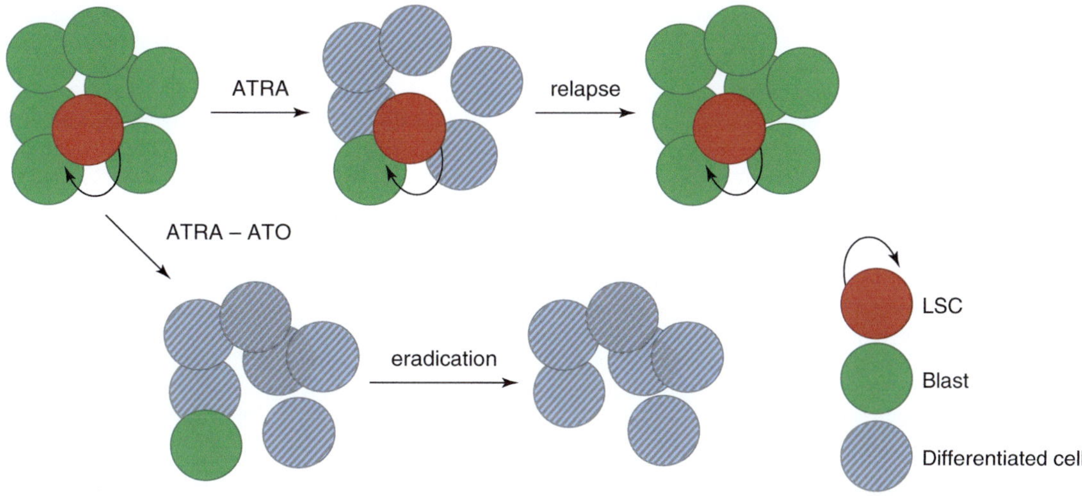

Fig. 3.2 LSC targeting is required for complete APL eradication. Treatment with pharmacological doses of ATRA is sufficient to induce rapid blast differentiation but is not effective against LSCs, which eventually results in leukemia relapse (*upper part* of the scheme). In contrast, the combinatorial use of ATRA and ATO synergizes in PML-RARα degradation, LSC eradication, and blast terminal differentiation, providing a definitive cure for APL patients (*lower part* of the scheme)

LSC eradication and APL complete remission (Fig. 3.2, upper part of the scheme). On the contrary, when ATRA and ATO are used in combination, they synergize in provoking marked disease regression and LSC eradication [78]. In more detail, the two drugs cooperate to trigger proteasome-dependent PML-RARα degradation and reactivation of RARα target genes. This in turn leads to terminal differentiation of leukemic blasts and the restoration of the physiological PML nuclear bodies (Fig. 3.2, lower part of the scheme) [80].

Investigation of residual normal HSCs in AML samples revealed that many patients harbor a population of HSCs bearing some of the mutations present in the corresponding leukemic cells. This so-called preleukemic HSCs are present both at diagnosis and relapse, and their proportion in the stem compartment is correlated with poor prognosis [81, 82]. This finding is clinically relevant because relapses in AML patients could arise both through selection of preexisting and resistant leukemic clones or through the evolution of preleukemic HSCs through the acquisition of additional mutations. Moreover, preleukemic mutations have been found in healthy individuals. The resulting clonal hematopoiesis is increasing with aging, and it is associated with higher risk of hematological cancer development [83]. Hopefully, in the next years, evaluation of preleukemic HSCs could be used for early detection of hematological malignancies and to refine patients risk stratification in clinical trials and therapy decisional processes.

References

1. Reya T, Morrison SJ, Clarke MF, Weissman IL. Stem cells, cancer, and cancer stem cells. Nature. 2001;414(6859):105–11.
2. Clarke MF, Dick JE, Dirks PB, Eaves CJ, Jamieson CH, Jones DL, et al. Cancer stem cells—perspectives on current status and future directions: AACR Workshop on cancer stem cells. Cancer Res. 2006;66(19):9339–44.
3. Beck B, Blanpain C. Unravelling cancer stem cell potential. Nat Rev Cancer. 2013;13(10):727–38.
4. Park CH, Bergsagel DE, McCulloch EA. Mouse myeloma tumor stem cells: a primary cell culture assay. J Natl Cancer Inst. 1971;46(2):411–22.
5. Salsbury AJ. The significance of the circulating cancer cell. Cancer Treat Rev. 1975;2(1):55–72.
6. Southam CM, Brunschwig A. Quantitative studies of autotransplantation of human cancer. Preliminary report. Cancer. 1961;14(5):971–8.
7. Kreso A, Dick JE. Evolution of the cancer stem cell model. Cell Stem Cell. 2014;14(3):275–91.

8. Sell S. On the stem cell origin of cancer. Am J Pathol. 2010;176(6):2584–494.
9. Pierce GB Jr, Dixon FJ Jr, Verney EL. Teratocarcinogenic and tissue-forming potentials of the cell types comprising neoplastic embryoid bodies. Lab Investig. 1960;9:583–602.
10. Bonnet D, Dick JE. Human acute myeloid leukemia is organized as a hierarchy that originates from a primitive hematopoietic cell. Nat Med. 1997;3(7):730–7.
11. Lapidot T, Sirard C, Vormoor J, Murdoch B, Hoang T, Caceres-Cortes J, et al. A cell initiating human acute myeloid leukaemia after transplantation into SCID mice. Nature. 1994;367(6464):645–8.
12. Taussig DC, Miraki-Moud F, Anjos-Afonso F, Pearce DJ, Allen K, Ridler C, et al. Anti-CD38 antibody-mediated clearance of human repopulating cells masks the heterogeneity of leukemia-initiating cells. Blood. 2008;112(3):568–75.
13. Taussig DC, Vargaftig J, Miraki-Moud F, Griessinger E, Sharrock K, Luke T, et al. Leukemia-initiating cells from some acute myeloid leukemia patients with mutated nucleophosmin reside in the CD34(-) fraction. Blood. 2010;115(10):1976–84.
14. Eppert K, Takenaka K, Lechman ER, Waldron L, Nilsson B, van Galen P, et al. Stem cell gene expression programs influence clinical outcome in human leukemia. Nat Med. 2011;17(9):1086–93.
15. Sarry JE, Murphy K, Perry R, Sanchez PV, Secreto A, Keefer C, et al. Human acute myelogenous leukemia stem cells are rare and heterogeneous when assayed in NOD/SCID/IL2Rgammac-deficient mice. J Clin Invest. 2011;121(1):384–95.
16. Al-Hajj M, Wicha MS, Benito-Hernandez A, Morrison SJ, Clarke MF. Prospective identification of tumorigenic breast cancer cells. Proc Natl Acad Sci U S A. 2003;100(7):3983–8.
17. Singh SK, Hawkins C, Clarke ID, Squire JA, Bayani J, Hide T, et al. Identification of human brain tumour initiating cells. Nature. 2004;432(7015):396–401.
18. O'Brien CA, Pollett A, Gallinger S, Dick JE. A human colon cancer cell capable of initiating tumour growth in immunodeficient mice. Nature. 2007;445(7123):106–10.
19. Quintana E, Shackleton M, Sabel MS, Fullen DR, Johnson TM, Morrison SJ. Efficient tumour formation by single human melanoma cells. Nature. 2008;456(7222):593–8.
20. Quintana E, Shackleton M, Foster HR, Fullen DR, Sabel MS, Johnson TM, et al. Phenotypic heterogeneity among tumorigenic melanoma cells from patients that is reversible and not hierarchically organized. Cancer Cell. 2010;18(5):510–23.
21. Roesch A, Fukunaga-Kalabis M, Schmidt EC, Zabierowski SE, Brafford PA, Vultur A, et al. A temporarily distinct subpopulation of slow-cycling melanoma cells is required for continuous tumor growth. Cell. 2010;141(4):583–94.
22. Visvader JE, Lindeman GJ. Cancer stem cells: current status and evolving complexities. Cell Stem Cell. 2012;10(6):717–28.
23. Agliano A, Martin-Padura I, Mancuso P, Marighetti P, Rabascio C, Pruneri G, et al. Human acute leukemia cells injected in NOD/LtSz-scid/IL-2Rgamma null mice generate a faster and more efficient disease compared to other NOD/scid-related strains. Int J Cancer. 2008;123(9):2222–7.
24. Visvader JE. Cells of origin in cancer. Nature. 2011;469(7330):314–22.
25. Cozzio A, Passegue E, Ayton PM, Karsunky H, Cleary ML, Weissman IL. Similar MLL-associated leukemias arising from self-renewing stem cells and short-lived myeloid progenitors. Genes Dev. 2003;17(24):3029–35.
26. Huntly BJ, Shigematsu H, Deguchi K, Lee BH, Mizuno S, Duclos N, et al. MOZ-TIF2, but not BCR-ABL, confers properties of leukemic stem cells to committed murine hematopoietic progenitors. Cancer Cell. 2004;6(6):587–96.
27. Wiseman DH, Greystoke BF, Somervaille TC. The variety of leukemic stem cells in myeloid malignancy. Oncogene. 2014;33(24):3091–8.
28. Morrison SJ, Uchida N, Weissman IL. The biology of hematopoietic stem cells. Annu Rev Cell Dev Biol. 1995;11:35–71.
29. Morrison SJ, Weissman IL. The long-term repopulating subset of hematopoietic stem cells is deterministic and isolatable by phenotype. Immunity. 1994;1(8):661–73.
30. Bhatia M, Wang JC, Kapp U, Bonnet D, Dick JE. Purification of primitive human hematopoietic cells capable of repopulating immune-deficient mice. Proc Natl Acad Sci U S A. 1997;94(10):5320–5.
31. Patel S, Zhang Y, Cassinat B, Zassadowski F, Ferre N, Cuccuini W, et al. Successful xenografts of AML3 samples in immunodeficient NOD/shi-SCID IL2Rgamma(-)/(-) mice. Leukemia. 2012;26(11):2432–5.
32. Brown D, Kogan S, Lagasse E, Weissman I, Alcalay M, Pelicci PG, et al. A PMLRARalpha transgene initiates murine acute promyelocytic leukemia. Proc Natl Acad Sci U S A. 1997;94(6):2551–6.
33. Grisolano JL, Wesselschmidt RL, Pelicci PG, Ley TJ. Altered myeloid development and acute leukemia in transgenic mice expressing PML-RAR alpha under control of cathepsin G regulatory sequences. Blood. 1997;89(2):376–87.
34. Early E, Moore MA, Kakizuka A, Nason-Burchenal K, Martin P, Evans RM, et al. Transgenic expression of PML/RARalpha impairs myelopoiesis. Proc Natl Acad Sci U S A. 1996;93(15):7900–4.
35. Pollock JL, Westervelt P, Kurichety AK, Pelicci PG, Grisolano JL, Ley TJ. A bcr-3 isoform of RARalpha-PML potentiates the development of PML-RARalpha-driven acute promyelocytic leukemia. Proc Natl Acad Sci U S A. 1999;96(26):15103–8.
36. Kelly LM, Kutok JL, Williams IR, Boulton CL, Amaral SM, Curley DP, et al. PML/RARalpha and FLT3-ITD induce an APL-like disease in a mouse model. Proc Natl Acad Sci U S A. 2002;99(12):8283–8.

37. Kogan SC, Brown DE, Shultz DB, Truong BT, Lallemand-Breitenbach V, Guillemin MC, et al. BCL-2 cooperates with promyelocytic leukemia retinoic acid receptor alpha chimeric protein (PMLRARalpha) to block neutrophil differentiation and initiate acute leukemia. J Exp Med. 2001;193(4):531–43.
38. Westervelt P, Lane AA, Pollock JL, Oldfather K, Holt MS, Zimonjic DB, et al. High-penetrance mouse model of acute promyelocytic leukemia with very low levels of PML-RARalpha expression. Blood. 2003;102(5):1857–65.
39. Wojiski S, Guibal FC, Kindler T, Lee BH, Jesneck JL, Fabian A, et al. PML-RARalpha initiates leukemia by conferring properties of self-renewal to committed promyelocytic progenitors. Leukemia. 2009;23(8):1462–71.
40. Guibal FC, Alberich-Jorda M, Hirai H, Ebralidze A, Levantini E, Di Ruscio A, et al. Identification of a myeloid committed progenitor as the cancer-initiating cell in acute promyelocytic leukemia. Blood. 2009;114(27):5415–25.
41. Minucci S, Monestiroli S, Giavara S, Ronzoni S, Marchesi F, Insinga A, et al. PML-RAR induces promyelocytic leukemias with high efficiency following retroviral gene transfer into purified murine hematopoietic progenitors. Blood. 2002;100(8):2989–95.
42. Grignani F, Valtieri M, Gabbianelli M, Gelmetti V, Botta R, Luchetti L, et al. PML/RAR alpha fusion protein expression in normal human hematopoietic progenitors dictates myeloid commitment and the promyelocytic phenotype. Blood. 2000;96(4):1531–7.
43. Matsushita H, Yahata T, Sheng Y, Nakamura Y, Muguruma Y, Matsuzawa H, et al. Establishment of a humanized APL model via the transplantation of PML-RARA-transduced human common myeloid progenitors into immunodeficient mice. PLoS One. 2014;9(11):e111082.
44. Edwards RH, Wasik MA, Finan J, Rodriguez R, Moore J, Kamoun M, et al. Evidence for early hematopoietic progenitor cell involvement in acute promyelocytic leukemia. Am J Clin Pathol. 1999;112(6):819–27.
45. Turhan AG, Lemoine FM, Debert C, Bonnet ML, Baillou C, Picard F, et al. Highly purified primitive hematopoietic stem cells are PML-RARA negative and generate nonclonal progenitors in acute promyelocytic leukemia. Blood. 1995;85(8):2154–61.
46. Grimwade D, Enver T. Acute promyelocytic leukemia: where does it stem from? Leukemia. 2004;18(3):375–84.
47. Reinisch A, Thomas D, Corces MR, Zhang X, Gratzinger D, Hong WJ, et al. A humanized bone marrow ossicle xenotransplantation model enables improved engraftment of healthy and leukemic human hematopoietic cells. Nat Med. 2016;22(7):812–21.
48. Pece S, Tosoni D, Confalonieri S, Mazzarol G, Vecchi M, Ronzoni S, et al. Biological and molecular heterogeneity of breast cancers correlates with their cancer stem cell content. Cell. 2010;140(1):62–73.
49. van Rhenen A, Feller N, Kelder A, Westra AH, Rombouts E, Zweegman S, et al. High stem cell frequency in acute myeloid leukemia at diagnosis predicts high minimal residual disease and poor survival. Clin Cancer Res. 2005;11(18):6520–7.
50. Ginestier C, Hur MH, Charafe-Jauffret E, Monville F, Dutcher J, Brown M, et al. ALDH1 is a marker of normal and malignant human mammary stem cells and a predictor of poor clinical outcome. Cell Stem Cell. 2007;1(5):555–67.
51. Pearce DJ, Taussig D, Zibara K, Smith LL, Ridler CM, Preudhomme C, et al. AML engraftment in the NOD/SCID assay reflects the outcome of AML: implications for our understanding of the heterogeneity of AML. Blood. 2006;107(3):1166–73.
52. Jung N, Dai B, Gentles AJ, Majeti R, Feinberg AP. An LSC epigenetic signature is largely mutation independent and implicates the HOXA cluster in AML pathogenesis. Nat Commun. 2015;6:8489.
53. Ng SW, Mitchell A, Kennedy JA, Chen WC, McLeod J, Ibrahimova N, et al. A 17-gene stemness score for rapid determination of risk in acute leukaemia. Nature. 2016;540(7633):433–7.
54. Graham SM, Jorgensen HG, Allan E, Pearson C, Alcorn MJ, Richmond L, et al. Primitive, quiescent, Philadelphia-positive stem cells from patients with chronic myeloid leukemia are insensitive to STI571 in vitro. Blood. 2002;99(1):319–25.
55. Ishikawa F, Yoshida S, Saito Y, Hijikata A, Kitamura H, Tanaka S, et al. Chemotherapy-resistant human AML stem cells home to and engraft within the bone-marrow endosteal region. Nat Biotechnol. 2007;25(11):1315–21.
56. Saito Y, Uchida N, Tanaka S, Suzuki N, Tomizawa-Murasawa M, Sone A, et al. Induction of cell cycle entry eliminates human leukemia stem cells in a mouse model of AML. Nat Biotechnol. 2010;28(3):275–80.
57. Chan SM, Thomas D, Corces-Zimmerman MR, Xavy S, Rastogi S, Hong WJ, et al. Isocitrate dehydrogenase 1 and 2 mutations induce BCL-2 dependence in acute myeloid leukemia. Nat Med. 2015;21(2):178–84.
58. Lagadinou ED, Sach A, Callahan K, Rossi RM, Neering SJ, Minhajuddin M, et al. BCL-2 inhibition targets oxidative phosphorylation and selectively eradicates quiescent human leukemia stem cells. Cell Stem Cell. 2013;12(3):329–41.
59. Liu G, Yuan X, Zeng Z, Tunici P, Ng H, Abdulkadir IR, et al. Analysis of gene expression and chemoresistance of CD133+ cancer stem cells in glioblastoma. Mol Cancer. 2006;5:67.
60. Bao S, Wu Q, McLendon RE, Hao Y, Shi Q, Hjelmeland AB, et al. Glioma stem cells promote radioresistance by preferential activation of the DNA damage response. Nature. 2006;444(7120):756–60.
61. Viale A, De Franco F, Orleth A, Cambiaghi V, Giuliani V, Bossi D, et al. Cell-cycle restriction limits DNA damage and maintains self-renewal of leukaemia stem cells. Nature. 2009;457(7225):51–6.
62. Diehn M, Cho RW, Lobo NA, Kalisky T, Dorie MJ, Kulp AN, et al. Association of reactive oxygen species levels and radioresistance in cancer stem cells. Nature. 2009;458(7239):780–3.

63. Tanei T, Morimoto K, Shimazu K, Kim SJ, Tanji Y, Taguchi T, et al. Association of breast cancer stem cells identified by aldehyde dehydrogenase 1 expression with resistance to sequential Paclitaxel and epirubicin-based chemotherapy for breast cancers. Clin Cancer Res. 2009;15(12):4234–41.
64. Shlush LI, Chapal-Ilani N, Adar R, Pery N, Maruvka Y, Spiro A, et al. Cell lineage analysis of acute leukemia relapse uncovers the role of replication-rate heterogeneity and microsatellite instability. Blood. 2012;120(3):603–12.
65. Guan Y, Gerhard B, Hogge DE. Detection, isolation, and stimulation of quiescent primitive leukemic progenitor cells from patients with acute myeloid leukemia (AML). Blood. 2003;101(8):3142–9.
66. Hope KJ, Jin L, Dick JE. Acute myeloid leukemia originates from a hierarchy of leukemic stem cell classes that differ in self-renewal capacity. Nat Immunol. 2004;5(7):738–43.
67. Lechman ER, Gentner B, Ng SW, Schoof EM, van Galen P, Kennedy JA, et al. miR-126 regulates distinct self-renewal outcomes in normal and malignant hematopoietic stem cells. Cancer Cell. 2016;29(2):214–28.
68. Jaiswal S, Jamieson CH, Pang WW, Park CY, Chao MP, Majeti R, et al. CD47 is upregulated on circulating hematopoietic stem cells and leukemia cells to avoid phagocytosis. Cell. 2009;138(2):271–85.
69. Majeti R, Chao MP, Alizadeh AA, Pang WW, Jaiswal S, Gibbs KD Jr, et al. CD47 is an adverse prognostic factor and therapeutic antibody target on human acute myeloid leukemia stem cells. Cell. 2009;138(2):286–99.
70. Peiper SC, Ashmun RA, Look AT. Molecular cloning, expression, and chromosomal localization of a human gene encoding the CD33 myeloid differentiation antigen. Blood. 1988;72(1):314–21.
71. Breccia M, Cimino G, Diverio D, Gentilini F, Mandelli F, Lo CF. Sustained molecular remission after low dose gemtuzumab-ozogamicin in elderly patients with advanced acute promyelocytic leukemia. Haematologica. 2007;92(9):1273–4.
72. Lo-Coco F, Cimino G, Breccia M, Noguera NI, Diverio D, Finolezzi E, et al. Gemtuzumab ozogamicin (Mylotarg) as a single agent for molecularly relapsed acute promyelocytic leukemia. Blood. 2004;104(7):1995–9.
73. Walter RB, Appelbaum FR, Estey EH, Bernstein ID. Acute myeloid leukemia stem cells and CD33-targeted immunotherapy. Blood. 2012;119(26):6198–208.
74. Petersdorf SH, Kopecky KJ, Slovak M, Willman C, Nevill T, Brandwein J, et al. A phase 3 study of gemtuzumab ozogamicin during induction and postconsolidation therapy in younger patients with acute myeloid leukemia. Blood. 2013;121(24):4854–60.
75. Stein EM, Stein A, Walter RB, Fathi AT, Lancet JE, Kovacsovics TJ, et al. Interim analysis of a phase 1 trial of SGN-CD33A in patients with CD33-positive acute myeloid leukemia (AML). Blood. 2014;124(21):623.
76. Vermeulen L, de Sousa e Melo F, Richel DJ, Medema JP. The developing cancer stem-cell model: clinical challenges and opportunities. Lancet Oncol. 2012;13(2):e83–9.
77. Theise ND, Wilmut I. Cell plasticity: flexible arrangement. Nature. 2003;425(6953):21.
78. Nasr R, Guillemin MC, Ferhi O, Soilihi H, Peres L, Berthier C, et al. Eradication of acute promyelocytic leukemia-initiating cells through PML-RARA degradation. Nat Med. 2008;14(12):1333–42.
79. Coombs CC, Tavakkoli M, Tallman MS. Acute promyelocytic leukemia: where did we start, where are we now, and the future. Blood Cancer J. 2015;5:e304.
80. Ablain J, Nasr R, Bazarbachi A, de The H. The drug-induced degradation of oncoproteins: an unexpected Achilles' heel of cancer cells? Cancer Discov. 2011;1(2):117–27.
81. Corces-Zimmerman MR, Hong WJ, Weissman IL, Medeiros BC, Majeti R. Preleukemic mutations in human acute myeloid leukemia affect epigenetic regulators and persist in remission. Proc Natl Acad Sci U S A. 2014;111(7):2548–53.
82. Shlush LI, Zandi S, Mitchell A, Chen WC, Brandwein JM, Gupta V, et al. Identification of pre-leukaemic haematopoietic stem cells in acute leukaemia. Nature. 2014;506(7488):328–33.
83. Genovese G, Kahler AK, Handsaker RE, Lindberg J, Rose SA, Bakhoum SF, et al. Clonal hematopoiesis and blood-cancer risk inferred from blood DNA sequence. N Engl J Med. 2014;371(26):2477–87.

Molecular Genetics of Acute Promyelocytic Leukemia

4

Lourdes Mendez, Ming Chen, and Pier Paolo Pandolfi

Introduction

In 1957, Dr. L.K. Hillestad published a case series describing three patients with a rapidly lethal form of acute myeloid leukemia characterized by the accumulation of promyelocytes in the peripheral blood and bone marrow and coagulopathy, leading to hemorrhage, which he termed acute promyelocytic leukemia (APL) [1]. The first signal of disease control came in the 1970s with the application of anthracyclines to the treatment of APL. *All-trans*-retinoic acid (ATRA) entered the stage in 1985 [2–4] and was followed shortly thereafter by mapping of the hallmark genetic translocation t(15;17) to the retinoic acid receptor alpha (RARα) [5–10]; thus, commenced an era of molecular genetic study into APL. Arsenic trioxide (ATO) entered the clinic in 1994 [11–14] and laid the foundation for the seminal Phase II trial of ATRA and ATO by Estey and colleagues [15] followed by the landmark Phase III trial of the combination by Lo-Coco and colleagues in 2013 [16]. APL is an unparalleled story—the first example of a malignancy cured by targeted therapy. Alongside profound molecular insights lies a history rooted in traditional Chinese medicine with therapy informing science and science informing therapy leading to phenomenal success against this once-fatal disease.

L. Mendez, M.D., Ph.D. • M. Chen, Ph.D.
P.P. Pandolfi, M.D., Ph.D. (✉)
Department of Medicine and Pathology, Cancer Research Institute, Beth Israel Deaconess Cancer Center, Beth Israel Deaconess Medical Center, Harvard Medical School, Boston, MA 02215, USA
e-mail: ppandolf@bidmc.harvard.edu

PML-RARα/RARα-PML and Other APL Translocations in Leukemogenesis

APL is associated with balanced and reciprocal translocations characterized by involvement of the RARα gene on chromosome 17 [5, 17–19]. To date, nine different translocation partners have been identified (atlastgeneticsoncology.org) including fusions with PLZF t(11;17) (q23;q21) [20], NPM1 t(5;17)(q32q21) [21], and NuMA t(11;17)(q13,q21) [22], the so-called "X" partner genes for RARα [23]. PML is by far the dominant partner gene with t(15;17) being present in 98% of cases (Fig. 4.1) [20]. An early question in the field was whether the oncoproteins encoded by such translocations were necessary and sufficient for leukemogenesis. Transgenic mouse models of APL were instrumental in addressing this fundamental question [24–28]. This approach was also utilized to address the role of reciprocal translocations, such as RARα-PML and RARα-PLZF, in the initiation and progression of disease [29–31].

In 1997 multiple groups successfully recapitulated the salient features of human APL in

O. Abla et al. (eds.), *Acute Promyelocytic Leukemia*, https://doi.org/10.1007/978-3-319-64257-4_4

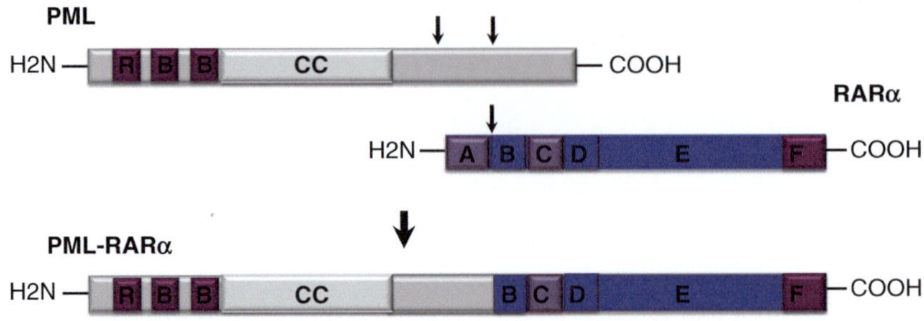

Fig. 4.1 Schematic of the PML-RARα fusion oncoprotein with functional domains. For PML, the RING (R), B boxes (B), and coiled-coil (CC) domains are indicated. For RARα, the DNA-binding domain (C) and ligand-binding domain (E) are indicated, and A, B, D, and F represent additional motifs

transgenic mouse models engineered to express the fusion PML-RARα oncoprotein under the control of myeloid-specific promoters, thus demonstrating that PML-RARα mediates leukemogenesis [24–26]. Interestingly, the models displayed a long latency and incomplete penetrance in developing acute leukemia suggesting that a "second hit" was involved; as we discuss below, RARα-X, the reciprocal product of the translocation, can act as a "second hit." The preleukemic stage in these transgenic models was characterized by myeloproliferation with the accumulation of myeloid progenitors in the bone marrow and spleen. Few additional genetic hits were identified in these models consistent with the notion that PML-RARα is the main driver of the disease, albeit not sufficient. This is coherent with a unique feature of APL, the consistent incidence of the disease across ages, which suggests that a single genetic event drives transformation [32]. Additional oncogenic events such as activation of fms-related tyrosine kinase through the FLT3-ITD mutation, NRAS mutation, and MYC overexpression promote disease penetrance or progression in mice and humans [33].

That the X-RARα translocations are disease-defining events was first hinted at by the differential response to ATRA and chemotherapy observed in patients harboring t(11;17) compared to t(15;17) APL, poor and favorable, respectively [34, 35]. That a distinct biology is prescribed by t(11;17) was also captured in the PLZF-RARα transgenic mouse model which developed disease reminiscent of a myeloproliferative neoplasm (Fig. 4.2); myeloid precursors retained the ability to terminally differentiate, and myeloid cells at different stages of maturation accumulated in the bone marrow and spleen [25]. This was cemented by seminal, preclinical studies showing that ATRA, ATO, and ATRA plus ATO prolonged survival in PML-RARα transgenic mice, whereas PLZF-RARα transgenic mice fail to attain complete remission in response to any of the three treatments (Fig. 4.2) [36]. Subsequent generation of the NPM-RARα TM allowed comparison with the PML- and PLZF-RARα TMs. In addition to cytomorphologic differences, the NPM-RARα TM also responded to treatment with ATRA or ATO like the PML-RARα TM, but different from the PLZF-RARα TMs. Interestingly, the NPM-RARα fusion oncoprotein was localized to the nucleolus suggesting possible interference with native NPM function [28]. Thus, X-RARα translocations and the encoded fusion proteins drive distinct biologic programs, and this translates into differential response to therapy.

As previously noted, translocations in APL are balanced and reciprocal. This begs the question—does RARα-X play an active role in leukemogenesis or is it merely a passenger? TMs again provided insights into the biologic role of RARα-Xs (Fig. 4.2). As with X-RARα, one size does not fit all. RARα-PML/PML-RARα TM displays increased penetrance of disease [29] consistent with an oncogenic role for RARα-PML. As noted above, PLZF-RARα TM develops disease that is MPN-like and falls short of leukemia;

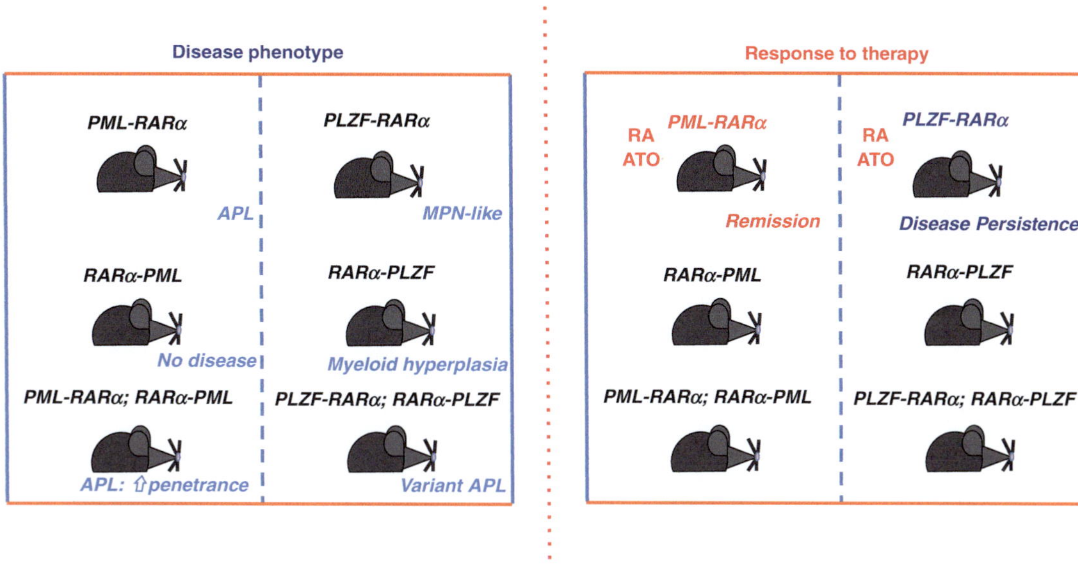

Fig. 4.2 Murine X-RARα and RARα-X transgenic models (TMs) recapitulate human APL and predict response to curative combination therapy. TMs bearing X-RARα, RARα-X, or both were generated (where X is either PML or PLZF). TMs reveal that the X partner protein modulates disease phenotype and dictates response to therapy

RARα-PLZF TM develop myeloid hyperplasia, but strikingly RARα-PLZF/PLZF-RARα TM develop APL-like disease [30]. In this regard, it is worth noting that RARα-PLZF expression is pervasive in t(11;17) human APL [34, 37].

Another layer of molecular detail was added by studies investigating whether transcriptional repression or activation by PML-RARα is required for leukemogenesis. Interestingly, the breakpoint for the RARα gene is consistently within the same intron [38] and results in preservation of the DNA-binding, ligand-binding, and RXR-binding domains. With multiple translocations involving RARα leading to the same phenotypic disease, the classical model of APL pathogenesis centers on suppression of RA signaling through repression of RARα target genes by a PML-RARα with dominant-negative activity. This model is in line with RARα regulation of myeloid differentiation, the block in differentiation seen in APL cells, and the ensuing differentiation of APL cells in response to pharmacologic retinoic acid. In support of this model, X-RARα proteins retain the ability to heterodimerize with RXR and bind to DNA RARE and the RA ligand, like the native RARα protein [39, 40]. Lending further support to the model, multiple lines of evidence indicated that X-RARα act as "super repressors" secondary to increased affinity for nuclear corepressors and histone deacetylases (HDAC) [41–43]. At pharmacologic doses of RA, the PML-RARα oncoprotein dissociates from corepressors/HDAC and transactivates RARα target genes (Fig. 4.3). And again, X-RARα specificity was observed since RA did not disrupt the PLZF-RARα interaction with corepressors. Interestingly, HDAC inhibitors did overcome transcription repression in the case of both PML-RARα and PLZF-RARα [41–43]. Investigators searched for the molecular basis for the observed "super repressor" activity of X-RARα. Oligomerization of X-RARα emerged as key to the repressive activity [44–46], and this was postulated to be due to more effective competition with native RARα for RXR binding as well as recruitment of X-moiety corepressors in the case of PML [47, 48].

The pivotal role of the X-moiety of the fusion oncoprotein in APL pathogenesis was further highlighted by studies by Kogan and

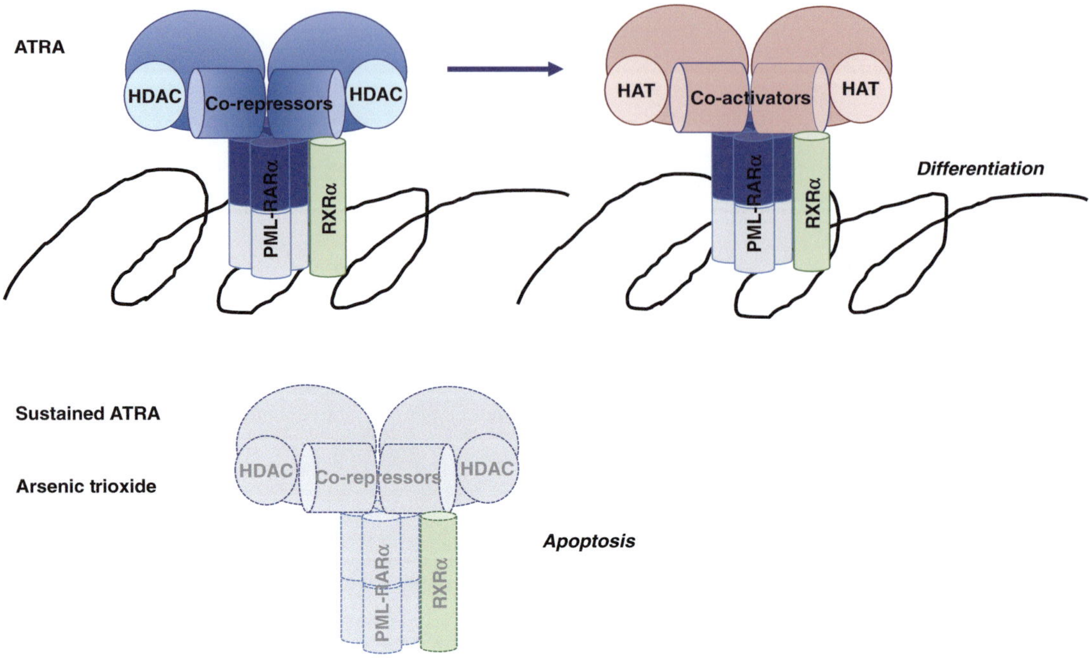

Fig. 4.3 ATRA and arsenic trioxide converge on PML-RARα to eliminate APL. ATRA prompts exchange of corepressors for coactivators and results in blast differentiation. Both ATRA and arsenic trioxide induce PML-RARα degradation, which is required for eradication of disease

colleagues demonstrating that transgenic mice expressing mutant RARα, unable to bind RA and thus activate transcription, do not develop leukemia challenging an RARα-centric paradigm. The same RARα mutation when engineered into PML-RARα resulted in myeloid leukemia albeit with differences compared to the original PML-RARα transgenic mice and unresponsive to RA-induced differentiation; this study demonstrated that lack of or aberrant activation of RARα target genes is not sufficient for the development of APL. However, the RARα mutant studies by Kogan et al. did not exclude the possibility that "super repression" of basal transcription levels of RARα targets in hematopoietic cells is the central transcriptional event in APL [23]; future studies would further elaborate this issue (discussed below). In PML-RARα, the functional domains of PML, the RING finger and coiled-coil domains, are retained suggesting that the PML moiety of the oncoprotein plays a specific and critical role in oncogenesis. Notably, the impressive clinical activity of single agent ATO, which does not lead to transactivation of RARα target genes [33], signaled that APL pathogenesis extended beyond an aberrant RARα pathway.

Multiple lines of evidence indicate that a central aspect of APL pathogenesis is functional impairment of PML. PML-RARα dominant-negative activity renders APL cells resistant to multiple apoptotic pathways mediated by the native PML protein [49]. A hallmark of t(15;17) APL cells is disruption of PML-NBs with reconstitution of the NBs upon treatment with RA or ATO [50–53]. Disruption of PML-NBs is a major mechanism by which PML-RARα results in functional impairment of PML with implications on p53 signaling, the PTEN-Akt pathway and other pathway, as we will also discuss below [54–58]. In an elegant proof of principle, Rego and colleagues demonstrated that homozygous or heterozygous deletion of PML accelerates the onset and increase the penetrance of leukemia in the PML-RARα TM [59]. Likewise, homozygous genetic deletion of PLZF had a profound effect on the phenotype of the PLZF-RARα TM, which now did display arrest at the promyelocyte stage of differentiation [30, 60]. Collectively, these genetic experiments provided evidence that APL pathogenesis and, specifically, the signature block at the promyelocytic stage of differentiation involve disruption of both native X and RARα activity.

More recently, several lines of evidence point to gain-of-function PML-RARα activity. Using ChIP-seq, Martens and colleagues profiled PML-RARα genomic binding sites in human APL and described a landscape characterized by the acquisition of de novo DNA binding sites by a heterotetramer composed of PML-RARα and RXRα. Many of the de novo binding sites overlapped with sites recognized by other nuclear receptors known to play a role in myeloid differentiation and stem cell self-renewal such as RARγ, the thyroid hormone receptor, and the vitamin D receptor [61]. Moreover, most RXRα was bound to PML-RARα raising the possibility that sequestration of RXRα, which has been implicated in myeloid lineage determination [62], plays an important role in the pathogenesis of APL. Transcriptional output by the PML-RARα oncoprotein is additionally regulated at the level of posttranslational modification. Sumoylation of the PML moiety, which has been shown to participate in APL initiation [63], results in transcriptional repression by the oncoprotein, and this may be mediated by sumoylation-dependent recruitment of cofactors such as the death domain-associated protein (DAXX) [64, 65]. Ex vivo, DAXX is required for immortalization and transcription repression [63]. As far as posttranslational modification of the RARα moiety, phosphorylation adds multiple layers of regulation including a possible nexus at S369 for cross talk with the MAPK signaling pathway with S369 being phosphorylated by RA-activated MSK1 [66].

Oncoprotein-Mediated Response to Therapy and Beyond

Transgenic models of APL demonstrated that the fusion oncoprotein is necessary for leukemogenesis. They also established that the specific X-RARα oncoprotein confers response or lack thereof to RA-induced differentiation. As in human t(15;17) APL, administration of RA to the hCG-PML-RARα TM, at a dose comparable to what would be used in patients, resulted in a transient complete remission with blast differentiation observed in vitro and in vivo [24–26]. The hCG-PLZF-RARα by contrast never achieved a complete remission upon treatment with RA [36, 41] nor with single agent ATO or the combination of ATO and RA, which in the hCG-PML-RARα TM induced complete remission and prolonged survival, respectively (Fig. 4.2). These studies revealed the power of these TMs as tools to [1] obtain mechanistic insights into APL biology and [2] model the response to therapy.

ATRA is able to evoke degradation of the PML-RARα oncoprotein through the RARα moiety as the RA-elicited negative feedback mechanism is preserved (Fig. 4.3) [67]. Liposomal preparations of ATRA, which yield sustained higher levels of intracellular ATRA than the conventional preparation, result in improved rates of cure for patients. This suggests that prolonged exposure to ATRA is required for elimination of the oncoprotein in patients [68, 69], which may be mediated via a low affinity interaction with the 26S proteasome subunit, SUG1 [70]. Zhu et al. found that RARα point mutations abrogating RXR binding and mutation of the AF-2 domain disrupted RA-prompted RARα degradation and surmised that an allosteric signal is sent from the DNA-binding domain to the AF-2 domain, consistent with a model in which degradation is couple to transcriptional activation. On the other hand, when synthetic retinoids are utilized as agonists, PML-RARα transactivation is uncoupled from proteolysis, and this allowed Ablain and colleagues to make the critical observation that transactivation in the absence of proteolysis accomplishes differentiation, but not elimination of disease. Strikingly, retinoid-differentiated APL blasts, which still possess PML-RARα, retain leukemia-initiating capacity in serial transplantation experiments.

We recently reported on a novel aspect of ATRA-induced PML-RARα proteolysis involving binding, inactivation, and degradation of the prolyl isomerase, Pin1. Pin1 regulates the prolyl isomerization of many oncogenes and tumor suppressors and, in so doing, integrates multiple pathways toward the development of cancer exerting proto-oncogenic roles. Surprisingly, ATRA emerged as the top hit in a high-throughput screen for Pin1 inhibitors. Pin1, itself, appears to dock at PML-RARα's pS581-proline motif, which was previously demonstrated to be required for PML-RARα proteolysis, resulting in stabilization of the oncoprotein. Multiple approaches were used to abrogate Pin1 activity: Pin1 silencing, ATRA, additional Pin1 inhibitors, in both murine APL and human APL cell lines, and all resulted in PML-RARα degradation in vitro and in vivo. Finally, silencing Pin1 or pharmacologic inhibition of Pin1 in vivo resulted in increased disease-free survival and/or significant reduction in disease burden in APL mouse models [71].

Retinoic Acid Signaling

The field of retinoic acid signaling is inextricably bound to the story of PML-RARα. RA acts principally by signaling through its receptor, RARα. RA is obtained directly from the extracellular medium or converted through a set of oxidative steps, from vitamin A. All-trans-retinoic acid is the most common isomer of RA. CYP26 members carry out the degradation of RA, and the intracellular availability of RA is further regulated by protein binding such as to CRABPs in the cytosol [72]. RARs, that is, RARα, RARβ, and RARγ, belong to the retinoid subfamily nuclear receptor superfamily of steroid hormones along with retinoic acid X receptor (RXR). Nuclear receptors function as intracellular receptors with some encountering their ligand in the cytoplasm and others in the nucleus. Their functional domains include ligand-independent activation function (AF-1), a DNA-binding domain and ligand-binding domain (LBD), a dimerization domain, and a ligand-dependent AF-2 domain involved in co-regulator binding and transactivation. The receptors bind to hormone-response elements on their target genes, and in the classic model, ligand binding results in exchange of corepressors for coactivators and, in so doing, leads to target gene activation. On DNA, RARα is found as a heterodimer with the retinoic acid X receptor alpha (RXRα); efficient binding of DNA requires dimerization with RXR. Together they bind to RA-responsive elements (RAREs) [73]. Interestingly, receptor-independent mechanisms of action of RA have also been described such as direct activation of kinases in the cytoplasm by RA [74]. In addition, the recent finding of inhibition and degradation of the prolyl isomerase, Pin1 [71], by RA raises the possibility that signaling pathways relying on proline-directed phosphorylation may be indirectly regulated by RA.

Posttranslational modification of RARα by phosphorylation is a further layer of control with resulting changes in conformation and activity [66, 75, 76]. In the absence of ligand, DNA-bound RARα represses transcription of its target genes. RA engages the ligand-binding domain of RARα prompting a conformational change and the exchange of corepressors such as SMRT/NCoR for coactivators [77, 78]. Steroid hormone receptor signaling is coupled with a negative self-regulatory function in which prolonged exposure to hormone results in catabolism of the receptor. Notably, RA-receptor engagement also prompts a negative feedback mechanism resulting in proteasome-mediated RARα degradation [67, 79].

Early on, scientists observed that the pro-differentiating activity of RA is retained with certain cancer cell lines [80, 81] including APL cell lines [82]. Remarkably, treatment of APL blasts from patients induces terminal differentiation into granulocytes [83]. Starting in the 1980s, in a transformative step for the field, APL patients were treated with all-trans-retinoic acid (ATRA) and saw improved remission rates and survival [2–4]. Subsequently, Longo et al. mapped the breakpoint in t(15;17) [5, 19] to the RARα gene which had recently been cloned [84, 85], and t(15;17) was shown to produce an aberrant form of RARα [10] opening the floodgates of investigation into the role of RARα in the pathogenesis of APL [5–10].

Promyelocytic Leukemia Gene

The promyelocytic leukemia gene, *PML* (also called *MYL*, *RNF71*, *PP8675*, or *TRIM19*), was originally identified based on its involvement in the t(15;17) chromosomal translocation of APL [7–10]. However, the discovery of the PML-RARα oncoprotein quickly led to the study of PML in its own right. *PML* encodes a homo- or hetero-multimeric protein with wide tissue expression and is required for the proper assembly of subnuclear macromolecular structures, called PML nuclear bodies (PML-NBs) [56, 86]. PML-NBs are discrete nuclear foci, 0.2–1.0 μm wide, with a typical number 1–30 bodies per nucleus, and are dynamic and heterogeneous structures [87]. The observation that the oncogenic PML-RARα protein disrupts PML-NBs in a treatment-reversible manner with two clinically effective therapies, retinoic acid (RA) and arsenic, drew instant excitement from the scientific community [50, 51, 53, 88], and it was later concluded that the restoration of tumor suppressive function of PML-NBs by RA and arsenic is essential for APL regression [36, 50, 57, 58, 89, 90]. Through its scaffold properties, PML recruits an ever-growing number of partner proteins (in the range of 70–100) into PML-NBs, including p53 [55], AKT [57], mTOR [91], PTEN [58], and SIRT1 [92], providing a possible explanation for the involvement of PML in many aspects of normal physiology and pathology, including senescence, apoptosis, stem cell self-renewal, metabolism, and, importantly, tumor suppression. PML and PML-NBs have been proposed to concentrate the partner proteins together with many posttranslational modifying enzymes facilitating their posttranslational modifications, notably sumoylation, leading to partner activation, degradation, and sequestration (Fig. 4.4) [93, 94].

The physiological roles of PML and PML-NBs are still a matter of debate, and the related

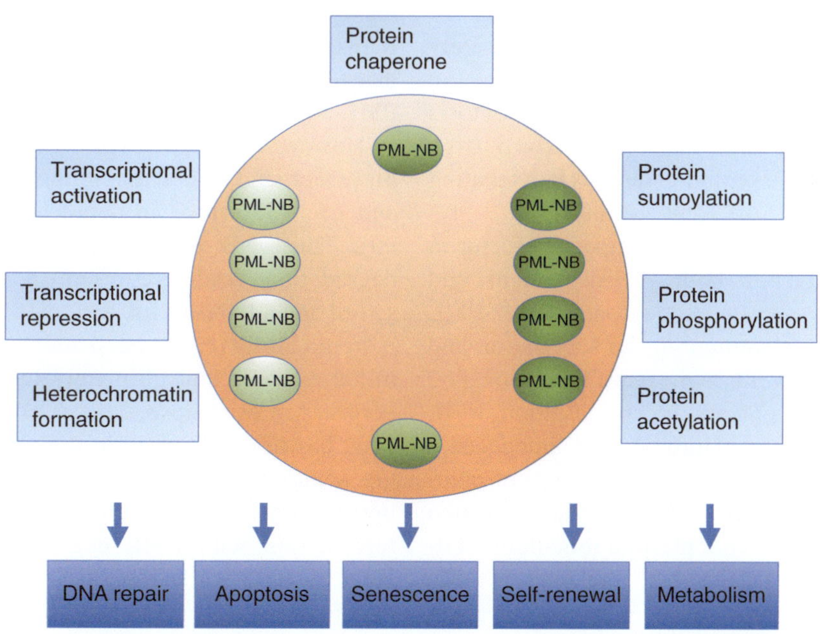

Fig. 4.4 The functions of PML and PML-NBs. PML and PML-NBs have been described as structures that regulate several, diverse cellular functions, including DNA repair, apoptosis, cellular senescence, stem cell self-renewal, and metabolism. The biochemical means used by PML and PML-NBs to regulate so many functions are varied and can be categorized into three main groups: protein chaperone activity, posttranslational modification of proteins, and regulation of nuclear activities such as transcriptional regulation and chromatin organization

research was greatly facilitated by the generation and analysis of Pml knockout (*Pml*$^{-/-}$) mice and cells that have provided direct genetic evidence and experimental tools linking Pml to a variety of biological processes [88]. Although *Pml*$^{-/-}$ mice are viable, they are more susceptible to cancer-promoting and stress-related insults and exhibit resistance to p53-dependent and p53-independent apoptosis [88, 95, 96].

Furthermore, PML and NBs are frequently lost in both leukemia and solid tumors [97], consistent with their prevalent tumor suppressive functions. Surprisingly, however, recent data have also demonstrated a selective pro-self-renewal and pro-survival role of PML in specific contexts, mainly due to its role in maintaining normal hematopoietic (HSC) and neuronal stem cell pool or leukemia-initiating cells (LICs) [92, 98, 99].

Here we briefly summarize PML functions in APL pathogenesis and response to therapy as well as the recent new findings on this multifunctional protein. The functions of PML and PML-NBs in other contexts and mechanisms underlying arsenic-mediated degradation of PML and PML/RARα have been extensively reviewed elsewhere [93, 94].

PML has a well-established role in apoptosis and cell senescence. The cells derived from *Pml*$^{-/-}$ mice have profound defects in executing cell death by different stimuli [90, 96]. Mechanistically, PML is an important factor in the regulation of both p53-dependent and p53-independent apoptotic pathways. PML activates p53 by promoting its acetylation and phosphorylation through recruitment of p53 into PML-NBs [54, 95, 96]. In addition, PML can induce apoptosis through p53-independent mechanisms. A discrete accumulation of cytoplasmic PML at the mitochondria-associated membranes of the endoplasmic reticulum facilitates transfer of calcium to the mitochondria and induces apoptosis in a p53-indepenent manner [90]. Moreover, PML can contribute to Fas-induced apoptosis through recruitment of FLICE-associated huge protein (FLASH) into PML-NBs [100]. It is therefore possible that NB disruption by PML/RARα could promote leukemia cell survival by inhibiting apoptosis. Along with apoptosis, PML regulates cellular senescence in both p53-dependent and p53-independent manner [55, 101]. PML was also implicated in the induction of premature senescence because Ras-induced senescence depends on PML-promoted p53 acetylation and subsequent activation [55]. Interestingly, recent studies have showed that among PML isoforms, only PML IV activates p53, leading to senescence when overexpressed due to its specific C-terminus motif that interacts with ARF and protects p53 from MDM2-driven degradation [102].

Furthermore, a newly defined PML/PP1α/Rb pathway is involved in the induction of senescence in a p53-independent manner [101]. The role of PML in the regulation of apoptosis and cell senescence is critical not only for understanding APL initiation but also the basis of response to therapy. Indeed, NB reformation in response to RA or arsenic treatments tightly correlates with enhanced cellular apoptosis and senescence. Importantly, this specific response is highly specific for PML/RARα, but not PLZF/RARα-driven APL [36, 103, 104], suggesting that restoration of normal function of PML and PML-NBs is critical for APL clearance.

However, it is also worth noting that PML plays a crucial role in maintaining normal HSC and LIC (described in detail below) [92, 98, 99]. Thus, NB reformation uncoupled from degradation could represent a double-edge sword and a liability for APL clearance, in that it would allow for the persistence of leukemia-initiating cells and ultimately lead to disease persistence or relapse. This is consistent with what has been observed in the clinic with single agent ATO leading to high rates of cure presumably because arsenic triggers initial NB reformation with PML degradation immediately ensuing while RA does not affect PML degradation and, in the clinic, leads to transient responses.

The role of PML in HSC self-renewal was first suggested by ex vivo studies in which PML-RARα resulted in increased self-renewal of myeloid progenitors [105]. PML has now been demonstrated to play an important role in normal hematopoiesis and in non-APL myeloid neoplasms. Our group and others have shown that PML is required for the maintenance of cancer-initiating cells [98, 106, 107]. In bone marrow mononuclear cells, PML is most highly expressed in the stem cell/progenitor compartment. Deletion of PML initially leads to normal HSC and LIC cycling and expansion of these pools. However, over time, both in vitro and in vivo, loss of PML leads to exhaustion of HSC and LICs [98].

Chronic myeloid leukemia is a paradigmatic stem cell disorder and consistent with prior observations that leukemia-initiating cells co-opt normal stem cell self-renewal mechanisms, in a retroviral BCR-ABL murine model, CML leukemia-initiating cells (LIC) collapse in the absence of PML or upon pharmacologic ablation of PML via arsenic trioxide [98]. Subsequent studies revealed that PML mediates stem cell maintenance by regulating lipid metabolism, thus revealing a specific HSC metabolic requirement. PML accomplishes this by acting upstream of a PPARδ-fatty acid oxidation pathway required for asymmetric division of HSC [99]. These interesting findings raise the possibility that LIC exhaustion in myeloid malignancies, including APL, could be induced by interfering with fatty acid metabolism, through PPAR-directed therapy or PML targeting drugs, such as ATO.

A metabolic dimension to PML-regulated cell biology in solid tumors was also recently uncovered. In breast cancer, a PML-PPARα-fatty acid oxidation pathway allows cells to withstand metabolic stress and survive loss of attachment. In primary patient samples, high PML expression is correlated with high-grade histology and reduced disease-free survival; accordingly, poor prognosis, triple negative breast cancers are enriched in the PML group. Consistent with the molecular studies, tumors with elevated PML levels exhibited an activated PPARα signaling gene expression signature [92]. The above described metabolic function of Pml in breast cancer suggests that in a subset of solid tumors, targeting Pml-directed metabolic programs may open new therapeutic avenues for patients.

Conclusions

The story of APL has by now paved the way to contemporary molecular oncology. It represents a paradigmatic example of a journey of discovery toward the cure, where genetic and molecular analyses, mouse modeling efforts, and preclinical and clinical trials converged toward disease eradication. This paradigm has by now inspired a generation of investigators and oncologists and has been exported above and beyond leukemia to any realm of cancer research and care.

Acknowledgments We would like to thank current members of the Pandolfi laboratory for critical discussion and Lauren Southwood and Elizabeth Stack for editing and administrative support. This work is supported in part by funding from the National Cancer Institute (R01CA142874 and R35-CA197529 to P.P.P.).

References

1. Hillestad LK. Acute promyelocytic leukemia. Acta Med Scand. 1957;159(3):189–94.
2. Huang ME, Ye YC, Chen SR, Chai JR, Lu JX, Zhoa L, et al. Use of all-trans retinoic acid in the treatment of acute promyelocytic leukemia. Blood. 1988;72(2):567–72.
3. Castaigne S, Chomienne C, Daniel MT, Ballerini P, Berger R, Fenaux P, et al. All-trans retinoic acid as a differentiation therapy for acute promyelocytic leukemia. I. Clinical results. Blood. 1990;76(9):1704–9.
4. Fenaux P, Chastang C, Chomienne C, Degos L. Tretinoin with chemotherapy in newly diagnosed acute promyelocytic leukaemia. European APL Group. Lancet (London, England). 1994;343(8904):1033.
5. Longo L, Donti E, Mencarelli A, Avanzi G, Pegoraro L, Alimena G, et al. Mapping of chromosome 17 breakpoints in acute myeloid leukemias. Oncogene. 1990;5(10):1557–63.
6. de The H, Chomienne C, Lanotte M, Degos L, Dejean A. The t(15;17) translocation of acute promyelocytic leukaemia fuses the retinoic acid receptor alpha gene to a novel transcribed locus. Nature. 1990;347(6293):558–61.
7. Goddard AD, Borrow J, Freemont PS, Solomon E. Characterization of a zinc finger gene disrupted by the t(15;17) in acute promyelocytic leukemia. Science (New York, NY). 1991;254(5036):1371–4.
8. Pandolfi PP, Grignani F, Alcalay M, Mencarelli A, Biondi A, LoCoco F, et al. Structure and origin of the

acute promyelocytic leukemia myl/RAR alpha cDNA and characterization of its retinoid-binding and trans-activation properties. Oncogene. 1991;6(7):1285–92.
9. Kakizuka A, Miller WH Jr, Umesono K, Warrell RP Jr, Frankel SR, Murty VV, et al. Chromosomal translocation t(15;17) in human acute promyelocytic leukemia fuses RAR alpha with a novel putative transcription factor, PML. Cell. 1991;66(4):663–74.
10. de The H, Lavau C, Marchio A, Chomienne C, Degos L, Dejean A. The PML-RAR alpha fusion mRNA generated by the t(15;17) translocation in acute promyelocytic leukemia encodes a functionally altered RAR. Cell. 1991;66(4):675–84.
11. Chen GQ, Shi XG, Tang W, Xiong SM, Zhu J, Cai X, et al. Use of arsenic trioxide (As2O3) in the treatment of acute promyelocytic leukemia (APL): I. As2O3 exerts dose-dependent dual effects on APL cells. Blood. 1997;89(9):3345–53.
12. Chen GQ, Zhu J, Shi XG, Ni JH, Zhong HJ, Si GY, et al. In vitro studies on cellular and molecular mechanisms of arsenic trioxide (As2O3) in the treatment of acute promyelocytic leukemia: As2O3 induces NB4 cell apoptosis with downregulation of Bcl-2 expression and modulation of PML-RAR alpha/PML proteins. Blood. 1996;88(3):1052–61.
13. Powell BL, Moser B, Stock W, Gallagher RE, Willman CL, Stone RM, et al. Arsenic trioxide improves event-free and overall survival for adults with acute promyelocytic leukemia: North American Leukemia Intergroup Study C9710. Blood. 2010;116(19):3751–7.
14. Soignet SL, Maslak P, Wang ZG, Jhanwar S, Calleja E, Dardashti LJ, et al. Complete remission after treatment of acute promyelocytic leukemia with arsenic trioxide. N Engl J Med. 1998;339(19):1341–8.
15. Estey E, Garcia-Manero G, Ferrajoli A, Faderl S, Verstovsek S, Jones D, et al. Use of all-trans retinoic acid plus arsenic trioxide as an alternative to chemotherapy in untreated acute promyelocytic leukemia. Blood. 2006;107(9):3469–73.
16. Lo-Coco F, Avvisati G, Vignetti M, Thiede C, Orlando SM, Iacobelli S, et al. Retinoic acid and arsenic trioxide for acute promyelocytic leukemia. N Engl J Med. 2013;369(2):111–21.
17. Rowley JD, Golomb HM, Dougherty C. 15/17 translocation, a consistent chromosomal change in acute promyelocytic leukaemia. Lancet (London, England). 1977;1(8010):549–50.
18. Mattei MG, Petkovich M, Mattei JF, Brand N, Chambon P. Mapping of the human retinoic acid receptor to the q21 band of chromosome 17. Hum Genet. 1988;80(2):186–8.
19. Longo L, Pandolfi PP, Biondi A, Rambaldi A, Mencarelli A, Lo Coco F, et al. Rearrangements and aberrant expression of the retinoic acid receptor alpha gene in acute promyelocytic leukemias. J Exp Med. 1990;172(6):1571–5.
20. Chen Z, Brand NJ, Chen A, Chen SJ, Tong JH, Wang ZY, et al. Fusion between a novel Kruppel-like zinc finger gene and the retinoic acid receptor-alpha locus due to a variant t(11;17) translocation associated with acute promyelocytic leukaemia. EMBO J. 1993;12(3):1161–7.
21. Redner RL, Rush EA, Faas S, Rudert WA, Corey SJ. The t(5;17) variant of acute promyelocytic leukemia expresses a nucleophosmin-retinoic acid receptor fusion. Blood. 1996;87(3):882–6.
22. Wells RA, Catzavelos C, Kamel-Reid S. Fusion of retinoic acid receptor alpha to NuMA, the nuclear mitotic apparatus protein, by a variant translocation in acute promyelocytic leukaemia. Nat Genet. 1997;17(1):109–13.
23. Pandolfi PP. In vivo analysis of the molecular genetics of acute promyelocytic leukemia. Oncogene. 2001;20(40):5726–35.
24. Grisolano JL, Wesselschmidt RL, Pelicci PG, Ley TJ. Altered myeloid development and acute leukemia in transgenic mice expressing PML-RAR alpha under control of cathepsin G regulatory sequences. Blood. 1997;89(2):376–87.
25. He LZ, Tribioli C, Rivi R, Peruzzi D, Pelicci PG, Soares V, et al. Acute leukemia with promyelocytic features in PML/RARalpha transgenic mice. Proc Natl Acad Sci U S A. 1997;94(10):5302–7.
26. Brown D, Kogan S, Lagasse E, Weissman I, Alcalay M, Pelicci PG, et al. A PMLRARalpha transgene initiates murine acute promyelocytic leukemia. Proc Natl Acad Sci U S A. 1997;94(6):2551–6.
27. Sukhai MA, Wu X, Xuan Y, Zhang T, Reis PP, Dube K, et al. Myeloid leukemia with promyelocytic features in transgenic mice expressing hCG-NuMA-RARalpha. Oncogene. 2004;23(3):665–78.
28. Rego EM, Ruggero D, Tribioli C, Cattoretti G, Kogan S, Redner RL, et al. Leukemia with distinct phenotypes in transgenic mice expressing PML/RAR alpha, PLZF/RAR alpha or NPM/RAR alpha. Oncogene. 2006;25(13):1974–9.
29. Pollock JL, Westervelt P, Kurichety AK, Pelicci PG, Grisolano JL, Ley TJ. A bcr-3 isoform of RARalpha-PML potentiates the development of PML-RARalpha-driven acute promyelocytic leukemia. Proc Natl Acad Sci U S A. 1999;96(26):15103–8.
30. He LZ, Bhaumik M, Tribioli C, Rego EM, Ivins S, Zelent A, et al. Two critical hits for promyelocytic leukemia. Mol Cell. 2000;6(5):1131–41.
31. Rego EM, Pandolfi PP. Reciprocal products of chromosomal translocations in human cancer pathogenesis: key players or innocent bystanders? Trends Mol Med. 2002;8(8):396–405.
32. Ablain J, de The H. Retinoic acid signaling in cancer: the parable of acute promyelocytic leukemia. Int J Cancer. 2014;135(10):2262–72.
33. de The H, Chen Z. Acute promyelocytic leukaemia: novel insights into the mechanisms of cure. Nat Rev Cancer. 2010;10(11):775–83.
34. Licht JD, Chomienne C, Goy A, Chen A, Scott AA, Head DR, et al. Clinical and molecular characterization of a rare syndrome of acute promyelocytic leukemia associated with translocation (11;17). Blood. 1995;85(4):1083–94.

35. Jansen JH, Lowenberg B. Acute promyelocytic leukemia with a PLZF-RARalpha fusion protein. Semin Hematol. 2001;38(1):37–41.
36. Rego EM, He LZ, Warrell RP Jr, Wang ZG, Pandolfi PP. Retinoic acid (RA) and As2O3 treatment in transgenic models of acute promyelocytic leukemia (APL) unravel the distinct nature of the leukemogenic process induced by the PML-RARalpha and PLZF-RARalpha oncoproteins. Proc Natl Acad Sci U S A. 2000;97(18):10173–8.
37. Grimwade D, Gorman P, Duprez E, Howe K, Langabeer S, Oliver F, et al. Characterization of cryptic rearrangements and variant translocations in acute promyelocytic leukemia. Blood. 1997;90(12):4876–85.
38. Redner RL. Variations on a theme: the alternate translocations in APL. Leukemia. 2002;16(10):1927–32.
39. Melnick A, Licht JD. Deconstructing a disease: RARalpha, its fusion partners, and their roles in the pathogenesis of acute promyelocytic leukemia. Blood. 1999;93(10):3167–215.
40. He LZ, Merghoub T, Pandolfi PP. In vivo analysis of the molecular pathogenesis of acute promyelocytic leukemia in the mouse and its therapeutic implications. Oncogene. 1999;18(38):5278–92.
41. He LZ, Guidez F, Tribioli C, Peruzzi D, Ruthardt M, Zelent A, et al. Distinct interactions of PML-RARalpha and PLZF-RARalpha with co-repressors determine differential responses to RA in APL. Nat Genet. 1998;18(2):126–35.
42. Lin RJ, Nagy L, Inoue S, Shao W, Miller WH Jr, Evans RM. Role of the histone deacetylase complex in acute promyelocytic leukaemia. Nature. 1998;391(6669):811–4.
43. Grignani F, De Matteis S, Nervi C, Tomassoni L, Gelmetti V, Cioce M, et al. Fusion proteins of the retinoic acid receptor-alpha recruit histone deacetylase in promyelocytic leukaemia. Nature. 1998;391(6669):815–8.
44. Minucci S, Maccarana M, Cioce M, De Luca P, Gelmetti V, Segalla S, et al. Oligomerization of RAR and AML1 transcription factors as a novel mechanism of oncogenic activation. Mol Cell. 2000;5(5):811–20.
45. Salomoni P, Pandolfi PP. Transcriptional regulation of cellular transformation. Nat Med. 2000;6(7):742–4.
46. Lin RJ, Evans RM. Acquisition of oncogenic potential by RAR chimeras in acute promyelocytic leukemia through formation of homodimers. Mol Cell. 2000;5(5):821–30.
47. Wu WS, Vallian S, Seto E, Yang WM, Edmondson D, Roth S, et al. The growth suppressor PML represses transcription by functionally and physically interacting with histone deacetylases. Mol Cell Biol. 2001;21(7):2259–68.
48. Khan MM, Nomura T, Kim H, Kaul SC, Wadhwa R, Shinagawa T, et al. Role of PML and PML-RARalpha in Mad-mediated transcriptional repression. Mol Cell. 2001;7(6):1233–43.
49. Wang ZG, Ruggero D, Ronchetti S, Zhong S, Gaboli M, Rivi R, et al. PML is essential for multiple apoptotic pathways. Nat Genet. 1998;20(3):266–72.
50. Daniel MT, Koken M, Romagne O, Barbey S, Bazarbachi A, Stadler M, et al. PML protein expression in hematopoietic and acute promyelocytic leukemia cells. Blood. 1993;82(6):1858–67.
51. Dyck JA, Maul GG, Miller WH Jr, Chen JD, Kakizuka A, Evans RM. A novel macromolecular structure is a target of the promyelocyte-retinoic acid receptor oncoprotein. Cell. 1994;76(2):333–43.
52. Koken MH, Puvion-Dutilleul F, Guillemin MC, Viron A, Linares-Cruz G, Stuurman N, et al. The t(15;17) translocation alters a nuclear body in a retinoic acid-reversible fashion. EMBO J. 1994;13(5):1073–83.
53. Weis K, Rambaud S, Lavau C, Jansen J, Carvalho T, Carmo-Fonseca M, et al. Retinoic acid regulates aberrant nuclear localization of PML-RAR alpha in acute promyelocytic leukemia cells. Cell. 1994;76(2):345–56.
54. Guo A, Salomoni P, Luo J, Shih A, Zhong S, Gu W, et al. The function of PML in p53-dependent apoptosis. Nat Cell Biol. 2000;2(10):730–6.
55. Pearson M, Carbone R, Sebastiani C, Cioce M, Fagioli M, Saito S, et al. PML regulates p53 acetylation and premature senescence induced by oncogenic Ras. Nature. 2000;406(6792):207–10.
56. Salomoni P, Pandolfi PP. The role of PML in tumor suppression. Cell. 2002;108(2):165–70.
57. Trotman LC, Alimonti A, Scaglioni PP, Koutcher JA, Cordon-Cardo C, Pandolfi PP. Identification of a tumour suppressor network opposing nuclear Akt function. Nature. 2006;441(7092):523–7.
58. Song MS, Salmena L, Carracedo A, Egia A, Lo-Coco F, Teruya-Feldstein J, et al. The deubiquitinylation and localization of PTEN are regulated by a HAUSP-PML network. Nature. 2008;455(7214):813–7.
59. Rego EM, Wang ZG, Peruzzi D, He LZ, Cordon-Cardo C, Pandolfi PP. Role of promyelocytic leukemia (PML) protein in tumor suppression. J Exp Med. 2001;193(4):521–9.
60. Barna M, Hawe N, Niswander L, Pandolfi PP. Plzf regulates limb and axial skeletal patterning. Nat Genet. 2000;25(2):166–72.
61. Martens JH, Brinkman AB, Simmer F, Francoijs KJ, Nebbioso A, Ferrara F, et al. PML-RARalpha/RXR alters the epigenetic landscape in acute promyelocytic leukemia. Cancer Cell. 2010;17(2):173–85.
62. Taschner S, Koesters C, Platzer B, Jorgl A, Ellmeier W, Benesch T, et al. Down-regulation of RXRalpha expression is essential for neutrophil development from granulocyte/monocyte progenitors. Blood. 2007;109(3):971–9.
63. Zhu J, Zhou J, Peres L, Riaucoux F, Honore N, Kogan S, et al. A sumoylation site in PML/RARA is essential for leukemic transformation. Cancer Cell. 2005;7(2):143–53.
64. Stielow B, Sapetschnig A, Kruger I, Kunert N, Brehm A, Boutros M, et al. Identification of SUMO-dependent chromatin-associated transcriptional repression components by a genome-wide RNAi screen. Mol Cell. 2008;29(6):742–54.

65. Garcia-Dominguez M, Reyes JC. SUMO association with repressor complexes, emerging routes for transcriptional control. Biochim Biophys Acta. 2009;1789(6–8):451–9.
66. Bruck N, Vitoux D, Ferry C, Duong V, Bauer A, de The H, et al. A coordinated phosphorylation cascade initiated by p38MAPK/MSK1 directs RARalpha to target promoters. EMBO J. 2009;28(1):34–47.
67. Zhu J, Gianni M, Kopf E, Honore N, Chelbi-Alix M, Koken M, et al. Retinoic acid induces proteasome-dependent degradation of retinoic acid receptor alpha (RARalpha) and oncogenic RARalpha fusion proteins. Proc Natl Acad Sci U S A. 1999;96(26):14807–12.
68. Estey EH, Giles FJ, Kantarjian H, O'Brien S, Cortes J, Freireich EJ, et al. Molecular remissions induced by liposomal-encapsulated all-trans retinoic acid in newly diagnosed acute promyelocytic leukemia. Blood. 1999;94(7):2230–5.
69. Tsimberidou AM, Tirado-Gomez M, Andreeff M, O'Brien S, Kantarjian H, Keating M, et al. Single-agent liposomal all-trans retinoic acid can cure some patients with untreated acute promyelocytic leukemia: an update of The University of Texas M. D. Anderson Cancer Center Series. Leuk Lymphoma. 2006;47(6):1062–8.
70. vom Baur E, Zechel C, Heery D, Heine MJ, Garnier JM, Vivat V, et al. Differential ligand-dependent interactions between the AF-2 activating domain of nuclear receptors and the putative transcriptional intermediary factors mSUG1 and TIF1. EMBO J. 1996;15(1):110–24.
71. Wei S, Kozono S, Kats L, Nechama M, Li W, Guarnerio J, et al. Active Pin1 is a key target of all-trans retinoic acid in acute promyelocytic leukemia and breast cancer. Nat Med. 2015;21(5):457–66.
72. Napoli JL. Biosynthesis and metabolism of retinoic acid: roles of CRBP and CRABP in retinoic acid: roles of CRBP and CRABP in retinoic acid homeostasis. J Nutr. 1993;123(2 Suppl):362–6.
73. Leid M, Kastner P, Lyons R, Nakshatri H, Saunders M, Zacharewski T, et al. Purification, cloning, and RXR identity of the HeLa cell factor with which RAR or TR heterodimerizes to bind target sequences efficiently. Cell. 1992;68(2):377–95.
74. Al Tanoury Z, Piskunov A, Rochette-Egly C. Vitamin A and retinoid signaling: genomic and nongenomic effects. J Lipid Res. 2013;54(7):1761–75.
75. Gaillard E, Bruck N, Brelivet Y, Bour G, Lalevee S, Bauer A, et al. Phosphorylation by PKA potentiates retinoic acid receptor alpha activity by means of increasing interaction with and phosphorylation by cyclin H/cdk7. Proc Natl Acad Sci U S A. 2006;103(25):9548–53.
76. Rochette-Egly C, Adam S, Rossignol M, Egly JM, Chambon P. Stimulation of RAR alpha activation function AF-1 through binding to the general transcription factor TFIIH and phosphorylation by CDK7. Cell. 1997;90(1):97–107.
77. Nagy L, Schwabe JW. Mechanism of the nuclear receptor molecular switch. Trends Biochem Sci. 2004;29(6):317–24.
78. Glass CK, Rosenfeld MG. The coregulator exchange in transcriptional functions of nuclear receptors. Genes Dev. 2000;14(2):121–41.
79. Kopf E, Plassat JL, Vivat V, de The H, Chambon P, Rochette-Egly C. Dimerization with retinoid X receptors and phosphorylation modulate the retinoic acid-induced degradation of retinoic acid receptors alpha and gamma through the ubiquitin-proteasome pathway. J Biol Chem. 2000;275(43):33280–8.
80. Sidell N. Retinoic acid-induced growth inhibition and morphologic differentiation of human neuroblastoma cells in vitro. J Natl Cancer Inst. 1982;68(4):589–96.
81. Strickland S, Mahdavi V. The induction of differentiation in teratocarcinoma stem cells by retinoic acid. Cell. 1978;15(2):393–403.
82. Breitman TR, Selonick SE, Collins SJ. Induction of differentiation of the human promyelocytic leukemia cell line (HL-60) by retinoic acid. Proc Natl Acad Sci U S A. 1980;77(5):2936–40.
83. Breitman TR, Collins SJ, Keene BR. Terminal differentiation of human promyelocytic leukemic cells in primary culture in response to retinoic acid. Blood. 1981;57(6):1000–4.
84. Petkovich M, Brand NJ, Krust A, Chambon P. A human retinoic acid receptor which belongs to the family of nuclear receptors. Nature. 1987;330(6147):444–50.
85. Giguere V, Ong ES, Segui P, Evans RM. Identification of a receptor for the morphogen retinoic acid. Nature. 1987;330(6149):624–9.
86. Ishov AM, Sotnikov AG, Negorev D, Vladimirova OV, Neff N, Kamitani T, et al. PML is critical for ND10 formation and recruits the PML-interacting protein daxx to this nuclear structure when modified by SUMO-1. J Cell Biol. 1999;147(2):221–34.
87. Dellaire G, Bazett-Jones DP. PML nuclear bodies: dynamic sensors of DNA damage and cellular stress. Bioessays. 2004;26(9):963–77.
88. Wang ZG, Delva L, Gaboli M, Rivi R, Giorgio M, Cordon-Cardo C, et al. Role of PML in cell growth and the retinoic acid pathway. Science (New York, NY). 1998;279(5356):1547–51.
89. Zhu J, Koken MH, Quignon F, Chelbi-Alix MK, Degos L, Wang ZY, et al. Arsenic-induced PML targeting onto nuclear bodies: implications for the treatment of acute promyelocytic leukemia. Proc Natl Acad Sci U S A. 1997;94(8):3978–83.
90. Giorgi C, Ito K, Lin HK, Santangelo C, Wieckowski MR, Lebiedzinska M, et al. PML regulates apoptosis at endoplasmic reticulum by modulating calcium release. Science (New York, NY). 2010;330(6008):1247–51.
91. Bernardi R, Guernah I, Jin D, Grisendi S, Alimonti A, Teruya-Feldstein J, et al. PML inhibits HIF-1alpha

translation and neoangiogenesis through repression of mTOR. Nature. 2006;442(7104):779–85.

92. Carracedo A, Weiss D, Leliaert AK, Bhasin M, de Boer VC, Laurent G, et al. A metabolic prosurvival role for PML in breast cancer. J Clin Invest. 2012;122(9):3088–100.
93. Bernardi R, Pandolfi PP. Structure, dynamics and functions of promyelocytic leukaemia nuclear bodies. Nat Rev Mol Cell Biol. 2007;8(12):1006–16.
94. Lallemand-Breitenbach V, de The H. PML nuclear bodies. Cold Spring Harb Perspect Biol. 2010;2(5):a000661.
95. Bernardi R, Pandolfi PP. Role of PML and the PML-nuclear body in the control of programmed cell death. Oncogene. 2003;22(56):9048–57.
96. Takahashi Y, Lallemand-Breitenbach V, Zhu J, de The H. PML nuclear bodies and apoptosis. Oncogene. 2004;23(16):2819–24.
97. Gurrieri C, Capodieci P, Bernardi R, Scaglioni PP, Nafa K, Rush LJ, et al. Loss of the tumor suppressor PML in human cancers of multiple histologic origins. J Natl Cancer Inst. 2004;96(4):269–79.
98. Ito K, Bernardi R, Morotti A, Matsuoka S, Saglio G, Ikeda Y, et al. PML targeting eradicates quiescent leukaemia-initiating cells. Nature. 2008;453(7198):1072–8.
99. Ito K, Carracedo A, Weiss D, Arai F, Ala U, Avigan DE, et al. A PML-PPAR-delta pathway for fatty acid oxidation regulates hematopoietic stem cell maintenance. Nat Med. 2012;18(9):1350–8.
100. Milovic-Holm K, Krieghoff E, Jensen K, Will H, Hofmann TG. FLASH links the CD95 signaling pathway to the cell nucleus and nuclear bodies. EMBO J. 2007;26(2):391–401.
101. Vernier M, Bourdeau V, Gaumont-Leclerc MF, Moiseeva O, Begin V, Saad F, et al. Regulation of E2Fs and senescence by PML nuclear bodies. Genes Dev. 2011;25(1):41–50.
102. Ivanschitz L, Takahashi Y, Jollivet F, Ayrault O, Le Bras M, de The H. PML IV/ARF interaction enhances p53 SUMO-1 conjugation, activation, and senescence. Proc Natl Acad Sci U S A. 2015;112(46):14278–83.
103. Ablain J, Rice K, Soilihi H, de Reynies A, Minucci S, de The H. Activation of a promyelocytic leukemia-tumor protein 53 axis underlies acute promyelocytic leukemia cure. Nat Med. 2014;20(2):167–74.
104. Nasr R, Guillemin MC, Ferhi O, Soilihi H, Peres L, Berthier C, et al. Eradication of acute promyelocytic leukemia-initiating cells through PML-RARA degradation. Nat Med. 2008;14(12):1333–42.
105. Du C, Redner RL, Cooke MP, Lavau C. Overexpression of wild-type retinoic acid receptor alpha (RARalpha) recapitulates retinoic acid-sensitive transformation of primary myeloid progenitors by acute promyelocytic leukemia RARalpha-fusion genes. Blood. 1999;94(2):793–802.
106. Li W, Ferguson BJ, Khaled WT, Tevendale M, Stingl J, Poli V, et al. PML depletion disrupts normal mammary gland development and skews the composition of the mammary luminal cell progenitor pool. Proc Natl Acad Sci U S A. 2009;106(12):4725–30.
107. Regad T, Bellodi C, Nicotera P, Salomoni P. The tumor suppressor Pml regulates cell fate in the developing neocortex. Nat Neurosci. 2009;12(2):132–40.

5 Acute Promyelocytic Leukemia Coagulopathy

Anna Falanga, Laura Russo, and Pau Montesinos

Introduction

Hemorrhages occur frequently in patients with acute leukemias and significantly affect morbidity and mortality [1]. Besides thrombocytopenia due to bone marrow failure, alterations of the hemostatic system contribute to the bleeding diathesis in these patients. In particular, patients with acute promyelocytic leukemia (APL) very often present with a range of laboratory abnormalities consistent with the diagnosis of disseminated intravascular coagulation (DIC), with an excess fibrinolysis activation, and may show a variety of clinical manifestations ranging from diffuse life-threatening bleeding secondary to the consumption of coagulation factors and platelets to localized venous or arterial thrombosis [2, 3]. Bleeding and clotting manifestations may take place concomitantly as part of the same thrombohemorrhagic syndrome (THS). Indeed, a profound dysregulation of the hemostatic system, due to the imbalance between procoagulant, anticoagulant, and profibrinolytic mechanisms, occurs in these patients [4]. A hemorrhagic phenotype prevails when the consumption of clotting factors and platelets and activation of fibrinolysis dominate the picture. A THS can occur to different extent in all acute myeloid leukemia subtypes [5, 6]; however, in patients with APL, hemorrhage is usually predominant and is relevant for mortality rates [7]. In recent years, the APL-associated coagulopathy has received new interest, due to the enhanced understanding of the biology of this unique myeloid differentiation disorder and to the greater sensitivity of diagnostic laboratory tests for coagulation abnormalities. In addition, most importantly, the development of new and very efficacious therapeutic drugs for APL remission induction, i.e., *all-trans*-retinoic acid (ATRA) and arsenic trioxide (ATO), has attracted much attention for the beneficial effects of these therapies on the coagulation disorder. ATRA-induced differentiation of leukemic promyelocytes with remission of APL is indeed accompanied by prompt improvement of the hemorrhagic symptoms [4]. Both ATRA and ATO, as single agents, induce the molecular remission of APL and a simultaneous rapid resolution of the related coagulopathy.

A. Falanga, M.D. (✉) • L. Russo, Ph.D.
Department of Immunohematology and Transfusion Medicine and the Hemostasis and Thrombosis Center, Hospital Papa Giovanni XXIII, Piazza OMS, 1, 24127 Bergamo, Italy
e-mail: annafalanga@yahoo.com

P. Montesinos, M.D., Ph.D.
Department of Hematology, Hospital Universitari i Politecnic La Fe, Valencia, Spain

Centro de Investigación Biomédica en Red de Cáncer, Instituto Carlos III, Madrid, Spain

O. Abla et al. (eds.), *Acute Promyelocytic Leukemia*, https://doi.org/10.1007/978-3-319-64257-4_5

ATO combined to ATRA is effective in inducing APL remission in newly diagnosed patients and may provide an alternative to ATRA + chemotherapy in this disease, with less toxic effects [8].

In this chapter, we will focus on the clinical aspects, the pathogenesis, and the proposed treatments of the THS occurring in APL.

The Coagulopathy of APL

Clinical Manifestations

APL typically presents with a life-threatening hemorrhagic diathesis, the clinical and laboratory features of which are consistent with DIC [9]. The bleeding disorder is particularly severe in the microgranular variant of APL (M3v), characterized by marked hyperleukocytosis. Before the introduction of ATRA for remission induction, APL was distinguished by a high incidence of hemorrhagic death (20%), which significantly contributed to treatment failure [10].

Currently, standard treatment of APL with ATRA and chemotherapy results in more than 90% complete remission rates accompanied by a resolution of the coagulopathy, with a reduction of early hemorrhagic deaths to 2.4–6.5% [11, 12]. Despite this reduction, lethal or life-threatening hemorragic complications still occur, while the coagulopathy of APL is active. These complications are not only the most frequent cause of death early during induction therapy but can also occur before the diagnosis of APL has been made and therapy started. It should be noted that an undetermined number of patients will die before starting any differentiating agent, being acute bleeding the main cause of death in this setting. According to the data from the Swedish registry [13], 12 out of 105 patients (11.4%) had early hemorrhagic death before treatment, but this incidence is lower in the Spanish registry (3.5% out of more than 2000 cases, unpublished data). After the systematic introduction of ATRA, most early deaths have been recorded within the first 2–3 weeks [14]. A retrospective analysis showed that delays in starting ATRA led to increased early hemorrhagic death [15].

In spite of the dramatic amelioration in the rate of remission induction in patients with APL and overall improvement in survival, hemorrhage remains the most common cause of early death, accounting for 5% of the cases (37 of 736 evaluable patients) in two consecutive Programa Español de Tratamiento de las Hemopatias Malignas (PETHEMA) group studies—PETHEMA LPA96 and LPA99 [16]. Hemorrhagic deaths were almost exclusively due to intracranial (65%) and pulmonary hemorrhages (32%), with only one case of fatal gastrointestinal bleeding. It should be noted that 2 of the 24 patients with intracranial bleeding developed the hemorrhage over an extensive cerebral thrombosis. The results of a multivariate analysis of pretreatment characteristics predictive of fatal hemorrhage implicated an elevated white blood cell count (WBC > 10×10^9/L; $P < 0.0001$) and an abnormal creatinine level ($P < 0.0004$). Of note, in the LPA99 study, routine use of tranexamic acid prophylaxis (100 mg/kg/day by continuous infusion) aimed to inhibit excess fibrinolysis failed to alter the risk of hemorrhagic death (5% in both studies). Furthermore, the use of tranexamic acid was associated with a trend toward a statistically significant increase in the thrombosis rate (6% in LPA99 vs. 3% in LPA96 trial, in which tranexamic acid was not utilized; $P = 0.08$ in multivariate analysis). Fatal hemorrhagic events occurred from day 1 to day 23 with the majority noted in the first week (21, 57%); no lethal hemorrhages were documented beyond the fourth week of therapy.

There are no consistent data regarding the frequency of the coagulopathy accompanying APL at presentation, probably because there is no homogeneous definition for this complication. In this regard, the PETHEMA group analyzed the rate of coagulopathy in 921 patients registered in two protocols with ATRA and chemotherapy (unpublished data), using the following definition for DIC: presence of thrombocytopenia along with (1) prolonged prothrombin time and/or activated partial thromboplastin and (2) hypofibrinogenemia and/or increased levels of fibrin degradation products or D-dimer. They found that coagulopathy was present at diagnosis in

65% of patients, and additionally 12% developed this complication during induction. Specifically, hypofibrinogenemia was present in 46% of patients, and additionally 10% manifested decrease of fibrinogen levels below 170 mg/dL during induction period. The median time to resolution of DIC was 11 days from diagnosis (range, 1–53 days).

Concomitant to the bleeding diathesis, thrombotic events occur in APL patients with an incidence rate ranging from 2 to 15% [17–19]. Interestingly, ATRA increases the thrombotic risk in those patients who manifest accelerated differentiation, otherwise known as the "differentiation syndrome" [1, 20]. More recently, Mitrovic et al. described a thrombotic event rate of 20.6% (6.3% arterial and 14.3% venous) in 63 patients treated with AIDA regimens, and these events occurred mostly during induction [21]. Of note, the reported incidence of thrombo-ischemic events seems different depending on the prospective or retrospective design of the studies (Fig. 5.1). As the incidence ranges between 5 and 6% in the retrospective series [17, 22], it becomes higher in the prospective series, ranging from 13 to 20% [23]. As an example, the PETHEMA database was retrospectively analyzed for thrombotic events in 759 consecutive APL patients (LPA96 and LPA99 trials) [16, 22]. An incidence rate of thrombosis of 5.1% (39/759) was observed, and four cases were associated with the use of tranexamic acid: two patients with deep vein thrombosis, one case of hemorrhagic skin necrosis, and one of renal necrosis. In multivariate analysis, hypofibrinogenemia at presentation (<170 mg/dL) and the M3 variant subtype remained from the univariate analysis as independent prognostic factors. Thrombosis was observed to relate with a higher induction mortality (including deaths prior to the initiation of chemotherapy), 28% vs. 11%, $P < 0.01$ [22]. In contrast, the prospective study by the PETHEMA group performed on 921 patients (LPA2005 and LPA2012 trials) showed an incidence of 4.1% at presentation, while 9.3% developed during induction therapy (overall 13.4% incidence). The type of thrombosis was catheter-related (46%), deep venous (17%), cerebral stroke (12%), pulmonary embolism (12%), acute myocardial infarction (9%), and others (4%). Regarding the risk factors for thrombosis, the study by Breccia and colleagues showed that high WBC, BCR3 isoform, FLT3-ITD, CD2, and CD15 surface antigens were related with the development of

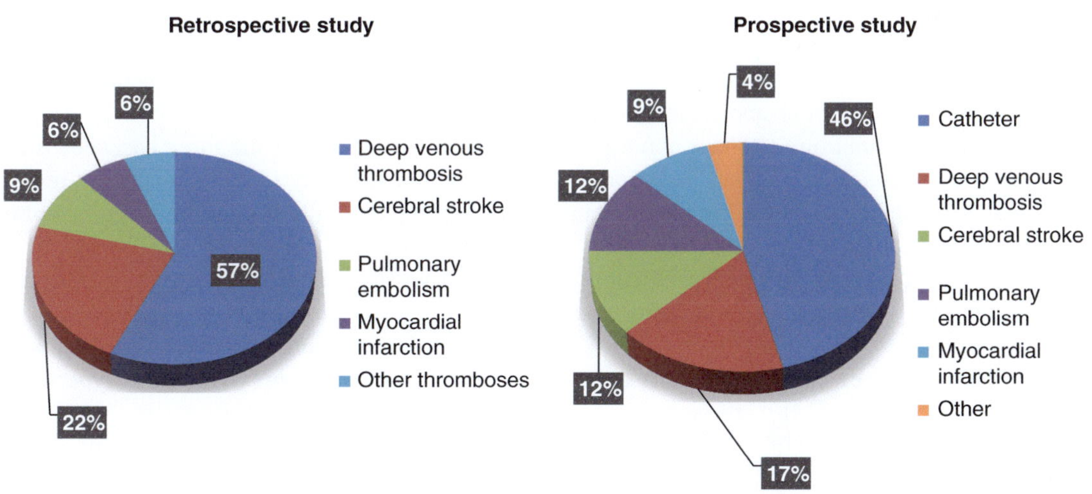

Fig. 5.1 Thrombotic events during induction therapy in retrospective and prospective studies (PETHEMA). The incidence of thrombo-ischemic events seems different depending on the prospective or retrospective design of the PETHEMA studies

this complication [17]. However, a large prospective study by Rodriguez-Veiga et al. showed the following risk factors for the development of non-catheter-related thrombosis at diagnosis or during induction: hypoalbuminemia, absence of hemorrhage at diagnosis, higher platelet counts, male sex, and worse performance status (ECOG scale) (unpublished data).

Hemostatic Abnormalities

Normal hemostatic mechanisms consist of three processes strictly connected: (1) primary hemostasis, in which platelet adhere to the vessel wall lesion and, upon activation and aggregation, generate a platelet plug; (2) the coagulation cascade activation, leading to fibrin formation and platelet plug establishment, which is finely regulated by natural inhibitors (i.e., antithrombin, protein C, protein S) that prevent excessive coagulation; and (3) fibrinolysis activation, triggered by fibrin itself, which determines the degradation and dissolution of cross-linked fibrin and final restoration of vessel wall integrity. In patients with APL, laboratory coagulation abnormalities show a profound dysregulation in all of these mechanisms at the onset of the disease. Besides thrombocytopenia, routine coagulation laboratory test alterations occur, including hypofibrinogenemia, increased circulating levels of fibrinogen-fibrin degradation products (FDPs), and prolonged prothrombin and thrombin times. These abnormalities can be accentuated by the initiation of cytotoxic chemotherapy, resulting in severe hemorrhagic complications [25]. As summarized in Table 5.1, the observed alterations of routine clotting tests are not specific of any hemostatic pathway.

Table 5.1 Lab abnormalities of hemostasis in APL patients

Test	Results
1. *Routine*	
Prothrombin time (PT)	↑
Thrombin time (TT)	↑
Fibrinogen	↓
Platelet count	↓
D-dimer	↑
Fibrin(ogen) degradation products (FDPs)	↑
2. *Markers of hypercoagulation*	
Prothrombin F 1+2	↑
Thrombin-antithrombin (TAT) complexes	↑
Fibrinopeptide A (FPA)	↑
3. *Markers of hyperfibrinolysis*	
Urokinase-type plasminogen activator (u-PA)	↑
Plasminogen	↓
α2-antiplasmin	↓
4. *Marker of non-specific proteolysis*	
Elastase-inhibitor complexes	↑

↑ = *Increased;* ↓ = *Decreased*

The results of more sensitive laboratory assays confirm the activation of all of these systems in APL. In fact, plasma levels of well-known markers of clotting activation, i.e., the prothrombin fragment F1 + 2 (F1 + 2), thrombin-antithrombin (TAT) complex, and fibrinopeptide A (FPA), are elevated in the majority of APL patients [9, 26, 27]. Additionally, plasma markers indicating ongoing hyperfibrinolysis, including high levels of FDPs and urokinase plasminogen activator (u-PA) together with low levels of plasminogen and 2-antiplasmin, are present [26, 28–30]. Finally, elevated plasma levels of leukocyte elastase and fibrinogen split products of elastase are detected, which demonstrate hyperactivity of non-specific proteases.

Activation of any of the three cascades (i.e., coagulation, fibrinolysis, or non-specific proteolysis) can potentially trigger the bleeding complications of APL. However, the detection of elevated levels of D-dimer, the lysis product of stabilized cross-linked fibrin, provides strong evidence for ongoing clotting activation and thrombin generation in vivo, with hyperfibrinolysis occurring secondarily to the generation of thrombin [26, 31–34]. Less evident is the occurrence of primary hyperfibrinolysis as the major event leading to the bleeding diathesis in APL [35–38]. Based on the laboratory tests currently available, it is difficult to prove the existence of primary systemic hyperfibrinolysis in APL. In fact, while reactive, or secondary, hyperfibrinolysis in response to clotting activation can be documented by the D-dimer level increment, there are no specific tests that define primary hyperfibrino(geno)lysis in vivo. The findings of profound reductions of 2-antiplasmin and plasminogen levels, sensitive to the therapeutic use of antifibrinolytic agents [35, 36], do not allow the distinction between primary and secondary hyperfibrinolysis. Menell and colleagues found that annexin II, a protein with high affinity for plasminogen (PA) and tissue-type plasminogen activator (tPA), is highly expressed by APL cells as compared to non-APL leukemic cells [37]. The expression of annexin II on circulating APL cell surface might be responsible for primary hyperfibrinolysis in vivo; however, in the same study, the assessment of systemic activation of fibrinolysis in patient plasma still relied on non-specific primary hyperfibrinolysis markers and on D-dimer levels, which rather stands for secondary hyperfibrinolysis.

In conclusion, the activation of coagulation leads to the development of a consumption coagulopathy with excess reactive activation of fibrinolysis, the mechanism of clot lysis, and dissolution. Clinical manifestations are diffuse hemorrhages, organ failure due to microthrombi, and sometimes thrombosis of large vessels. Primary hyperfibrinolysis may occur in specific districts (i.e., cerebral vessels) where annexin II is highly expressed and aggravates bleeding.

One laboratory finding that may distinguish the coagulopathy of APL from typical DIC complicating other clinical conditions (e.g., sepsis) is the maintenance of relatively normal levels of the coagulation inhibitors antithrombin (AT). This has raised some arguments against DIC, favoring the hypothesis of primary hyperfibrinolysis as the determinant of severe bleeding in acute leukemia [39]. Of interest, however, is that reduced levels of AT in patients with APL tend to occur in patients with hepatic dysfunction, while these levels are usually normal in those with normal liver function [40]. Therefore, normal levels of AT in APL patients do not exclude DIC but may emphasize other features of this coagulopathy.

Pathogenesis of the Coagulopathy of APL

Many exogenous factors, including cytotoxic chemotherapy and concomitant infections, can impair the normal delicate balance between procoagulant and anticoagulant forces in the hemostatic system of patients with APL. However, the major determinants of coagulopathy in these patients are the intrinsic hemostatic properties of leukemic cells and their interactions with the host coagulation system, as well as the host vascular cells. These properties include (1) expression of procoagulant factors and the release of procoagulant microparticles, (2) expression of fibrinolytic proteins and proteolytic enzymes, and (3) secretion of inflammatory cytokines [i.e., interleukin-1b (IL-1β) and tumor necrosis factor (TNFα)] and expression of adhesion molecules to bind to vascular endothelium and other blood cells (Fig. 5.2).

Increasing evidence from molecular studies of experimental models of human cancers shows that oncogene and repressor gene-mediated neoplastic transformation activate the clotting system as an integral feature of neoplastic transformation [41]. Triggering signaling pathways by one or more of these genes results in activation of the coagulation cascade and platelet function and/or suppression of fibrinolysis, which altogether can produce thrombosis and/or DIC in these models [42–44]. Along this line, oncogenic events may drive the expression of cellular procoagulant activities in APL cells, in which the typical *PML/RARα* genetic lesion is associated with the overexpression of cellular procoagulant activities and the appearance of the coagulopathy, while cellular differentiation leads to the loss of cellular procoagulant potential [1].

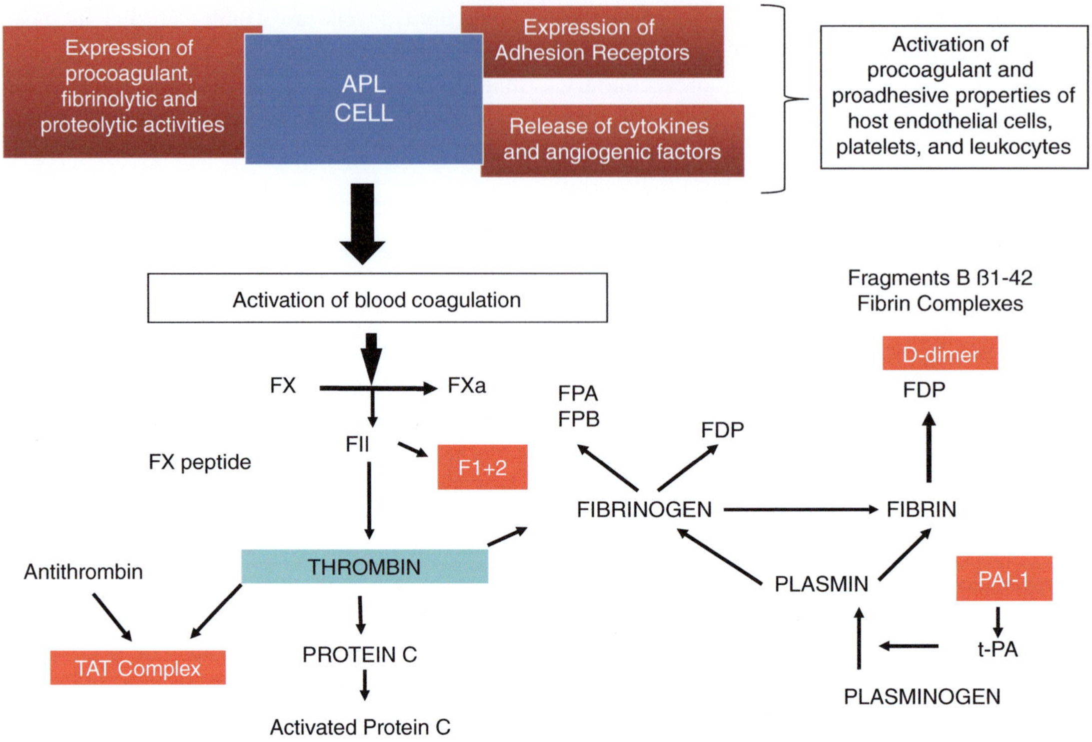

Fig. 5.2 Pathogenesis of coagulopathy in APL. APL cells interact with the host hemostatic system by (1) the expression of procoagulant, fibrinolytic, and proteolytic activities; (2) the release of inflammatory cytokines and angiogenic factors and the expression of cell membrane adhesion receptors, which induce the procoagulant and proadhesive properties of normal vascular cells and mediate APL cell-vascular cell direct interaction. All these events reflect in the peripheral blood with alterations in the levels of circulating biomarkers of hypercoagulation, hyperfibrinolysis, proteolysis, and inflammation. *TAT* thrombin-antithrombin complex, *F1 + 2* prothrombin fragment 1 + 2, *FPA* fibrinopeptide A, *FPB* fibrinopeptide B, *FDP* fibrinogen-fibrin degradation product, *tPA* tissue-type plasminogen activator, *PAI-1* plasminogen activator inhibitor 1

Procoagulant Activity

The principal cancer cell-associated clotting activating mechanisms include the expression of procoagulant factors: tissue factor (TF) and cancer procoagulant (CP). These proteins are highly expressed by APL cells.

TF is a transmembrane glycoprotein that is the primary initiator of normal blood coagulation. TF forms a complex with factor VIIa (TF/FVIIa) to trigger blood coagulation by proteolytically activating FIX and FX. Normal cells, including endothelial cells (EC) and monocyte-macrophages, do not express TF, unless they are adequately stimulated [45]. Differently, a constitutive TF expression characterizes numerous malignant tumor tissues, including APL. TF was identified in the NB4 cell line, the first human APL cell line containing the typical t(15;17) chromosomal balanced translocation. Thereafter TF has been characterized in APL cells by several laboratories [26, 27, 46–49]. The underlying molecular mechanisms are unclear; however in vitro the TF promoter is active in the PML-RARα-positive NB4 APL cell line, and it is possible that this relates to the fusion protein. Furthermore, bone marrow cells from mice transgenic for the fusion genes PLZF-RARα or NPM-RARα do express the TF gene, whereas cells derived from mice without those fusion genes do not express the TF gene [50]. A strong link is found between the regulation of TF gene expression in APL cells and the malignant transforming events. Additionally, increased levels of

TF-bearing microparticles (TF-MPs) have been described in APL patients [51]. As in solid tumors, the TF-MPs found in APL exhibit procoagulant activity as shown by thrombin generation measurements [52].

CP is a cysteine protease that directly activates factor X in the absence of activated factor VII. CP is synthesized by malignant cells, and its activity has been found in extracts of different tumors [53–55]. CP is expressed in patient leukemic blasts of various phenotypes and is found at the highest levels in APL blasts. Accordingly, it is highly expressed in the NB4 cell line APL [56]. In APL cells, at the onset of disease, the levels of CP are found elevated compared to cells obtained from patients at the time of complete remission, confirming the association of a procoagulant protein expression with the malignant phenotype [57].

Fibrinolytic and Proteolytic Properties

Leukemic cells can express on their surface all constituents of the fibrinolytic system, which are relevant for maintenance of proper hemostasis. There are specific receptors that support the assembly of all fibrinolysis proteins on leukemic cells thus facilitating the activation of the fibrinolytic cascade [58].

APL cells are capable to interact with the host fibrinolytic system, owing to the expression of plasminogen activators (u-PA and tPA); their inhibitors, i.e., plasminogen activator inhibitor 1 and 2 (PAI-1 and PAI-2); and receptors such as u-PAR and annexin II (a co-receptor for PA and tPA) [59–61]. Annexin II is overexpressed on t(15;17)-positive APL cells [37, 62] and can cause a marked increase in tPA-dependent plasmin generation compared to non-APL cells in vitro [62]. However, the study of 26 patients failed to show any correlation between increased cellular annexin II expression and increased systemic fibrinolytic activity measured by FDP, plasminogen, and fibrinogen levels [62]. Increased levels of MPs expressing annexin II and tPA have been found in the circulation of patients with APL [51]. Abnormalities of the fibrinolytic system have been proposed to play a major role in the pathogenesis of the APL coagulopathy and to be responsible for the commonly observed hemorrhagic complications. Likely, the increased expression of annexin II on cerebral endothelial cells [63] may contribute to the high incidence of intracranial hemorrhage in APL [64]. Relevant in this context are also changes in other fibrinolytic proteins in APL, including increased expression of u-PA, tPA, and the urokinase-type plasminogen activator receptor (u-PAR) [65].

In addition, an increased proteolysis by nonspecific proteases, such as elastase, can occur in APL. Increased plasma levels of elastase, detected as elastase-inhibitor complex, are found in these patients [66, 67]. These enzymes can interfere with coagulation by degrading clotting factors and cleaving inhibitors of fibrinolysis [67, 68]. Elastase can degrade fibrinogen, producing a pattern of FDPs different from those produced by plasmin cleavage [69, 70]. Varieties of proteases, which can be elaborated by APL cells, have been implicated in the pathogenesis of the bleeding syndrome. In an in vitro study, freshly isolated APL blasts expressed lower fibrinolytic and proteolytic activities compared to mature neutrophils. Plasma elastase levels are elevated at the onset of APL, most likely as the result of cell degranulation and lysis [31].

Cytokine Release and Adhesive Properties

Several cytokines are secreted by APL cells, including interleukin (IL)-1β and tumor necrosis factor alpha (TNFα) [71]. Both TNFα and IL-1β induce a procoagulant endothelium by upregulating the expression of TF and downregulating the expression of the anticoagulant thrombomodulin (TM) on endothelial cells (EC) [72]. In addition, these cytokines increase the production of endothelial PAI-1, the inhibitor of fibrinolysis. Upregulation of TF and PAI-1 and downregulation of TM lead the shift of the vessel wall to a prothrombotic phenotype. An increased secretion of IL-1β has been observed in leukemic promyelocytes from patients with DIC compared to patients without DIC [73].

The expression on the surface of leukemic cells of adhesion molecules and/or their counter-receptors permits the direct interaction of these cells with the host endothelial cells (EC), platelets, and leukocytes. The attachment of malignant cells to vascular EC favors the localization of clotting activation to the vessel wall with on-site release of cytokines and the activation of the endothelium. This, in turn, increases the expression of endothelial counter-receptors, i.e., ICAM-1 or VCAM-1, which bind to the leukemic cell membrane adhesion integrins, such as LFA-1 and Mac-1. Attachment of leukemic cells to the vessel wall via these adhesion mechanisms, and subsequent trans-endothelial migration, represents one potential mechanism to explain the higher incidence of vascular complications in association with high WBC count. Experimental evidence supports the concept that adhesive mechanisms of APL cells promote the localization of clotting activation to the vessel wall, WBC and platelet aggregation, thrombin generation (and hyperfibrinolysis), and further endothelium activation. Accordingly, leukemic cells can activate platelets by cell-cell interaction, generation of thrombin, and secretion of platelet-activating molecules. Recent data show that podoplanin, a type I transmembrane sialomucin-like glycoprotein expressed by several tumor cells and capable to induce platelet aggregation [74], is aberrantly expressed by APL promyelocytes. This might contribute to abnormal platelet aggregation and possibly to APL-related bleeding [75]. Due to the leukemia-related severe thrombocytopenia, the relevance of this mechanism in APL coagulopathy remains to be clarified.

The Effects of ATRA and ATO on the Coagulopathy of APL

Differentiating therapy with ATRA and ATO for remission induction therapy exerts overall beneficial effects on the APL-associated coagulopathy. Several studies document the decrease or normalization of clotting variables, such as F1 + 2, TAT, FPA, and D-dimer, during therapy with ATRA. Additionally, ATRA inhibits fibrinolysis by inducing the synthesis of PAI-1 and by reducing the synthesis of annexin II (with consequent reduction of receptor-bound PA) [26, 31–33]. Furthermore, the proteolysis of von Willebrand factor (vWF) is reduced by ATRA treatment [76]. These beneficial effects of ATRA on markers of coagulation, fibrinolysis, and proteolysis activation are associated with improvement in clinical signs of bleeding in the same patients. The benefits persist when ATRA is given in combination with chemotherapy. Induction therapy with ATRA has a long-term benefit on both disease-free and overall survival in APL, while serious bleeding at the time of presentation remains a negative prognostic finding [77]. Rapid reversal of the coagulopathy with ATRA may improve survival in some of those poor prognosis patients.

In vitro studies show that ATRA interferes with APL procoagulant and fibrinolytic mechanisms. ATRA-induced APL cell differentiation in vitro causes loss of expression of procoagulant proteins like CP [78] and TF [79, 80]. This occurs also in vivo, in the bone marrow cells of APL patients given ATRA for remission induction therapy [26]. Reduction of leukemic cell procoagulant activity by ATRA appears to be one important mechanism involved in the resolution of the coagulopathy. An in vitro study demonstrated that, after ATRA treatment, CP activity is downregulated only in those NB4 cells that are sensitive to ATRA-induced cytodifferentiation, and not in ATRA-resistant cells that do not differentiate. However, TF activity was significantly reduced in all cell lines in response to ATRA, regardless of sensitivity to ATRA-induced differentiation [81]. TF expression can be downregulated by ATRA in both APL cells and in other types of leukemic cells [82] and also in normally differentiated cells [83–86]. Nuclear run-on experiments in human monocytes and monocytic leukemia cells support the concept that ATRA inhibits induction of TF expression at the level of transcription [85] but independently of the common transcription factors AP-1 or NF-kB [85]. The destabilization of TF mRNA induced by ATRA in NB4 cells is partially dependent upon protein synthesis [86], and ATRA induces synthesis of a protein in NB4 cells that selectively degrades PML/RARα fusion protein [87]. Therefore, one or more proteins induced by ATRA in leukemic cells may also destabilize TF mRNA [88]. Additionally these data provide strong support for the hypothesis that downregulation of TF gene expression is a direct result of the mechanism of the ATRA effect on oncogene expression. Recently, Fang et al. demonstrated that ATRA treatment of NB4 APL cells leads to reduced microparticle delivery of TF to endothelial cells, underlying the importance of immediate treatment with ATRA [89]. Similarly, circulating markers of clotting activation are downregulated after induction therapy with ATRA [26, 27].

Concerning fibrinolysis, ATRA inhibits the expression of annexin II by APL blasts [62]. Furthermore, retinoids induce a rapid increase of u-PA activity on APL cell surface, which is however promptly downregulated by an increased production of PA inhibitors, including PAI-1 and PAI-2 [90]. Overall, these mechanisms can contribute to a reduction of fibrinolytic activity in APL cells in response to ATRA. These results agree with the findings of normal plasma fibrinolytic activity, measured by the assay of "euglobulin lysis area," in APL patients receiving ATRA [26]. In conclusion, hyperfibrinolysis may reflect activation of the fibrinolytic system on the surface of the leukemic cells, where specific receptors favor the assembly of all the fibrinolytic components. ATRA acts initially to enhance this fibrinolytic activity by increasing the synthesis of u-PA. Thereafter, however, ATRA-induced synthesis of PA inhibitors and inhibition of annexin II synthesis may be favored, contributing to the downregulation of receptor-bound plasminogen activators. On balance, therefore, no change in plasma total fibrinolytic activity occurs in most patients in response to ATRA.

No relation has been observed between plasma elastase concentration and the levels of D-dimer or other hemostatic variables during treatment with ATRA. These data, together with the data of De Stefano et al. [80], cast doubt on the earlier hypothesis that elastase makes an important contribution to the bleeding disorder of patients with APL [66].

Further, ATRA upregulates the ability of leukemic cells to produce cytokines [72]. This effect should shift the balance at the endothelium to the prothrombotic side of the equation. However, ATRA also appears to protect the endothelium in vitro against the prothrombotic assault of inflammatory cytokines, because ATRA prevents both the downregulation of TM and the upregulation of TF induced by TNFα [83] and by IL-1β in the endothelial cells [84]. Therefore, although ATRA increases cytokine synthesis by APL cells, it appears to protect the endothelium against the prothrombotic stimulus of these mediators through a complex set of interactions.

Finally, ATRA increases the adhesion capacity of APL cells to the endothelium in vitro [91], although pretreatment of ECs with ATRA reverses this effect and actually results in impaired adhesion of APL cells to ECs, due to the downregulation of EC counter-receptors by ATRA. Perhaps ATRA is unable to exert this same protective effect on the specialized endothelium of the lung, thus explaining the unusual features of the differentiation syndrome, occurring in APL patients with elevated WBC count under ATRA treatment. Both early mortality and the differentiation syndrome (characterized by unexplained fever, weight gain, respiratory distress, interstitial pulmonary infiltrates, pleural and pericardial effusions, episodic hypotension, and acute renal failure) are correlated with high WBC count, the expression of adhesion molecules, and/or the release of cytokines [92–96]. It seems likely that a further understanding of the pathogenesis of the differentiation syndrome and its prevention, as well as a better strategy for the treatment of the consumptive coagulopathy of APL, will evolve from an improved appreciation of the biological properties of the fusion proteins of PML-RARα [97].

ATO induces apoptosis and differentiation of APL cells [98]. Current data show that ATO, as well as ATRA, can reduce TF expression and

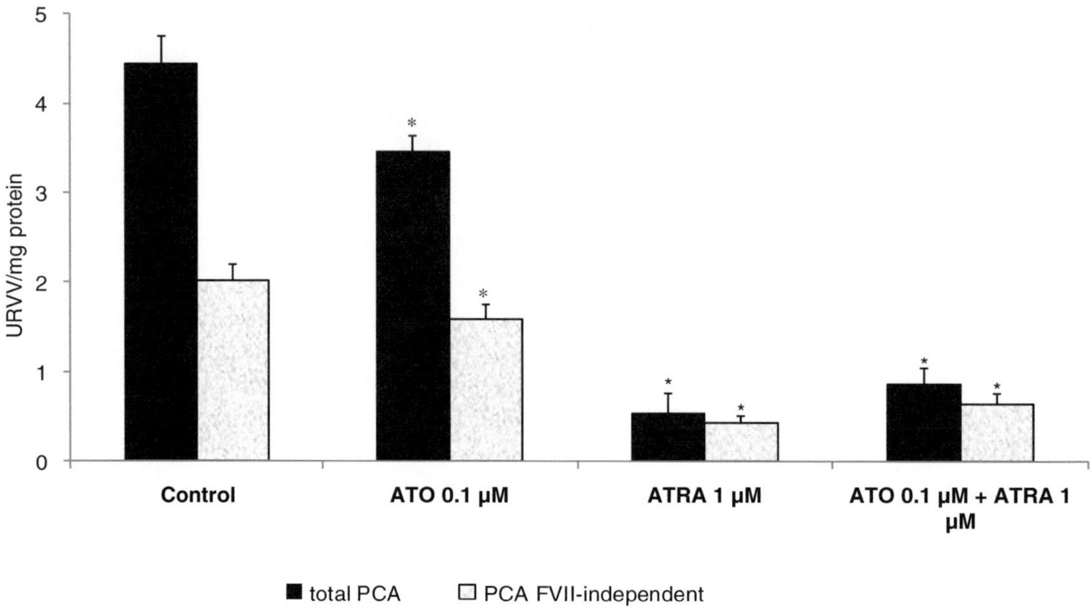

Fig. 5.3 Modulation of procoagulant activity of NB4 cells by ATO and ATRA. NB4 cells were incubated for 96 h with ATO (0.1 μM) +/− ATRA (1 μM), while control cells received the vehicle alone (DMSO). Total procoagulant activity and FVII-independent procoagulant activity were evaluated by the clotting assays of normal human plasma (NHP) and FVII-deficient plasma (FVII-DP). Results are expressed as mean ± SD of three separate experiments performed in duplicate. * = $P < 0.01$ vs. controls, by Student's *t*-test on paired samples

procoagulant activity of APL blast cells in vitro and in vivo. ATO treatment induces rapid loss of membrane procoagulant activity and TF mRNA leading to beneficial effects in vivo on the coagulopathy of APL patients [99, 100]. Data from our laboratory show that ATO alone reduces both TF and CP expression in NB4 cells, although to a lesser extent than ATRA. Additionally, the ATO + ATRA combination is as effective as ATRA alone in reducing the procoagulant activity, suggesting no additive effect between the two drugs (Fig. 5.3). A dual role for the ATO molecular-targeted therapy for the control of both the disease remission and the APL-associated coagulopathy can be investigated and support the importance of ATO in the cure of APL.

Management of the Coagulopathy

APL is a medical emergency, and aggressive measures to support the bleeding complications should begin at first suspicion of APL. Modern recommendations indicate that three simultaneous actions must be immediately undertaken when a diagnosis of APL is suspected: (1) start ATRA or ATO therapy, (2) administer supportive care, and (3) confirm genetic diagnosis [101] (Fig. 5.4).

The main strategy in the management of APL coagulopathy is early initiation of ATRA or ATO, which results in resolution of the bleeding tendency and rapid normalization of coagulation tests and fibrinogen level. It is mandatory to start as soon as possible ATRA therapy and supportive measures aimed at counteracting the coagulopathy. In high-risk patients, a delay in ATRA administration appears to contribute to bleeding and early death rate [15].

The responses to the supportive treatments for DIC in APL are the most disparate. The most important supportive tool is the judicious use of platelet transfusion, whereas the use of anticoagulants and antifibrinolytic agents remains a hotly debated issue [102–104]. The advent of ATRA treatment has ushered in a new era in the management of the coagulopathy of APL.

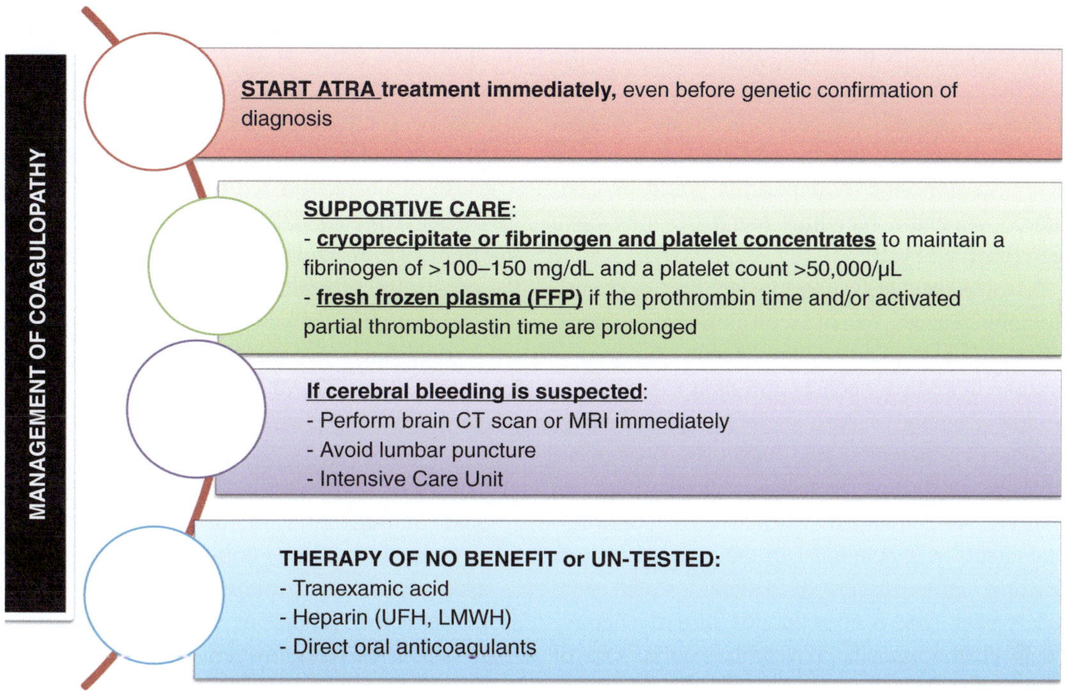

Fig. 5.4 Schematics of the current approaches to the APL coagulopathy. *LMWH* low-molecular-weight heparin, *UFH* unfractionated heparin

Platelet Transfusions, Heparin, and Antifibrinolytic Agents

Platelet transfusions represent an essential part of the modern supportive care for APL patients, even if there is no study that specifically addressed the threshold for platelet transfusion. Prophylactic transfusion of platelets has resulted in a significant decrease in the incidence of fatal bleeding and, therefore, a prolongation of survival. In patients with APL, the bleeding risk and platelet transfusion requirements remain high even in the ATRA era [1, 105]. Current recommendations for patients with APL suggest that platelets should be transfused to maintain the platelet count above 30×10^9/L in patients not actively bleeding and above 50×10^9/L in those with active bleeding [102, 105].

In order to maintain the fibrinogen level above 100–150 mg/dL, transfusion of frozen plasma, fibrinogen, and/or cryoprecipitate has been recommended [106, 107]. These and other supportive measures should be rapidly instituted and maintained until disappearance of all clinical and laboratory signs of coagulopathy. Routine use of heparin, tranexamic acid, or other anticoagulant or antifibrinolytic therapies is not recommended. The role of heparin therapy in the treatment of the coagulopathy complicating APL is uncertain and has never been ruled out in a prospective randomized trial. Before the ATRA era, several studies concluded that the use of heparin reduced the rate of hemorrhagic death and improved long-term survival. However, the GIMEMA group, in a large retrospective analysis of 268 APL patients, demonstrated no benefit for the prevention of early hemorrhagic deaths or overall survival [108]. Additionally, in a series of 65 adults with APL, the complete remission rate was higher in patients transfused intensively with platelets and not given heparin suggesting that the correction of thrombocytopenia with platelet transfusion is of special importance and may obviate the need for heparin therapy [109]. Although markers of coagulation activation and fibrinolysis decrease rapidly, following the start of ATRA, there appears to be a slower resolution of the clinical manifestations, suggesting the persistence of a prothrombotic state during the initial period of treatment. These evidences suggest that prophylactic use of low-molecular-weight heparin (LMWH) or even the factor Xa inhibitor fondaparinux could be considered once the bleeding manifestations have been resolved [110].

It would seem logical to consider the use of antifibrinolytic agents such as epsilon-aminocaproic acid (EACA, Amicar) or tranexamic acid and/or protease inhibitors, such as aprotinin (Trasylol) in the management of APL patients with bleeding, because of a potential role played by fibrinolytic activators and other proteases. Although several small studies concluded that the use of antifibrinolytic agents was beneficial in the management of bleeding, large studies of patients treated with ATRA have shown no reduction in early hemorrhagic deaths associated with the routine use of these agents. In addition, a PETHEMA retrospective study performed on 759 patients showed that the use of prophylactic tranexamic acid was an independent risk factor for thrombosis (odds ratio 1.96). Thus, it has been suggested that antifibrinolytic agents should be reserved for patients with retinal or intracranial and other life-threatening bleeding [7, 110].

The role of factor VIIa and prothrombin complex concentrates to treat or prevent the hemorrhagic episodes is controversial, as they may enhance the thrombotic risk. Some anecdotal use of recombinant factor VIIa in patients with APL was reported, being effective for life-threatening hemorrhages [111, 112]. The use of prothrombin complex to correct coagulopathy, instead of fresh frozen plasma, could be recommended only in patients with fluid overload or DS. In any case, the use of recombinant factor VIIa or prothrombin complex should be restricted to clinical trials.

The treatment of thrombotic episodes occurring in APL patients remains a challenge, especially because this complication mainly occur during induction phase, in a patient that presents concomitant DIC and severe thrombocytopenia. In fact, no ad hoc studies or guidelines are available for the management of such complication. However, the clinician should have in mind that the hemorrhagic risk is predominant in APL, as it is the major cause of death. When a catheter-related thrombosis occurs, the central venous line should be removed as soon as possible, and a catheter-associated infection must be ruled out. The use of unfractionated heparin could be recommended in case of cerebral stroke, in view of the high risk of hemorrhagic transformation and the possibility of rapid reversion using protamine sulfate. If a standard low-molecular-weight heparin is used, the dose could be adapted to the platelet counts (e.g., 70–80% if $<70 \times 10^9$/L, 50% if $<50 \times 10^9$/L, stop if $<30 \times 10^9$/L).

Conclusions

The pathogenesis of the coagulopathy in patients with APL is complex and multifactorial. A prominent role is played by leukemic cell-specific properties interfering with the patient hemostatic system. In APL, bleeding manifestations prevail, although localized thrombosis of large vessels can coexist. ATRA and ATO treatments for remission induction have improved hemorrhagic accident rates and overall mortality in APL patients. However, early hemorrhagic death still remains one of the major causes of induction treatment failures. Low fibrinogen levels, prolongation of the PT and TT, and abnormal plasma levels of markers of hypercoagulation, hyperfibrinolysis, and non-specific proteolysis characterize the coagulopathy of APL. The nearly ubiquitous presence of elevated levels of fibrin D-dimer clearly demonstrates the occurrence of secondary or reactive hyperfibrinolysis in response to activation of blood coagulation and thrombin generation. Primary mechanisms of hyperfibrinolysis may take place in some specific districts, particularly in the cerebral tissues.

Reducing the bleeding-related mortality is an important task and remains a major challenge in the cure of APL. The immediate start of ATRA and the use of prophylactic platelet transfusions are highly recommended. In contrast, the routine use of anticoagulants and/or antifibrinolytic agents in the control or prevention of DIC cannot be recommended at this time.

References

1. Falanga A, Rickles FR. Pathogenesis and management of the bleeding diathesis in acute promyelocytic leukaemia. Best Pract Res Clin Haematol. 2003;16(3):463–82.
2. Falanga A. Predicting APL lethal bleeding in the ATRA era. Blood. 2017;129(13):1739–40.
3. Levi M. Cancer-related coagulopathies. Thromb Res. 2014;133(Suppl 2):S70–5.
4. Falanga A, Russo L, Tartari CJ. Pathogenesis and treatment of thrombohemorrhagic diathesis in acute promyelocytic leukemia. Mediterr J Hematol Infect Dis. 2011;3(1):e2011068.
5. Falanga A, Marchetti M. Venous thromboembolism in the hematologic malignancies. J Clin Oncol. 2009;27(29):4848–57.
6. Libourel EJ, et al. Disseminated intravascular coagulation at diagnosis is a strong predictor for both arterial and venous thrombosis in newly diagnosed acute myeloid leukemia. Blood. 2016.
7. Tallman MS, Abutalib SA, Altman JK. The double hazard of thrombophilia and bleeding in acute promyelocytic leukemia. Semin Thromb Hemost. 2007;33(4):330–8.
8. Lo-Coco F, et al. Retinoic acid and arsenic trioxide for acute promyelocytic leukemia. N Engl J Med. 2013;369(2):111–21.
9. Tallman MS, Kwaan HC. Reassessing the hemostatic disorder associated with acute promyelocytic leukemia. Blood. 1992;79(3):543–53.
10. Fenaux P. Management of acute promyelocytic leukemia. Eur J Haematol. 1993;50(2):65–73.
11. Barbui T, Finazzi G, Falanga A. The impact of all-trans-retinoic acid on the coagulopathy of acute promyelocytic leukemia. Blood. 1998;91(9):3093–102.
12. Castaigne S, et al. All-trans retinoic acid as a differentiation therapy for acute promyelocytic leukemia. I. Clinical results. Blood. 1990;76(9):1704–9.
13. Lehmann S, et al. Continuing high early death rate in acute promyelocytic leukemia: a population-based report from the Swedish Adult Acute Leukemia Registry. Leukemia. 2011;25(7):1128–34.
14. Breccia M, Lo Coco F. Thrombo-hemorrhagic deaths in acute promyelocytic leukemia. Thromb Res. 2014;133(Suppl 2):S112–6.
15. Altman JK, et al. Administration of ATRA to newly diagnosed patients with acute promyelocytic leukemia is delayed contributing to early hemorrhagic death. Leuk Res. 2013;37(9):1004–9.
16. de la Serna J, et al. Causes and prognostic factors of remission induction failure in patients with acute promyelocytic leukemia treated with all-trans retinoic acid and idarubicin. Blood. 2008;111(7):3395–402.
17. Breccia M, et al. Occurrence of thrombotic events in acute promyelocytic leukemia correlates with consistent immunophenotypic and molecular features. Leukemia. 2007;21(1):79–83.
18. Chang H, et al. Acute promyelocytic leukemia-associated thrombosis. Acta Haematol. 2013;130(1):1–6.
19. Rashidi A, et al. Thrombosis in acute promyelocytic leukemia. Thromb Res. 2013;131(4):281–9.
20. Montesinos P, et al. Differentiation syndrome in patients with acute promyelocytic leukemia treated with all-trans retinoic acid and anthracycline chemotherapy: characteristics, outcome, and prognostic factors. Blood. 2009;113(4):775–83.
21. Mitrovic M, et al. Thrombotic events in acute promyelocytic leukemia. Thromb Res. 2015;135(4):588–93.
22. Montesinos P, de la Serna J, Vellenga E, Rayon C, Bergua J, Parody R, Esteve J, Gonzalez M, Brunet S, Sanz M. Incidence and Risk Factors for Thrombosis in Patients with Acute Promyelocytic Leukemia. Experience of the PETHEMA LPA96 and LPA99 Protocols. Blood. 2006;108:1503.
23. De Stefano V, et al. The risk of thrombosis in patients with acute leukemia: occurrence of thrombosis at diagnosis and during treatment. J Thromb Haemost. 2005;3(9):1985–92.
24. Falanga A. Mechanisms of hypercoagulation in malignancy and during chemotherapy. Haemostasis. 1998;28(Suppl 3):50–60.
25. Falanga A, et al. Loss of blast cell procoagulant activity and improvement of hemostatic variables in patients with acute promyelocytic leukemia administered all-trans-retinoic acid. Blood. 1995;86(3):1072–81.
26. Tallman MS, et al. Effects of all-trans retinoic acid or chemotherapy on the molecular regulation of systemic blood coagulation and fibrinolysis in patients with acute promyelocytic leukemia. J Thromb Haemost. 2004;2(8):1341–50.
27. Booth NA, Bennett B. Plasmin-alpha 2-antiplasmin complexes in bleeding disorders characterized by primary or secondary fibrinolysis. Br J Haematol. 1984;56(4):545–56.
28. Reddy VB, et al. Global and molecular hemostatic markers in acute myeloid leukemia. Am J Clin Pathol. 1990;94(4):397–403.
29. Speiser W, et al. Hemostatic and fibrinolytic parameters in patients with acute myeloid leukemia: activation of blood coagulation, fibrinolysis and unspecific proteolysis. Blut. 1990;61(5):298–302.
30. Dombret H, et al. Coagulation disorders associated with acute promyelocytic leukemia: corrective effect of all-trans retinoic acid treatment. Leukemia. 1993;7(1):2–9.
31. Dombret H, et al. In vivo thrombin and plasmin activities in patients with acute promyelocytic leukemia (APL): effect of all-trans retinoic acid (ATRA) therapy. Leukemia. 1995;9(1):19–24.
32. Kawai Y, et al. Rapid improvement of coagulopathy by all-trans retinoic acid in acute promyelocytic leukemia. Am J Hematol. 1994;46(3):184–8.
33. Watanabe R, et al. Long-term follow-up of hemostatic molecular markers during remission induction therapy with all-trans retinoic acid for acute promyelocytic leukemia. Keio Hematology-Oncology Cooperative Study Group (KHOCS). Thromb Haemost. 1997;77(4):641–5.

34. Avvisati G, et al. Acquired alpha-2-antiplasmin deficiency in acute promyelocytic leukaemia. Br J Haematol. 1988;70(1):43–8.
35. Schwartz BS, et al. Epsilon-aminocaproic acid in the treatment of patients with acute promyelocytic leukemia and acquired alpha-2-plasmin inhibitor deficiency. Ann Intern Med. 1986;105(6):873–7.
36. Menell JS, et al. Annexin II and bleeding in acute promyelocytic leukemia. N Engl J Med. 1999;340(13):994–1004.
37. Kwaan HC. The unique hemostatic dysfunction in acute promyelocytic leukemia. Semin Thromb Hemost. 2014;40(3):332–6.
38. Avvisati G. Coagulopathy in APL: a step forward? Blood. 2012;120(1):4–6.
39. Rodeghiero F, et al. Liver dysfunction rather than intravascular coagulation as the main cause of low protein C and antithrombin III in acute leukemia. Blood. 1984;63(4):965–9.
40. Falanga A, Barbui T, Rickles FR. Hypercoagulability and tissue factor gene upregulation in hematologic malignancies. Semin Thromb Hemost. 2008; 34(2):204–10.
41. Boccaccio C, et al. The MET oncogene drives a genetic programme linking cancer to haemostasis. Nature. 2005;434(7031):396–400.
42. Rong Y, et al. PTEN and hypoxia regulate tissue factor expression and plasma coagulation by glioblastoma. Cancer Res. 2005;65(4):1406–13.
43. Yu JL, et al. Oncogenic events regulate tissue factor expression in colorectal cancer cells: implications for tumor progression and angiogenesis. Blood. 2005;105(4):1734–41.
44. Furie B, Furie BC. Mechanisms of thrombus formation. N Engl J Med. 2008;359(9):938–49.
45. Andoh K, et al. Tissue factor activity in leukemia cells. Special reference to disseminated intravascular coagulation. Cancer. 1987;59(4):748–54.
46. Gouault Heilmann M, et al. The procoagulant factor of leukaemic promyelocytes: demonstration of immunologic cross reactivity with human brain tissue factor. Br J Haematol. 1975;30(2):151–8.
47. Bauer KA, et al. Tissue factor gene expression in acute myeloblastic leukemia. Thromb Res. 1989;56(3):425–30.
48. Hair GA, et al. Tissue factor expression in human leukemic cells. Leuk Res. 1996;20(1):1–11.
49. Cheng GX, et al. Distinct leukemia phenotypes in transgenic mice and different corepressor interactions generated by promyelocytic leukemia variant fusion genes PLZF-RARalpha and NPM-RARalpha. Proc Natl Acad Sci U S A. 1999;96(11):6318–23.
50. Kwaan HC, Rego EM. Role of microparticles in the hemostatic dysfunction in acute promyelocytic leukemia. Semin Thromb Hemost. 2010;36(8):917–24.
51. Ma G, et al. Increased promyelocytic-derived microparticles: a novel potential factor for coagulopathy in acute promyelocytic leukemia. Ann Hematol. 2013;92(5):645–52.
52. Falanga A, Gordon SG. Isolation and characterization of cancer procoagulant: a cysteine proteinase from malignant tissue. Biochemistry. 1985;24(20):5558–67.
53. Donati MB, et al. Cancer procoagulant in human tumor cells: evidence from melanoma patients. Cancer Res. 1986;46(12 Pt 1):6471–4.
54. Mielicki W, et al. Procoagulant activity of human stomach and colon cancers. Oncology. 1990;47(4):299–302.
55. Falanga A, et al. A new procoagulant in acute leukemia. Blood. 1988;71(4):870–5.
56. Donati MB, et al. Cancer procoagulant in acute non lymphoid leukemia: relationship of enzyme detection to disease activity. Thromb Haemost. 1990;64(1):11–6.
57. Hajjar KA. Cellular receptors in the regulation of plasmin generation. Thromb Haemost. 1995;74(1):294–301.
58. Bennett B, et al. The bleeding disorder in acute promyelocytic leukaemia: fibrinolysis due to u-PA rather than defibrination. Br J Haematol. 1989;71(4):511–7.
59. Francis RB Jr, Seyfert U. Tissue plasminogen activator antigen and activity in disseminated intravascular coagulation: clinicopathologic correlations. J Lab Clin Med. 1987;110(5):541–7.
60. Stephens R, et al. Production of an active urokinase by leukemia cells: a novel distinction from cell lines of solid tumors. Leuk Res. 1988;12(5):419–22.
61. Liu Y, et al. The expression of annexin II and its role in the fibrinolytic activity in acute promyelocytic leukemia. Leuk Res. 2011;35(7):879–84.
62. Kwaan HC, Wang J, Weiss I. Expression of receptors for plasminogen activators on endothelial cell surface depends on their origin. J Thromb Haemost. 2004;2(2):306–12.
63. Stein E, et al. The coagulopathy of acute promyelocytic leukaemia revisited. Best Pract Res Clin Haematol. 2009;22(1):153–63.
64. Graf M, et al. High expression of urokinase plasminogen activator receptor (UPA-R) in acute myeloid leukemia (AML) is associated with worse prognosis. Am J Hematol. 2005;79(1):26–35.
65. Egbring R, et al. Demonstration of granulocytic proteases in plasma of patients with acute leukemia and septicemia with coagulation defects. Blood. 1977;49(2):219–31.
66. Nevo S, et al. Acute bleeding after bone marrow transplantation (BMT)- incidence and effect on survival. A quantitative analysis in 1,402 patients. Blood. 1998;91(4):1469–77.
67. Brower MS, Harpel PC. Proteolytic cleavage and inactivation of alpha 2-plasmin inhibitor and C1 inactivator by human polymorphonuclear leukocyte elastase. J Biol Chem. 1982;257(16):9849–54.
68. Sterrenberg L, et al. Anticoagulant properties of purified X-like fragments of human fibrinogen produced by degradation with leukocyte elastase. Thromb Haemost. 1984;51(3):398–402.
69. Sterrenberg L, Nieuwenhuizen W, Hermans J. Purification and partial characterization of a D-like fragment from human fibrinogen, produced

by human leukocyte elastase. Biochim Biophys Acta. 1983;755(2):300–6.
70. Griffin JD, et al. Secretion of interleukin-1 by acute myeloblastic leukemia cells in vitro induces endothelial cells to secrete colony stimulating factors. Blood. 1987;70(4):1218–21.
71. Khan MM, et al. Upregulation of tissue factor in monocytes by cleaved high molecular weight kininogen is dependent on TNF-alpha and IL-1beta. Am J Physiol Heart Circ Physiol. 2010;298(2):H652–8.
72. Cozzolino F, et al. Potential role of interleukin-1 as the trigger for diffuse intravascular coagulation in acute nonlymphoblastic leukemia. Am J Med. 1988;84(2):240–50.
73. Raica M, Cimpean AM, Ribatti D. The role of podoplanin in tumor progression and metastasis. Anticancer Res. 2008;28(5B):2997–3006.
74. Lavallée VP, Marquis M, Bordeleau ME, Chagraoui J, MacRae T, Boivin I, Boucher G, Gendron P, Lemieux S, Bonnefoy A, Rivard GE, Hébert J, Sauvageau G. Transcriptional landscape of APL identifies aberrant podoplanin expression as a defining feature and missing link for the bleeding disorder of this disease. Blood. 2016;128:1075.
75. Federici AB, et al. Proteolysis of von Willebrand factor is decreased in acute promyelocytic leukaemia by treatment with all-trans-retinoic acid. Br J Haematol. 1996;92(3):733–9.
76. Tallman MS, et al. All-trans retinoic acid in acute promyelocytic leukemia: long-term outcome and prognostic factor analysis from the North American Intergroup protocol. Blood. 2002;100(13):4298–302.
77. Falanga A, et al. Cancer procoagulant in the human promyelocytic cell line NB4 and its modulation by all-trans-retinoic acid. Leukemia. 1994;8(1):156–9.
78. Koyama T, et al. All-trans retinoic acid upregulates thrombomodulin and downregulates tissue-factor expression in acute promyelocytic leukemia cells: distinct expression of thrombomodulin and tissue factor in human leukemic cells. Blood. 1994;84(9):3001–9.
79. De Stefano V, et al. Effect of all-trans retinoic acid on procoagulant and fibrinolytic activities of cultured blast cells from patients with acute promyelocytic leukemia. Blood. 1995;86(9):3535–41.
80. Falanga A, et al. Cancer procoagulant and tissue factor are differently modulated by all-trans-retinoic acid in acute promyelocytic leukemia cells. Blood. 1998;92(1):143–51.
81. Saito T, et al. Anticoagulant effects of retinoic acids on leukemia cells. Blood. 1996;87(2):657–65.
82. Ishii H, et al. Retinoic acid counteracts both the downregulation of thrombomodulin and the induction of tissue factor in cultured human endothelial cells exposed to tumor necrosis factor. Blood. 1992;80(10):2556–62.
83. Falanga A, et al. All-trans-retinoic acid counteracts endothelial cell procoagulant activity induced by a human promyelocytic leukemia-derived cell line (NB4). Blood. 1996;87(2):613–7.
84. Oeth P, et al. Retinoic acid selectively inhibits lipopolysaccharide induction of tissue factor gene expression in human monocytes. Blood. 1998;91(8):2857–65.
85. Zhu J, et al. Tissue factors on acute promyelocytic leukemia and endothelial cells are differently regulated by retinoic acid, arsenic trioxide and chemotherapeutic agents. Leukemia. 1999;13(7):1062–70.
86. Raelson JV, et al. The PML/RAR alpha oncoprotein is a direct molecular target of retinoic acid in acute promyelocytic leukemia cells. Blood. 1996;88(8):2826–32.
87. Brand K, et al. Tissue factor mRNA in THP-1 monocytic cells is regulated at both transcriptional and posttranscriptional levels in response to lipopolysaccharide. Mol Cell Biol. 1991;11(9):4732–8.
88. Fang Y, et al. PML-RARa modulates the vascular signature of extracellular vesicles released by acute promyelocytic leukemia cells. Angiogenesis. 2016;19(1):25–38.
89. Tapiovaara H, et al. Induction of differentiation of promyelocytic NB4 cells by retinoic acid is associated with rapid increase in urokinase activity subsequently downregulated by production of inhibitors. Blood. 1994;83(7):1883–91.
90. Marchetti M, et al. All-trans-retinoic acid increases adhesion to endothelium of the human promyelocytic leukaemia cell line NB4. Br J Haematol. 1996;93(2):360–6.
91. Vahdat L, et al. Early mortality and the retinoic acid syndrome in acute promyelocytic leukemia: impact of leukocytosis, low-dose chemotherapy, PMN/RAR-alpha isoform, and CD13 expression in patients treated with all-trans retinoic acid. Blood. 1994;84(11):3843–9.
92. Di Noto R, et al. All-trans retinoic acid promotes a differential regulation of adhesion molecules on acute myeloid leukaemia blast cells. Br J Haematol. 1994;88(2):247–55.
93. Larson RS, Brown DC, Sklar LA. Retinoic acid induces aggregation of the acute promyelocytic leukemia cell line NB-4 by utilization of LFA-1 and ICAM-2. Blood. 1997;90(7):2747–56.
94. Dubois C, et al. Modulation of IL-8, IL-1 beta, and G-CSF secretion by all-trans retinoic acid in acute promyelocytic leukemia. Leukemia. 1994;8(10):1750–7.
95. Marchetti M, et al. All-trans retinoic acid modulates microvascular endothelial cell hemostatic properties. Haematologica. 2003;88(8):895–905.
96. Melnick A, Licht JD. Deconstructing a disease: RARalpha, its fusion partners, and their roles in the pathogenesis of acute promyelocytic leukemia. Blood. 1999;93(10):3167–215.
97. Emadi A, Gore SD. Arsenic trioxide—an old drug rediscovered. Blood Rev. 2010;24(4–5):191–9.
98. Zhou J, et al. Phosphatidylserine exposure and procoagulant activity in acute promyelocytic leukemia. J Thromb Haemost. 2010;8(4):773–82.
99. Zhang X, et al. [The impact of arsenic trioxide or all-trans retinoic acid treatment on coagulopathy in

acute promyelocytic leukemia]. Zhonghua Nei Ke Za Zhi. 2001;40(12):829–33.
100. Watts JM, Tallman MS. Acute promyelocytic leukemia: what is the new standard of care? Blood Rev. 2014;28(5):205–12.
101. Squizzato A, et al. Supportive management strategies for disseminated intravascular coagulation. An international consensus. Thromb Haemost. 2016;115(5):896–904.
102. Sanz MA, Lo-Coco F. Modern approaches to treating acute promyelocytic leukemia. J Clin Oncol. 2011;29(5):495–503.
103. Sanz MA, et al. Risk-adapted treatment of acute promyelocytic leukemia with all-trans retinoic acid and anthracycline monochemotherapy: long-term outcome of the LPA 99 multicenter study by the PETHEMA Group. Blood. 2008;112(8):3130–4.
104. Rickles FR, et al. Bleeding and thrombosis in acute leukemia: what does the future of therapy look like? Thromb Res. 2007;120(Suppl 2):S99–106.
105. Sanz MA, Montesinos P. Open issues on bleeding and thrombosis in acute promyelocytic leukemia. Thromb Res. 2010;125(Suppl 2):S51–4.
106. Sanz MA, et al. Management of acute promyelocytic leukemia: recommendations from an expert panel on behalf of the European LeukemiaNet. Blood. 2009;113(9):1875–91.
107. Rodeghiero F, et al. Early deaths and anti-hemorrhagic treatments in acute promyelocytic leukemia. A GIMEMA retrospective study in 268 consecutive patients. Blood. 1990;75(11):2112–7.
108. Bassan R, et al. Short-term treatment for adult hypergranular and microgranular acute promyelocytic leukemia. Leukemia. 1995;9(2):238–43.
109. Arbuthnot C, Wilde JT. Haemostatic problems in acute promyelocytic leukaemia. Blood Rev. 2006;20(6):289–97.
110. Zver S, Andoljsek D, Cernelc P. Effective treatment of life-threatening bleeding with recombinant activated factor VII in a patient with acute promyelocytic leukaemia. Eur J Haematol. 2004;72(6):455–6.
111. Alimoghaddam K, Ghavamzadeh A, Jahani M. Use of Novoseven for arsenic trioxide-induced bleeding in PML. Am J Hematol. 2006;81(9):720.

6 Early Death in Acute Promyelocytic Leukemia

Sören Lehmann

Introduction

Already in the first report by Hillestad in 1957, APL was described as a form of leukemia characterized by a high risk of early mortality [1]. Ever since, APL has been known as a medical emergency [2]. With the remarkable improvement in cure rates due to the introduction of all-*trans* retinoic acid (ATRA) and arsenic trioxide (ATO), APL has gone from being one of the most fatal forms of acute leukemia to be the most curable [3]. As a result of these improvements and rarity of treatment resistance, early death (ED) now constitutes the major obstacle to cure in APL. Thus, we can expect to see an increased focus on ED and the APL-related coagulopathy in the future. It is still unclear to what extent the introduction of ATO treatment will affect this coagulopathy and the subsequent thrombo-hemorrhagic complications. Infection-related ED may decrease due to the less myelosuppressive effects of ATO [4, 5].

Causes of ED include APL-specific complications such as hemorrhagic and thrombotic events and the differentiation syndrome (DS) as well as complications shared with other types of acute leukemia such as infections due to the myelosuppression as a result of the disease or cytotoxic treatment. Measures to prevent ED have focused on early suspicion of the diagnosis, immediate start of ATRA treatment at the first suspicion of APL, vigilant surveillance of coagulopathy, and aggressive blood product transfusions [6]. Despite these measures and the increased awareness of ED, high ED rates seem to persist in population-based studies. This chapter will give a historical background as well as a review of the current knowledge regarding the incidence, causes, risk factors, and preventive treatment strategies of ED in APL.

S. Lehmann, M.D., Ph.D.
Department of Medical Sciences, Uppsala University, Uppsala University Hospital, Entrance 40, 5th Floor, 751 85 Uppsala, Sweden
e-mail: Soren.Lehmann@ki.se

Definition and Timing of Early Death

Early death is commonly defined as death from any cause within 30 days from diagnosis [4, 8–14], but many clinical trials use a less strict definition with deaths that occur at any time during the induction therapy and the aplasia period [15–21]. However, other definitions are also used, especially in earlier studies where ED was defined as death within 5, 7, 10, 14, 28, or 40 days from diagnosis [2, 7, 22–25]. Earlier studies often discriminate between fatal bleeding that occurs within 5 days from diagnosis and subsequent death during aplasia [2, 7, 16]. This distinction partly reflects the true clinical picture with the immediate threat of bleeding in contrast to

O. Abla et al. (eds.), *Acute Promyelocytic Leukemia*, https://doi.org/10.1007/978-3-319-64257-4_6

death from infections that typically occurs later during induction. However, the situation is more complex and includes other causes of ED such as thrombotic events, DS, multiorgan failure, etc. Moreover, nonhemorrhagic death may occur very early, and a fatal bleeding may occur also after the first week.

The starting time point from which the occurrence of ED is calculated, often defined as "day 0," also differs between studies [9, 11, 12, 14, 26]. These differences are important to consider for very early deaths and when evaluating which EDs could be prevented as a result of earlier diagnosis, earlier start of ATRA treatment and aggressive transfusions once APL is highly suspected. In clinical trials, day 0 is often synonymous with the day of inclusion which usually coincides with the first day of ATRA treatment. However, in population- and hospital-based studies, day 0 is rather defined as the day of admission, the day when APL is initially suspected, the day of the first abnormal blood counts, the day of the diagnostic bone marrow, or the day of diagnosis. In such studies, the start of ATRA treatment is often later than day 0, and some studies even report deaths that occur before day 0 when patients die before diagnostic confirmation [11].

One of the most typical features of ED in APL is the immediate threat of a sudden death around the time of diagnosis. It is not uncommon that the presenting symptoms are due to bleeding that becomes rapidly fatal within a few days [26]. In a population-based study, early death rate was the highest at the day of the diagnostic bone marrow examination, followed by the successive 4 days [10]. In total, the 7-day mortality ranged between 4.9 and 22% of all patients diagnosed with APL, and up to 77% of all EDs occurred during the first week after diagnosis [10].

Early Death in the Pre-ATRA Era

Coagulopathy, hemorrhages, and the risk of immediate death were factors that contributed to the discovery of APL as a distinct subtype of acute myeloid leukemia (AML) [1, 33]. Already during those early years, there was a focus on the specific coagulopathy that occurred in APL and studies from that time included extensive characterization of patients' coagulopathy with measurement of coagulation factors such as fibrinogen, factor V, and prothrombin [33]. Didisheim et al. reviewed all 57 APL in the literature in 1964 and concluded that only three were alive after 4 months and that deaths were most commonly caused by fatal bleeding [33]. Earlier pre-ATRA studies report ED rates approaching 50%, while later studies showed somewhat lower rates between 18 and 43% [2, 7, 24, 27–32] (Table 6.1). Of note, the definition of ED in the pre-ATRA era was more heterogeneous between studies compared to the current definition (see above).

The introduction of daunorubicin (DNR) in the 1960s substantially increased the chances of a complete remission (CR) in APL. Also, hemorrhages occurring during the later stages of induction therapy decreased when DNR was introduced; however, this contrasted with the lack of improvement in the deaths that occurred at a very early time point [7]. Early start of DNR was recommended in the first studies in order to decrease fatal bleeding, since the clearance of promyelocytes decreased the risk of bleeding. On the other hand, the introduction of more intensive chemotherapy increased the risk of death from infections during the weeks following induction chemotherapy. The proportion of fatal bleedings as the cause of EDs was almost invariably over 60% and often above 80% during that era [2, 24, 27–32]. However, these early reports consisted of retrospective studies including consecutive patients from one or several centers, and these ED rates cannot be compared to those of more recent ATRA/ATO clinical trials that included selected APL populations with a lower risk of ED [2, 4, 5, 7, 15–22, 24–45]. Rather, the results of early pre-ATRA trials are more similar to recently published population-based studies [8–14, 23, 47] (Table 6.3) when it comes to patient selection.

Table 6.1 Early death rates in pre-ATRA studies

Study	*n*	Study years	Treatment	Age (median)	Gender (% female)	High-risk patients (%)	ED (%)	Death by bleeding (%)	Factors associated with ED
Bernard et al. (1973)	80	1963–1971	DNR (after 1969), 6-MP, prednisone, methotrexate methyl GAG[a]		56		25 (5 days) 50 (3 weeks)		WBC, fibrinogen
Drapkin et al. (1977)	24	1970–1976	Ara-C, 6-TG, DNR	39	46	33	54	85	
Cordonnier et al. (1985)	57	1972–1982	Ara-C and DNR	41[b]	49	23 (>15)	12 (5 days) 47	84 (until day 5) 41 (after day 5)	Renal failure, respiratory failure, active bleeding
Kantarjian et al. (1986)	60	1973–1984	Ara-C, Amsa, vincristine, prednisone, anthracyclines	34	47	30	26[c] 43	65 of all EDs	Platelets, fibrinogen, age hemoglobin
Hoyle et al. (1987)	115	1976–1986	DNR, Ara-C, 6-TG	<39	50		33	84	
Sanz et al (1988)	34	1976–1986	DNR	34.5	47	24	29	60	
Rodeghiero et al. (1990)	268	1984–1987	DNR, doxorubicin, Ara-C and VP-16	41		31	13 (10 days)	74	WBC
Cunningham et al. (1990)	57	1974–1984	Amsa, Ara-C, 6-TG	<39[d]	53	32	21	67	WBC, LDH
Thomas et al. (1991)	67	1974–1989	DNR, Ara-C, vincristine, 6-TG	40	52	28	30	63	Hyperuricemia, splenomegaly, anemia, LDH
Fenaux et al. (1991)	70	1975–1988	DNR alone or DNR + Ara-C	44	59	21	18	40 (until day 7) 0 (after day 7)	

Characteristics and data from studies performed before the introduction of ATRA (*DNR* daunorubicin, *6-TG* 6-thioguanine, *Amsa* amsacrine, *6-MP* 6-mercaptopurine, *Ara-C* cytarabine)

[a]Methylglyoxal-bis[guanylhydrazone]

[b]Mean age

[c]Fatal hemorrhage within 48 h

[d]Maximum age

Early Death in Clinical Trials vs. Population-Based Studies

The discovery of the beneficial effect of ATRA in the late 1980s was followed by a large number of clinical trials confirming the benefit of ATRA and successively of ATO in phase II and randomized phase III trials (Table 6.2) [4, 15, 16, 18, 22, 26, 34, 36, 39, 42, 48]. These clinical trials are usually large and typically report ED rates between 3 and 10% with only rare studies reporting ED rates >10% (Table 6.2). The median age in these studies ranged between 35 and 45 years, and the number of high-risk patients was between 21 and 28%. Compared to the pre-ATRA era, the proportion of hemorrhages as the cause of ED appeared somewhat lower.

Although inclusion criteria differed between these clinical trials, they almost invariably excluded patients with the highest risk of ED such as patients with poor performance status, the most elderly patients, those with severe infections and significant comorbidities [14, 26]. Also, patients with ongoing intracranial or pulmonary bleeding and patients that died before the inclusion or even before being considered for a clinical trial were routinely excluded [18, 26]. In a population-based study, up to 35% of patients suffering from ED did not receive ATRA [11]. Rahme et al. reported that up to one third of the patients might not be eligible for inclusion in clinical trials. The reasons for exclusion included refusal of the patient to enter the study, initial admissions to ICU, older age and/or comorbidities, previous cancers, and contraindications to anthracyclines as well as rapid death before start of treatment. In their study, the ED rate was 2.5% in patients included in clinical trials compared to 17% in patients that were not included. However, these figures excluded patients that died before the start of ATRA treatment which was reported to be 2.2% [14]. The age was higher in patients excluded from clinical trials, but other factors such as initial white blood cell (WBC) count did not differ.

The study by Rahme et al. aimed to include all APL patients in selected French centers with the goal of capturing also patients within the hospitals' catchment area who were not eligible for a clinical trial. The study showed a larger proportion of ineligible patients compared to reports from clinical trials where approximately 5% of the patients were ineligible [22, 25, 26]. The PETHEMA group showed that two thirds of the patients were ineligible due to intracranial hemorrhages or infections, while one third of the patient were considered too old or having a very poor performance status and/or severe comorbidities [26]. Poor performance status may also be a result of an intracerebral bleeding since these conditions may co-occur [45]. Other studies report lack of confirmed *PML-RARA* fusion by an appropriate method to be the most common reason for ineligibility into a trial [19]. In a study by Lengfelder et al., 2.6% of the patients were excluded from a clinical trial due to a fatal bleeding, and 9% were excluded for any reason [39].

As a consequence of exclusion criteria and deaths occurring before inclusion in a trial, we can expect clinical trials to underestimate ED rates compared to population-based or hospital-based studies, as well as compared to the experience in clinical practice. Table 6.3 shows characteristics and ED rates in population-based registries or in studies that include unselected consecutive APL patients in one or several hematological centers. Indeed, the ED rates in such studies ranged between 10 and 32% [8, 10–14, 23, 47] (Table 6.2). The age and the proportion of high-risk patients in these population-based studies were higher than in clinical trials, likely due to the fact that exclusion criteria are directly or indirectly linked to age and WBC as well as to factors discussed above. The highest ED rates, ranging between 26 and 32%, are reported in studies from Brazil, Sweden, and Stanford [10–12, 23]. The largest registry-based studies from the USA and Canada report rates between 17 and 21% [8, 13, 47], while some other hospital-based trials from Canada, USA, and France reported ED rates of 9–14% [9, 13, 14]. The difference in ED rates between these studies is unclear but may be due to several factors. Patients' selection may still differ due to differences in the actual coverage of the cohort in relation to all APL cases in the area, with biases that exclude patients with a higher or lower risk of ED. There may also

Table 6.2 Early deaths rates in clinical trials

	n	Study years	Induction treatment	Age (median)	Gender (% female)	High-risk patients (%)	ED (%)	Death by bleeding (%)	Risk factors for ED (univariate)
Di Bona et al. (2000)	123	1989–1993	IDA only	38			7.3 (D10) 16.2 (D40)	35	Peripheral blast count
Di Bona et al. (2000)	499	1993–1997	AIDA	39			3.8 (D10) 7.6 (D40)	50	Peripheral blast count, bleeding symptoms
Fenaux et al. (1993)	101	1991–1992	ATRA alone or CHEMO	40	47	28	9 vs. 8	67	WBC > 5, microgranular variant
Tallman et al. (1997)	346	1992–1996	ATRA alone or CHEMO	38	48	21	11 vs. 14% (D28)	53	
Asou et al. (1998)	196	1992–1994	ATRA[a]	46	55	26	9	94	
Avvisati et al. (1996)	20	1993	AIDA	35	60	25	10	50	
Lo Coco et al. (2010)	642	1993–2000	AIDA	38	45.6	27.6	5.5	37	
Lo Coco et al. (2010)	453	2000–2006	AIDA	41	49.5	28.5	5.6	32	
Fenaux et al. (1999)	413	1993–1996	ATRA alone or ATRA + CHEMO	46	49	39 (WBC > 5)	7	32	Age, WBC
Lengfelder et al. (2000)	51	1994–1999	ATRA + CHEMO	43	53	22	8	75	
Schlenk et al. (2004)	75	1995–2003	AIDA	43	46	22	9	71	WBC, +8 or abn(7q)
Sanz et al. (1999)	123	1996–1998	AIDA	42	42		9.8	67	

(continued)

Table 6.2 (continued)

	n	Study years	Induction treatment	Age (median)	Gender (% female)	High-risk patients (%)	ED (%)	Death by bleeding (%)	Risk factors for ED (univariate)
De la Serna et al. (2008)	732	1996–2005	AIDA	40	49	25	9.0	56	Creatinine, albumin, peripheral blasts, WBC, age, male gender, microgranular variant, coagulopathy
Powell et al. (2010)	481	1999–2005	ATRA + CHEMO		48	23	8		
Yanada et al. (2007)	279		ATRA[b]		44		3	89	
Lengfelder et al. (2009)	142	1994–2005	ATRA + CHEMO	40	41.5	26	7.7	67	WBC
Ghavamzadeh et al. (2011)	197	1999–2010	ATO	29	58	19	14.7	90	
Illand et al. (2012)	124	2004–2009	ATRA + ida + ATO	44	50	20	3.2	50	Age
Shen et al. (2004)	61	2001–2003	ATO vs. ATRA vs. ATRA + ATO	30, 40, 34	46	23	6.6	100	
Ravandi et al. (2009)	82	2002–2008	ATRA + ATO + GO for high risk	47	46	32	8.5		
Lo Coco et al. (2013)	162	2007–2010	ATRA + ATO vs. AIDA	44.6 vs. 46.6	49	0	0 vs. 5	0	
Burnett et al. (2015)	235	2009–2013	ATRA + ATO vs. AIDA	47	49	24	4 vs. 6 5 vs. 9 (60D)	0 with ATO 27 in AIDA	

Table shows characteristics and data from clinical trials with ATRA and ATO (*IDA* idarubicin, *AIDA* ATRA + idarubicin, *CHEMO* chemotherapy, *ATO* arsenic trioxide)

[a]Addition of daunorubicin and behenoyl cytarabine when WBC > 3.0×10^9/L

[b]Addition of CHEMO when WBC > 3.0×10^9/L

Table 6.3 Early death rates in population- or hospital-based studies

Study	*n*	Study years	Age (median)	Gender (% female)	High-risk patients (%)	ED (%)	Death before ATRA	Death by bleeding (%)	Risk factors associated with ED
Jacomo et al. (2007)	134	2003–2006	36[a]	54	35	13 (D5) 26 (D14) 32 (ind[b])	2	60.5	
Lehmann et al. (2011)	105	1997–2006	54	62	34	22 (D7) 29 (D30)	9.5	41	Age, PS, WBC, platelets, creatinine, C-reactive protein, albumin, LDH
Park et al. (2011)	1400	1992–2007	44	53		17.3 (1 month)			Age
McClellan (2012)	70	1997–2009	50	63	35	19 (D7) 26 (D30)	2.8	54	WBC, INR
Altman et al. (2013)	204	1992–2009	47.5	54	25	4.9 (D7) 11 (D30)	2.5	61	WBC, fibrinogen, PTT
Rahme et al. (2014)	399	2006–2011	51	48	27	9 (D30)	2.2	31	Age, admission to ICU
Paulsen et al. (2014)	399	1993–2007 (registry-based)		49		21.8 (D30)			
	131	1999–2009 (hospital-based)	47.9[a]	54	20.6	14.6 (D30)			
Abrahao et al. (2015)	722	1988–2011	0–39[c]			11(D7) 17 (D30)			Pre-ATRA period, Hispanic ethnicity, health insurance
Lehmann et al. (2017)	195	1997–2013	56	55	30	25 (D30)		46	Age, PS, WBC, platelets, creatinine

Characteristics and data from studies of early death performed in population-based studies

[a]Mean age

[b]Deaths during induction treatment

[c]Age range

be differences in the staff's experience and in treatment traditions. However, it is not clear from these reports what the most likely reasons for the variations between studies are. The aim of a population-based study is to include all APL patients diagnosed within a specific region or country, and such studies are ideally based on population-based registries with a good coverage. However, the coverage may also differ between registries depending on the methodology of case reporting. Center or hospital-based studies normally aim to cover all cases admitted to one or several centers, usually assuming that all patients within a hospital's catchment area are admitted to a specific hospital.

In conclusion, well-performed clinical trials constitute the major driver behind the tremendous success story of APL treatment. Nevertheless, focusing only on results from clinical trials will lead to an underestimation of the most significant unmet medical need in APL, such as early deaths. Thus, population-based APL registries and other studies of unselected APL patient cohorts will be crucial in defining and preventing one of the most significant challenges for APL in the future.

Causes of Early Death

Bleeding

Symptoms and/or signs of bleeding are present at presentation in 67–94% of APL patients [15, 19, 29, 30, 49]. The most common sites of such initial hemorrhages are the skin and mucous membranes. In contrast, fatal bleedings are dominated by intracranial hemorrhage (ICH) followed by pulmonary hemorrhage. Other sites of bleeding such as the gastrointestinal and the urogenital tracts are very rarely reported as being fatal [26]. Yanada et al. studied the occurrence of severe bleeding in 279 patients and found that 18 (6.4%) of the patients developed severe bleeding with a median of 7 days from diagnosis, and 9 (56%) of the patients with a severe bleeding suffered an early death [45]. A large study of 1009 patients included in clinical trials reported an incidence of hemorrhagic deaths of 3.7% [50]. One study showed that for patients with a severe but nonfatal bleeding who achieve a CR, no survival difference was reported compared to patients without a severe bleeding [45]. However, other studies have shown an increased risk of CNS relapse in patients who survive an ICH [51].

In Tables 6.1, 6.2, and 6.3, the proportion of the EDs caused by hemorrhages is shown from a large number of studies [2, 4, 5, 9–12, 14–32, 34–39, 42–47]. While the percentage varies considerably, most studies reported between 35 and 70% of the deaths to be attributed to bleeding and, invariably in these studies, ICH dominated as a cause of death. The proportion of bleedings appears higher in clinical trials compared to population-based studies, although comparisons are difficult due to the heterogeneity of the studies. The reason for a lower proportion in population-based studies may be the older age and poorer performance status; thus a larger proportion of deaths are due to infections, organ failures, and other nonhemorrhagic causes.

The majority of fatal bleeding events occur during the first week of treatment, and several studies show a median time of 4–7 days from diagnosis to fatal bleeding [9, 11, 26, 39]. Most patients who die from bleeding have a fulminant course with death occurring within 24 h [26]. Hemorrhages may occur up to week 4, although they become much less frequent after the first and second week. There are data to support that ICH tends to occur earlier compared to pulmonary bleeding, with a median time of 6 vs. 9 days, respectively [26]. Once the patient has achieved a CR, the risk of bleeding becomes comparable to that of other subtypes of AML, where thrombocytopenia resulting from intensive chemotherapy may cause bleeding.

Infections

Infections are the second most common cause of ED in APL occurring in 10–28% of ED cases. Compared to bleeding-related deaths, deaths due to infections occur later with a median time of 21 days after start of treatment [26]. Also, the age of the patients that succumb to infections is usually higher compared to that of patients who die from bleeding [11, 36, 39]. Pneumonia is reported to be the most common type of infection followed by septicemia, and the type of infection does not appear to be different from what is seen during induction treatment for other AML subtypes [26]. Some studies report lower rates of infections during induction therapy for APL compared to other AML subtypes. This is potentially due to the younger age of APL patients and a less myelosuppressive and cytarabine-free induction therapy, especially in low- and intermediate-risk APL. ATRA in combination with ATO during induction has shown to be significantly less myelotoxic compared to ATRA/chemotherapy regimens [4, 5]. Induction with ATO also decreases the number of fever episodes and the days of antibiotic therapy. Thus, infectious complications are expected to become less frequent with the introduction of ATO induction as first-line treatment, although it is still unclear whether this will translate into a decrease in the number of EDs due to infections.

Thrombosis

Thrombosis is reported to occur in 2–15% of APLs which represents a higher figure compared to other types of AML [52]. De Stefano et al. reported thromboembolic events in 9.6% of APL patients compared to 3.2% in patients with non-APL AML [26]. Indeed, the 3–9% of the ED cases caused by thromboembolic events might be an underestimation [53]. Fatal thrombosis is dominated by cerebral and cardiac ischemic events, although pulmonary emboli have been reported as well. Arterial thrombosis usually occurs early on during induction, whereas nonfatal deep vein thrombosis occurs more often during consolidation phases [52]. Cerebral thrombosis may also occur together with ICH, and it may sometimes be difficult to distinguish which of these causes is the primary cause of death. In one study, cerebral thrombosis was considered as the primary fatal event in 2 of 24 ICH events [26]. Myocardial infarctions are recurrently reported as a cause of death in larger ED studies [26, 52, 53], however, usually in low numbers. Nevertheless, thrombosis constitutes an important ant and potentially underestimated cause of death in APL.

Although still controversial, ATRA treatment has been implicated in the occurrence of thrombosis in APL. Furthermore, treatment with tranexamic acid to prevent lethal hemorrhages has also been linked to an increased risk of thrombosis and, in addition to the lack of proof of a beneficial effect of tranexamic acid, this is one of the reasons why the drug is not used routinely in APL. Thrombosis has also been associated with DS, while other risk factors linked to an increased risk of thrombosis in APL includes high WBC, presence of the *PML/RARA* bcr3 transcript, morphological variant M3 type, FLT3-ITD mutations, CD2 and CD15 expression, low fibrinogen level at baseline and high platelet count, male sex, and worse PS [52].

Differentiation Syndrome (DS)

DS is reported to occur in 2–31% of APL cases, although most studies report an incidence of around 20% [54]. Notably, the incidence can differ due to differences in the definition of DS [54]. In very early ATRA trials, before steroid treatment was established as a standard therapy for suspected DS, the death rate reached almost 30% [55]. In later reports, between 14 and 26% of patients experienced ED, although this was not always attributed to DS since patients with severe DS also have an increased risk of fatal bleeding [51]. The risk of ED increases primarily among patients with severe DS where ED has been reported in up to 40% of cases in clinical trials, while in moderate DS the risk of ED is not increased. Among all ED events, death due to differentiation syndrome occurs in between 3 and 16% of the patients. Usually, these deaths occur later during the induction course with a median of 17 days after start of ATRA treatment (range 1–28%) [26, 35]. There is no evidence that prophylactic steroids decrease the risk of death due to DS. Poor performance status and low albumin are risk factors for death due to DS in univariate as well as in multivariable analysis [26].

Organ Failure

Renal, respiratory, cardiac, and multiorgan failures are reported to a variable degree (Table 6.4). However, these situations are not always clearly distinguishable from each other or from other

Table 6.4 Causes of death

Cause	Percentage of ED (range)
Hemorrhage	31–64
Infection	10–28
Differentiation syndrome	3–16
Multiorgan failure	6–14
Pulmonary	9–12
Thrombosis	2–9
Myocardial infarction	3–8
Renal failure	4–6
Others or unknown	3–14

Percentages in relation to all early deaths

causes of death. Among organ failures, multiorgan failure is the most commonly reported with up to 16% of the EDs. Multiorgan failures are by nature complex and may be provoked by other potentially lethal events or a combination of life-threatening events. Infections and DS are not unlikely to be a primary event in such cases. Other specific organ failures such as renal and pulmonary organ failures are reported in some studies. In one pre-ATRA study, renal failure was reported as a significant risk factor for early death [2].

Early Death Risk Factors

Many factors have been reported to be associated with increased risk of ED in APL patients. Even though all newly diagnosed and suspected APL patients should be subjected to intensive surveillance and supportive care, knowing these risk factors is the first step in preventing early mortality. In addition, as studies suggest that ED risk remains high despite the current measures, one could anticipate a future ambition to find new approaches to prevent ED.

In the far right column in Tables 6.1, 6.2, and 6.3, factors associated with an increased risk of ED are listed for each APL study that included risk factor calculations. Although several factors are uniformly reported, there are differences between studies that partly could be explained by the fact that some data were not assessed and followed in all the studies. The factors reviewed here are based on assessments at presentation of the disease. In most studies, risk factor analyses are mainly based on univariate analyses while a minority of the studies also reported statistically independent risk factors (see below). Some studies also identified factors associated with a failure to achieve CR rather than the ED rate [18, 20, 34]. As primary ATRA resistance is extremely rare in APL, such figures are highly dependent on the ED rate and therefore, also the risk factors are similar to those for ED. However, only risk factors associated with death during the first weeks of treatment will be considered below.

The most commonly reported risk factors include initial WBC and peripheral blast counts, age, ECOG performance status, creatinine, albumin, male gender, microgranular variant, and signs of coagulopathy [2, 7–9, 16, 22, 26, 27, 29, 36, 38]. A high WBC is unanimously reported to be associated with an increased ED rate although rare studies do not report this [14, 38]. As the WBC count is defining the Sanz risk score, Sanz risk is also associated with an increased risk of ED, even though this risk score was primarily developed to predict relapse [56]. Consequently, patients with high-risk disease (WBC > 10×10^9/L) have a higher risk of ED compared to low and intermediate risk, but some studies also show intermediate-risk patients (platelets < 40×10^9/L) to have a higher risk of ED compared to those at low risk [11]. Nevertheless, there are also studies that fail to report Sanz score as a risk factor [13]. Though Sanz risk uses 10×10^9/L as a WBC threshold, the WBC limit that best predicts an increased risk of ED remains unclear. Thresholds from as low as 2.5×10^9/L ranging up to 30×10^9/L have been described. McClellan et al. specifically studied the optimal cutoff and found 17×10^9/L to be the best discriminator, whereas others report a WBC of 5 or 20×10^9/L as relevant cutoffs [10, 12, 16, 50]. The peripheral blast count, which is closely linked to the WBC count, is also repeatedly reported as a risk factor [22, 24, 26, 50].

Age is among the most frequently reported risk factors [11, 14, 16, 26, 47, 50], and it is usually but not invariably retained in multivariate analysis [26]. The performance status, measured as ECOG PS, is another risk factor that is commonly reported both in univariate and multivariate analysis [10, 11, 50]. However, PS is not assessed in all studies which explains why it is lacking as a risk factor in many studies. A frequently reported risk factor is the presence of the microgranular variant of APL [26, 39, 57, 58], while other disease-specific factors such as additional chromosomal abnormalities are anecdotally reported [42].

Blood chemistry values such as creatinine emerge as a risk factor for early death as well as for fatal bleeding although the mechanism behind the increased risk of bleeding remains elusive [10, 26]. Other lab chemistry risk factors that have been suggested include serum albumin, C-reactive protein (CRP), and lactate dehydrogenase (LDH); the latter is usually linked to the WBC count. Somewhat surprisingly, the platelet count at presentation seldom appears as a significant risk factor, although it is reported in some studies [10, 11]. However, individual studies suggest that deaths commonly occur when platelets are low during the initial period after diagnosis [2, 9]. On the other hand, McClellan et al. could not show an increased risk of ED when patients failed to reach the desired platelet level during the first 7 days after diagnosis [12]. To a variable degree, coagulation factors are reported as risk factors and most commonly the fibrinogen level. However, the majority of the studies do not find the fibrinogen level at presentation to be predictive of ED, and as such it clearly differs from more uniformly reported risk factors such as WBC, ECOG, and age. However, one study showed an association between the number of days below 1.0 g/L in fibrinogen and ED during the initial week after diagnosis [12]. Only few studies show fibrinogen as well as other coagulation parameters including PTT to be associated with ED [9].

In studies that specifically looked at clinical signs of bleeding at diagnosis, such signs are also reported as associated with ED. In PETHEMA studies, a hemorrhagic score was developed based on clinical signs of bleeding where hematoma, mucosal bleeding, and hematuria each gave 1 point. A hemorrhagic score of 3 was a significant risk of hemorrhagic death also in multivariate analysis [22]. A Californian study looked at ethnical and socioeconomic factors and found Hispanic ethnicity, but no other ethnic background, to be associated with a significantly increased risk of ED [33]. Another American study based on SEER data did not find an association between ED and any ethnicity [47]. Patients without health insurance showed a higher ED compared to patients with a private health insurance in the Californian study; however, patients with private versus public health insurance did not differ in ED rates [8].

Early death risk factors may vary depending on the cause of death. A review of PETHEMA studies has provided enough patients to calculate factors independently associated with deaths due to hemorrhages, infections, and DS [26]. They analyzed risk factors both in a univariable and a multivariable analysis, and in the multivariable analysis, patients that died from hemorrhages and infections shared risk factors such as older age and increased creatinine level, whereas hemorrhagic deaths were associated with high WBC, peripheral blast count, and coagulopathy at presentation. Early deaths due to infections were associated with fever at presentation and male gender, whereas ED due to DS was independently associated with ECOG PS score and serum albumin levels. In other studies including multivariate analysis, the following factors were most commonly reported as independently associated with an increased ED: WBC [10, 11, 26, 50], age [10, 11, 13, 26], PS [10, 11] time period, Hispanic ethnicity, type of health insurance, as well as peripheral blasts, creatinine, gender, and bleeding symptoms [22, 26].

Role of ATRA in Early Death

ATRA has been shown to reverse coagulopathy within days from onset of the treatment [16, 59, 60], and this reversal is faster compared to treatment with chemotherapy alone [16]. Fenaux et al. showed that coagulopathy was significantly improved within a median of 4 days from start of ATRA compared to 7 days during chemotherapy treatment. Thus, with the introduction of ATRA as standard therapy in APL, a treatment was introduced that specifically could target and counteract the APL-related coagulopathy which causes most of the early deaths. Several population-based studies showed higher ED rates in patients not receiving ATRA [9, 10, 12], but these were deaths that occurred before the start of treatment, and the studies did not inform about the role of ATRA for ED. In a study by Di Bona et al., ED was lower with a combination of ATRA and idarubicin compared to historical controls treated with idarubucin alone. Moreover, bleeding symptoms, the number of days with low platelet counts and fibrinogen levels were lower in the ATRA trial [22]. Other comparisons between studies performed before vs. after the introduction of ATRA have suggested that ED rates decreased with the introduction of ATRA. However, these studies did not compare treatment with and without ATRA in a controlled and randomized fashion. Rather, none of the randomized trials comparing ATRA and chemotherapy combinations to chemotherapy alone showed any significant difference in ED rate [16, 25]; thus, evidence regarding the role of ATRA in ED is lacking from randomized trials. However, these randomized trials generally showed low ED rates, likely due to exclusion of the patients with the highest risk of ED; thus, these studies do not confidently address the role of ATRA in ED prevention.

Several studies have evaluated the role of delay in ATRA treatment for the risk of ED, but most have failed to find such an association [9, 11, 12, 14]. However, while the population-based study by Altman et al. did not find a significant increase in ED with delays of ATRA treatment, they found an increase in the proportion of hemorrhages with delays. Also, when specifically studying high-risk patients, the risk of ED was 80% if ATRA administration was delayed until days 3–4 from first suspicion compared to 20% in those who received ATRA within 2 days. However, these observations are based on very few patients [9]. Delays in ATRA treatment once APL has been suspected seem generally infrequent [9–11, 14], and they are mainly caused by delays in suspecting the APL diagnosis. Nevertheless, delays from the time of symptoms to admission could potentially be linked to an increased risk of ED [9].

In conclusion, ATRA remains the most powerful tool in reversing the APL specific coagulopathy and minimizing the days with coagulopathy through early institution of ATRA is logical. Even though most studies cannot find a clear association between ED and delayed ATRA or even ATRA treatment at all, these studies have significant weaknesses and do not rule out a beneficial effect of ATRA. Thus, giving ATRA at the slightest suspicion of APL remains a cornerstone in the prevention of ED.

Early Death over Time

Several studies have assessed whether ED has changed over time during the last decades. The lack of improvement or the relatively slight improvements presented in such studies sharply contrasts to the remarkable improvements in survival and cure rates during the same period. A SEER study from 1977 to 2007 could not find a significant decrease in ED comparing the pre- and post-ATRA [12]. This is in contrast to an average decrease in 3-year mortality of 61% per decade in the same study. Another SEER study showed a significant decline between the periods 1992–1995 and 1996–2001, but when comparing 2002–2007 to the earliest period, this was not statistically significant [47]. In a Canadian registry study, there was no improvement in ED during the period 1993–2007. In parallel, the same group performed a hospital-based study covering five centers where they found a significant decrease in ED rate between 1999–2004 and 2005–2010 from 18.5 to 10.8% [13]. A Californian study showed a significant decrease in the 30-day ED between the pre-ATRA era and the ATRA from 26 to 14%; however, there was no change in 7-day mortality between the two periods. The same study could not show a significant difference between the early and late ATRA era [8]. An update from the Swedish registry showed no improvement of ED during the period of 1997–2013 despite increased awareness and early institution of ATRA treatment [10]. In conclusion, although some studies show a decrease in ED over time, several studies cannot confirm a statistically significant improvement.

Prevention of ED

Early deaths and the risk of fatal bleeding, as well as ED prevention methods, have been in focus since the first recognition of APL as a medical emergency. Treatment with heparin was previously widely used and often part of the standard treatment in the pre-ATRA era [7, 24, 29, 30]. However, since no clear benefit has been shown, heparin is not routinely recommended anymore [6, 24, 29, 61]. Similarly, antifibrinolytic agents, such as tranexamic acid, have not been shown to decrease the risk of ED [26], but rather to increase the risk of thrombotic events. In summary, there is no data to support a routine use of heparin, tranexamic acid, or any other anticoagulant therapy as part of the standard therapy of APL.

Once APL is suspected on clinical or morphological basis, ATRA should be started immediately in order to rapidly alleviate the coagulopathy. Since bleeding is the most common cause of early fatalities, aggressive blood product transfusions guided by frequent coagulation studies monitoring should start promptly. In general, the available guidelines recommend keeping a platelet count of 30–50 × 10^9/L and a fibrinogen level above or at least equal to 1.5 g/L. In order to adhere to these guidelines, platelets and coagulation blood chemistry should be followed at least daily and more frequently when needed, and this policy should remain until all clinical and laboratory signs of coagulopathy have disappeared [6].

Early start of chemotherapy is not considered as important as the immediate institution of ATRA. However, in high-risk disease and in the case of increasing WBC, chemotherapy should not be delayed when a chemotherapy-containing protocol is used. With a rapid increase in the use of ATO based-protocols, more data is urgently needed on the role of an early start of ATO in preventing ED. To date, it is still recommended that ATRA is started at the earliest suspicion of APL while ATO is started when the diagnosis has been confirmed. This recommendation is likely to remain until a beneficial role of early ATO simultaneously to ATRA has been documented. Cytotoxic therapy with oral hydroxyurea is recommended when WBC increases above 10 × 10^9/L during the initial ATO/ATRA treatment. However, there is no data to indicate that this leukocytosis would increase the risk of ED or that using hydroxyurea in this scenario would have an impact on the risk of ED.

As the differentiation syndrome represents one of the causes of ED, measures to prevent and treat DS are also among available measures to prevent ED. The prevention and treatment of DS is described in Chap. 21 of this book. Other measures that are common to any type of leukemia are treatment and prevention of infectious complications due to the disease or its treatment. In patients with hyperleukocytosis, leukapheresis is not recommended as it has been suggested to even exacerbate coagulopathy and lead to an increased risk of ED [55].

Conclusions

With improved antileukemic treatment in APL, prevention of early mortality is a key element in increasing the cure rate. Even though the challenges are substantial, the excellent prognosis of patients that do not succumb to ED underlines not only the need to adhere to current guidelines but also to find new ways to prevent early mortality.

References

1. Hillestad LK. Acute promyelocytic leukemia. Acta Med Scand. 1957;159(3):189–94.
2. Cordonnier C, Vernant JP, Brun B, Heilmann MG, Kuentz M, Bierling P, et al. Acute promyelocytic leukemia in 57 previously untreated patients. Cancer. 1985;55(1):18–25.
3. Cicconi L, Lo-Coco F. Current management of newly diagnosed acute promyelocytic leukemia. Ann Oncol. 2016;27(8):1474–81.
4. Burnett AK, Russell NH, Hills RK, Bowen D, Kell J, Knapper S, et al. Arsenic trioxide and all-trans retinoic acid treatment for acute promyelocytic leukaemia in all risk groups (AML17): results of a randomised, controlled, phase 3 trial. Lancet Oncol. 2015;16(13):1295–305.
5. Lo-Coco F, Avvisati G, Vignetti M, Thiede C, Orlando SM, Iacobelli S, et al. Retinoic acid and arsenic trioxide for acute promyelocytic leukemia. N Engl J Med. 2013;369(2):111–21.
6. Sanz MA, Grimwade D, Tallman MS, Lowenberg B, Fenaux P, Estey EH, et al. Management of acute

promyelocytic leukemia: recommendations from an expert panel on behalf of the European LeukemiaNet. Blood. 2009;113(9):1875–91.
7. Bernard J, Weil M, Boiron M, Jacquillat C, Flandrin G, Gemon MF. Acute promyelocytic leukemia: results of treatment by daunorubicin. Blood. 1973;41(4):489–96.
8. Abrahao R, Ribeiro RC, Medeiros BC, Keogh RH, Keegan TH. Disparities in early death and survival in children, adolescents, and young adults with acute promyelocytic leukemia in California. Cancer. 2015;121(22):3990–7.
9. Altman JK, Rademaker A, Cull E, Weitner BB, Ofran Y, Rosenblat TL, et al. Administration of ATRA to newly diagnosed patients with acute promyelocytic leukemia is delayed contributing to early hemorrhagic death. Leuk Res. 2013;37(9):1004–9.
10. Lehmann S, Deneberg S, Antunovic P, Rangert-Derolf A, Garelius H, Lazarevic V, et al. Early death rates remain high in high-risk APL: update from the Swedish Acute Leukemia Registry 1997-2013. Leukemia. 2017;31(6):1457–9.
11. Lehmann S, Ravn A, Carlsson L, Antunovic P, Deneberg S, Mollgard L, et al. Continuing high early death rate in acute promyelocytic leukemia: a population-based report from the Swedish Adult Acute Leukemia Registry. Leukemia. 2011;25(7):1128–34.
12. McClellan JS, Kohrt HE, Coutre S, Gotlib JR, Majeti R, Alizadeh AA, et al. Treatment advances have not improved the early death rate in acute promyelocytic leukemia. Haematologica. 2012;97(1):133–6.
13. Paulson K, Serebrin A, Lambert P, Bergeron J, Everett J, Kew A, et al. Acute promyelocytic leukaemia is characterized by stable incidence and improved survival that is restricted to patients managed in leukaemia referral centres: a pan-Canadian epidemiological study. Br J Haematol. 2014;166(5):660–6.
14. Rahme R, Thomas X, Recher C, Vey N, Delaunay J, Deconinck E, et al. Early death in acute promyelocytic leukemia (APL) in French centers: a multicenter study in 399 patients. Leukemia. 2014;28(12):2422–4.
15. Avvisati G, Lo Coco F, Diverio D, Falda M, Ferrara F, Lazzarino M, et al. AIDA (all-trans retinoic acid + idarubicin) in newly diagnosed acute promyelocytic leukemia: a Gruppo Italiano Malattie Ematologiche Maligne dell'Adulto (GIMEMA) pilot study. Blood. 1996;88(4):1390–8.
16. Fenaux P, Le Deley MC, Castaigne S, Archimbaud E, Chomienne C, Link H, et al. Effect of all transretinoic acid in newly diagnosed acute promyelocytic leukemia. Results of a multicenter randomized trial. European APL 91 Group. Blood. 1993;82(11):3241–9.
17. Lengfelder E, Reichert A, Schoch C, Haase D, Haferlach T, Loffler H, et al. Double induction strategy including high dose cytarabine in combination with all-trans retinoic acid: effects in patients with newly diagnosed acute promyelocytic leukemia. German AML Cooperative Group. Leukemia. 2000;14(8):1362–70.
18. Lo-Coco F, Avvisati G, Vignetti M, Breccia M, Gallo E, Rambaldi A, et al. Front-line treatment of acute promyelocytic leukemia with AIDA induction followed by risk-adapted consolidation for adults younger than 61 years: results of the AIDA-2000 trial of the GIMEMA Group. Blood. 2010;116(17):3171–9.
19. Mandelli F, Diverio D, Avvisati G, Luciano A, Barbui T, Bernasconi C, et al. Molecular remission in PML/RAR alpha-positive acute promyelocytic leukemia by combined all-trans retinoic acid and idarubicin (AIDA) therapy. Gruppo Italiano-Malattie Ematologiche Maligne dell'Adulto and Associazione Italiana di Ematologia ed Oncologia Pediatrica Cooperative Groups. Blood. 1997;90(3):1014–21.
20. Sanz MA, Martin G, Gonzalez M, Leon A, Rayon C, Rivas C, et al. Risk-adapted treatment of acute promyelocytic leukemia with all-trans-retinoic acid and anthracycline monochemotherapy: a multicenter study by the PETHEMA group. Blood. 2004;103(4):1237–43.
21. Sanz MA, Martin G, Rayon C, Esteve J, Gonzalez M, Diaz-Mediavilla J, et al. A modified AIDA protocol with anthracycline-based consolidation results in high antileukemic efficacy and reduced toxicity in newly diagnosed PML/RARalpha-positive acute promyelocytic leukemia. PETHEMA group. Blood. 1999;94(9):3015–21.
22. Di Bona E, Avvisati G, Castaman G, Luce Vegna M, De Sanctis V, Rodeghiero F, et al. Early haemorrhagic morbidity and mortality during remission induction with or without all-trans retinoic acid in acute promyelocytic leukaemia. Br J Haematol. 2000;108(4):689–95.
23. Jacomo RH, Melo RA, Souto FR, de Mattos ER, de Oliveira CT, Fagundes EM, et al. Clinical features and outcomes of 134 Brazilians with acute promyelocytic leukemia who received ATRA and anthracyclines. Haematologica. 2007;92(10):1431–2.
24. Rodeghiero F, Avvisati G, Castaman G, Barbui T, Mandelli F. Early deaths and anti-hemorrhagic treatments in acute promyelocytic leukemia. A GIMEMA retrospective study in 268 consecutive patients. Blood. 1990;75(11):2112–7.
25. Tallman MS, Andersen JW, Schiffer CA, Appelbaum FR, Feusner JH, Ogden A, et al. All-trans-retinoic acid in acute promyelocytic leukemia. N Engl J Med. 1997;337(15):1021–8.
26. de la Serna J, Montesinos P, Vellenga E, Rayon C, Parody R, Leon A, et al. Causes and prognostic factors of remission induction failure in patients with acute promyelocytic leukemia treated with all-trans retinoic acid and idarubicin. Blood. 2008;111(7):3395–402.
27. Cunningham I, Gee TS, Reich LM, Kempin SJ, Naval AN, Clarkson BD. Acute promyelocytic leukemia: treatment results during a decade at Memorial Hospital. Blood. 1989;73(5):1116–22.
28. Drapkin RL, Gee TS, Dowling MD, Arlin Z, McKenzie S, Kempin S, et al. Prophylactic heparin therapy in acute promyelocytic leukemia. Cancer. 1978;41(6):2484–90.

29. Hoyle CF, Swirsky DM, Freedman L, Hayhoe FG. Beneficial effect of heparin in the management of patients with APL. Br J Haematol. 1988;68(3):283–9.
30. Kantarjian HM, Keating MJ, Walters RS, Estey EH, McCredie KB, Smith TL, et al. Acute promyelocytic leukemia. M.D. Anderson Hospital experience. Am J Med. 1986;80(5):789–97.
31. Sanz MA, Jarque I, Martin G, Lorenzo I, Martinez J, Rafecas J, et al. Acute promyelocytic leukemia. Therapy results and prognostic factors. Cancer. 1988;61(1):7–13.
32. Thomas X, Archimbaud E, Treille-Ritouet D, Fiere D. Prognostic factors in acute promyelocytic leukemia: a retrospective study of 67 cases. Leuk Lymphoma. 1991;4(4):249–56.
33. Didisheim P, Trombold JS, Vandervoort LE, Mibashan RS. Acute promyelocytic leukemia with fibrinogen and factor V deficiencies. Blood. 1964;23:717–28.
34. Asou N, Adachi K, Tamura J, Kanamaru A, Kageyama S, Hiraoka A, et al. Analysis of prognostic factors in newly diagnosed acute promyelocytic leukemia treated with all-trans retinoic acid and chemotherapy. Japan Adult Leukemia Study Group. J Clin Oncol. 1998;16(1):78–85.
35. De Botton S, Dombret H, Sanz M, Miguel JS, Caillot D, Zittoun R, et al. Incidence, clinical features, and outcome of all trans-retinoic acid syndrome in 413 cases of newly diagnosed acute promyelocytic leukemia. The European APL Group. Blood. 1998;92(8):2712–8.
36. Fenaux P, Chastang C, Chevret S, Sanz M, Dombret H, Archimbaud E, et al. A randomized comparison of all transretinoic acid (ATRA) followed by chemotherapy and ATRA plus chemotherapy and the role of maintenance therapy in newly diagnosed acute promyelocytic leukemia. The European APL Group. Blood. 1999;94(4):1192–200.
37. Ghavamzadeh A, Alimoghaddam K, Rostami S, Ghaffari SH, Jahani M, Iravani M, et al. Phase II study of single-agent arsenic trioxide for the front-line therapy of acute promyelocytic leukemia. J Clin Oncol. 2011;29(20):2753–7.
38. Iland HJ, Bradstock K, Supple SG, Catalano A, Collins M, Hertzberg M, et al. All-trans-retinoic acid, idarubicin, and IV arsenic trioxide as initial therapy in acute promyelocytic leukemia (APML4). Blood. 2012;120(8):1570–80; quiz 752.
39. Lengfelder E, Haferlach C, Saussele S, Haferlach T, Schultheis B, Schnittger S, et al. High dose ara-C in the treatment of newly diagnosed acute promyelocytic leukemia: long-term results of the German AMLCG. Leukemia. 2009;23(12):2248–58.
40. Powell BL, Moser B, Stock W, Gallagher RE, Willman CL, Stone RM, et al. Arsenic trioxide improves event-free and overall survival for adults with acute promyelocytic leukemia: North American Leukemia Intergroup Study C9710. Blood. 2010;116(19):3751–7.
41. Ravandi F, Estey E, Jones D, Faderl S, O'Brien S, Fiorentino J, et al. Effective treatment of acute promyelocytic leukemia with all-trans-retinoic acid, arsenic trioxide, and gemtuzumab ozogamicin. J Clin Oncol. 2009;27(4):504–10.
42. Schlenk RF, Germing U, Hartmann F, Glasmacher A, Fischer JT, del Valle y Fuentes F, et al. High-dose cytarabine and mitoxantrone in consolidation therapy for acute promyelocytic leukemia. Leukemia. 2005;19(6):978–83.
43. Shen ZX, Shi ZZ, Fang J, Gu BW, Li JM, Zhu YM, et al. All-trans retinoic acid/As2O3 combination yields a high quality remission and survival in newly diagnosed acute promyelocytic leukemia. Proc Natl Acad Sci U S A. 2004;101(15):5328–35.
44. Tallman MS, Kwaan HC. Reassessing the hemostatic disorder associated with acute promyelocytic leukemia. Blood. 1992;79(3):543–53.
45. Yanada M, Matsushita T, Asou N, Kishimoto Y, Tsuzuki M, Maeda Y, et al. Severe hemorrhagic complications during remission induction therapy for acute promyelocytic leukemia: incidence, risk factors, and influence on outcome. Eur J Haematol. 2007;78(3):213–9.
46. Fenaux P, Pollet JP, Vandenbossche-Simon L, Morel P, Zandecki M, Jouet JP, et al. Treatment of acute promyelocytic leukemia: a report of 70 cases. Leuk Lymphoma. 1991;4(4):239–48.
47. Park JH, Qiao B, Panageas KS, Schymura MJ, Jurcic JG, Rosenblat TL, et al. Early death rate in acute promyelocytic leukemia remains high despite all-trans retinoic acid. Blood. 2011;118(5):1248–54.
48. Iland HJ, Collins M, Bradstock K, Supple SG, Catalano A, Hertzberg M, et al. Use of arsenic trioxide in remission induction and consolidation therapy for acute promyelocytic leukaemia in the Australasian Leukaemia and Lymphoma Group (ALLG) APML4 study: a non-randomised phase 2 trial. Lancet Haematol. 2015;2(9):e357–66.
49. Huang ME, Ye YC, Chen SR, Chai JR, Lu JX, Zhoa L, et al. Use of all-trans retinoic acid in the treatment of acute promyelocytic leukemia. Blood. 1988;72(2):567–72.
50. Mantha S, Goldman DA, Devlin SM, Lee JW, Zannino D, Collins M, et al. Determinants of fatal bleeding during induction therapy for acute promyelocytic leukemia in the ATRA era. Blood. 2017;129(13):1763–7.
51. Montesinos P, Bergua JM, Vellenga E, Rayon C, Parody R, de la Serna J, et al. Differentiation syndrome in patients with acute promyelocytic leukemia treated with all-trans retinoic acid and anthracycline chemotherapy: characteristics, outcome, and prognostic factors. Blood. 2009;113(4):775–83.
52. Breccia M, Avvisati G, Latagliata R, Carmosino I, Guarini A, De Propris MS, et al. Occurrence of thrombotic events in acute promyelocytic leukemia correlates with consistent immunophenotypic and molecular features. Leukemia. 2007;21(1):79–83.
53. Sanz MA, Montesinos P. Open issues on bleeding and thrombosis in acute promyelocytic leukemia. Thromb Res. 2010;125(Suppl 2):S51–4.
54. Montesinos P, Sanz MA. The differentiation syndrome in patients with acute promyelocytic leukemia: experience

of the pethema group and review of the literature. Mediterr J Hematol Infect Dis. 2011;3(1):e2011059.
55. Vahdat L, Maslak P, Miller WH Jr, Eardley A, Heller G, Scheinberg DA, et al. Early mortality and the retinoic acid syndrome in acute promyelocytic leukemia: impact of leukocytosis, low-dose chemotherapy, PMN/RAR-alpha isoform, and CD13 expression in patients treated with all-trans retinoic acid. Blood. 1994;84(11):3843–9.
56. Sanz MA, Lo Coco F, Martin G, Avvisati G, Rayon C, Barbui T, et al. Definition of relapse risk and role of nonanthracycline drugs for consolidation in patients with acute promyelocytic leukemia: a joint study of the PETHEMA and GIMEMA cooperative groups. Blood. 2000;96(4):1247–53.
57. Fenaux P. Management of acute promyelocytic leukemia. Eur J Haematol. 1993;50(2):65–73.
58. Rovelli A, Biondi A, Cantu Rajnoldi A, Conter V, Giudici G, Jankovic M, et al. Microgranular variant of acute promyelocytic leukemia in children. J Clin Oncol. 1992;10(9):1413–8.
59. Falanga A, Iacoviello L, Evangelista V, Belotti D, Consonni R, D'Orazio A, et al. Loss of blast cell procoagulant activity and improvement of hemostatic variables in patients with acute promyelocytic leukemia administered all-trans-retinoic acid. Blood. 1995;86(3):1072–81.
60. Grignani F, Fagioli M, Alcalay M, Longo L, Pandolfi PP, Donti E, et al. Acute promyelocytic leukemia: from genetics to treatment. Blood. 1994;83(1):10–25.
61. Goldberg MA, Ginsburg D, Mayer RJ, Stone RM, Maguire M, Rosenthal DS, et al. Is heparin administration necessary during induction chemotherapy for patients with acute promyelocytic leukemia? Blood. 1987;69(1):187–91.

7 Prognostic Factors in Acute Promyelocytic Leukemia

Javier de la Serna, Pau Montesinos, and Miguel A. Sanz

Introduction

The prognosis of acute promyelocytic leukemia (APL) has extraordinarily improved since the introduction of anthracycline-based chemotherapy [1], but especially after the advent of all-*trans* retinoic acid (ATRA) [2] and arsenic trioxide (ATO) [3]. In fact, following the optimization of frontline therapy with the use of a simultaneous combination of ATRA and anthracycline-based chemotherapy, primary resistance during induction therapy has virtually disappeared, with death during induction remaining as the only cause of failure [4]. In addition, using ATRA and anthracycline-based approaches, both in induction and post-remission therapy, several groups have reported a dramatic reduction in relapse rates to roughly 10% of patients who achieve first complete remission (CR) [5–9]. Such improvements in APL prognosis have also been reported with alternative treatments based on the addition of ATO to the conventional ATRA plus chemotherapy combination [10–15], but also with the combination of ATRA and ATO without or with minimal use of chemotherapy [16, 17].

Death during induction therapy and relapse are currently the major events involved in therapeutic failures in patients with APL. However, other less frequent but important late events, such as death while in first CR during post-remission therapy and the development of therapy-related neoplasms, have also an impact on patient outcome and, therefore, should be taken into account to design curative strategies for patients with APL. In this regard, the study of key characteristics associated with these events (prognostic factors) has always been considered a matter of great interest, since their recognition would translate into therapeutic improvements. In fact, over the past two decades, most therapeutic approaches have been designed following risk-adapted strategies in order to optimize the therapeutic efficacy by minimizing side effects, particularly in those patients considered at low risk of developing a given event.

In this chapter, in addition to review the prognostic factors of classical composite end points, such as CR rate, disease-free survival

J. de la Serna, M.D.
Department of Hematology, Hospital Universitario 12 de Octubre, Madrid, Spain

P. Montesinos, M.D., Ph.D.
Department of Hematology, Hospital Universitari i Politècnic La Fe, Valencia, Spain

Centro de Investigación Biomédica en Red de Cáncer, Instituto Carlos III, Madrid, Spain

M.A. Sanz, M.D. (✉)
Department of Medicine, Hospital Universitari i Politecnic La Fe, University of Valencia, Valencia, Spain

Centro de Investigacion Biomedica en Red de Cancer, Instituto Carlos III, Madrid, Spain
e-mail: msanz@uv.es

O. Abla et al. (eds.), *Acute Promyelocytic Leukemia*, https://doi.org/10.1007/978-3-319-64257-4_7

(DFS), event-free survival (EFS), and overall survival (OS), we will also discuss those patient and disease characteristics associated with specific events which determine the previously mentioned composite end points. Thus, for example, together with the recognition of prognostic factors of induction response, typically analyzed as a binary end point, the identification of predictive factors of the different causes of induction failure would provide an added value. The recognition of specific predictors of the different causes of induction failure would allow the design of tailored approaches according to the specific risk of death due to bleeding, infection, or differentiation syndrome (DS). Furthermore, assuming that the effectiveness of treatment is a major determinant in prognosis, this issue should be analyzed today in the context of the two principal therapeutic approaches currently used for APL, such as ATRA plus chemotherapy-based and ATRA plus ATO-based therapy.

Prognostic Factors of Induction Response

Classically, prognostic factors of induction response have been assessed considering only the binary option of CR versus induction failure, considering the latter as a whole. Table 7.1 shows the prognostic factors found in most representative series of patients with APL treated using modern therapeutic approaches. To analyze prognostic factors of induction response, the vast majority of these studies considered all causes of induction death as a single event.

The prognostic impact of WBC counts on induction response has been demonstrated in virtually all series (Table 7.1). Both in patients treated with ATRA plus anthracycline-based chemotherapy [4, 7, 18–24] and in those managed with ATO-based treatment [25, 26], WBC count is associated with a higher risk of induction failure. The cutoff point generally used for WBC count is 10×10^9/L at presentation. The prognostic impact of age is also an almost constant finding in series including sufficient patients with a wide age range, with older patients being those with a higher risk of induction failure.

Other patient and disease characteristics have also been reported less consistently as prognostic factors of induction failure. The presence of coagulopathy, abnormal serum creatinine, and albumin levels at presentation have been recognized as prognostic factors in two large series [4, 24].

A higher induction mortality rate in CD56-positive patients was originally suggested in a study based on a small series of patients not receiving a state-of-the-art treatment [27]. In a large study including 651 patients homogeneously treated with AIDA regimen [28], a multivariable analysis was able to demonstrate an independent prognostic value of CD56 positivity ($\geq$20% of leukemic cells) not only for relapse (which will be discussed below) but also as predictor of induction death. Despite of the association of CD56 expression with other recognized adverse factors for induction response [4], this phenotypic feature was selected to enter into the regression model together with abnormal creatinine level, WBC count greater than 10×10^9/L, age older than 60 years, male sex, and ECOG more than 1 [28].

Carriers of a functional variant in the core promoter of the CD95 cell death receptor gene, who were enrolled in the United Kingdom Medical Research Council (MRC) AML 12 trial, were more likely to die during remission induction and had a significantly worse overall survival [29]. To the best of our knowledge, this finding has not yet been validated in other studies.

A relationship between additional chromosomal abnormalities (ACA) and induction outcome in APL was first suggested in the 1990s in two retrospective studies carried out in small series of patients mostly treated with chemotherapy alone [30, 31]. More recently, also in a small cohort of patients managed with ATRA plus anthracycline-based induction therapy, the German AML Study Group [20] found that patients dying during induction therapy had significantly higher likelihood of trisomy 8 or abn(7q). However, other larger studies in patients with APL managed with state-of-the-art

Table 7.1 Studies of prognostic factors of induction response with modern induction therapy

Study	Group	Treatment	No. of patients	Age, median (range)	CR rate	Induction death rate	Prognostic factors identified in multivariable analysis
Fenaux et al. [22]	European APL	ATRA + Dauno/AraC	413	46 (1–83)	92	7	WBC count Age
Lo-Coco et al. [7]	GIMEMA	AIDA	1081	38–41 (18–81)	94	6	WBC count Platelets count Age
Sanz et al. [21]	PETHEMA	AIDA	426	39 (2–81)	90	9	WBC count Age
de la Serna et al. [4]	PETHEMA	AIDA	732	40 (2–83)	91	9	Creatinine level WBC count PB blast count Age Sex
Schlenk et al. [20]	AMLSG	AIDA	75	43 (16–60)	76 (+15)	9	WBC count Cytogenetics
Burnett et al. [18]	MRC	ATRA + Dauno/AraC ± other	120	NA	87	12	WBC count Age
Gale et al. [47]	MRC	ATRA + Dauno/AraC ± other	203	37 (1–60)	84	13	WBC count
Lengfelder et al. [23]	GAMLCG	ATRA + TAD/HAM	142	40 (16–60)	92	8	WBC count
Rego et al [24]	ICAL	ATRA + Dauno	180	34 (15–73)	85	15	WBC count Coagulopathy Creatinine level Albumin level
Ghavamzadeh et al. [25]	Single institution	ATO	197	29 (11–71)	86	15	WBC count
Ravandi et al. [26]	Single institution	ATRA + ATO ± GO	81	47 (14–81)	92	8	WBC count

Table 7.2 Prognostic factors of specific causes of induction death with modern induction therapy

					Prognostic factors identified in multivariable analysis		
Study	Group	No. of patients	CR rate	Induction death rate	Induction death due to bleeding	Induction death due to infection	Induction death due to DS
Di Bona et al. [19]	GIMEMA	499	92	8	Peripheral blast count[a] Hemorrhagic score[a]	Not analyzed	Not analyzed
de la Serna et al. [4]	PETHEMA	732	91	9	Creatinine level PB blast count Coagulopathy	Age Sex Fever	ECOG score Albumin level
De Botton et al. [36]	European APL	413	92	7	Not analyzed	Not analyzed	Not found
Yanada et al. [72]	JALSG	279	95	5	Fibrinogen level[b] WBC count[b] PS score[b]	Not analyzed	Not analyzed

[a]Prognostic factors of early death (<day 10)
[b]Prognostic factors of severe hemorrhage (half of them were not lethal)

treatments have not found such impact on induction outcome [32–35].

Some additional studies shown in Table 7.2 have analyzed separately specific induction outcomes instead of induction response as a whole. A study of the Italian GIMEMA group reported a significant association between peripheral blast counts, hemorrhagic score and early death (<day 10) [19]. On the other hand, a study of the European APL group was unable to find any pretreatment feature associated with mortality due to DS [36]. In contrast, a larger study of the PETHEMA-HOVON groups identified ECOG score >1 and low albumin levels to be associated with an increased risk of death due to this syndrome [4]. In addition, this analysis identified specific and distinct pretreatment set of characteristics associated with an increased risk of death due to hemorrhage (abnormal creatinine level, increased peripheral blast counts, and presence of coagulopathy) and infection (age > 60 years, male gender, and fever at presentation). This study provided clinically relevant information for practice and for designing risk-adapted strategies focused on reducing mortality from hemorrhage, infection, and DS during early treatment phases of APL.

An increased body mass index at diagnosis has also been associated with a higher risk of developing DS in APL patients treated with AIDA protocols, but not with an increased mortality due to this syndrome [37–39].

Although many prognostic factors that were recognized in the pre-ATO era have now been challenged in the era of ATO therapy [40], there is enough evidence demonstrating a poorer induction outcome for patients with elevated WBC count also when they are treated with ATO-based regimens. In fact, most current ATO-based approaches include the addition of anthracyclines or gemtuzumab ozogamicin for induction therapy in patients presenting hyperleukocytosis. The prognostic impact on induction outcome of other presenting features, such as age, gender, coagulopathy, CD56 expression, creatinine, and albumin levels, among others, should be confirmed in large series treated with ATO-based regimens.

Prognostic Factors of Induction Response in Children

A large retrospective study [41] has recently focused on determining the incidence and predictors of thrombo-hemorrhagic deaths during induction therapy in children and adolescents with APL treated with ATRA and chemotherapy by several international groups. This study has shown an incidence of early thrombo-hemorrhagic deaths of 4.7%, with CNS hemorrhage being the most common site for this lethal complication. High WBC (>10 × 10^9/L) and high PB blast (>30 × 10^9/L), M3v morphological subtype and black ethnicity were identified as predictors of hemorrhagic death during induction therapy in univariable analysis. However, in multivariable analysis, only high WBC count retained an independent prognostic value together with obesity, defined as a body mass index ≥95 percentile for age. As far as we know, no other studies have been reported regarding prognostic factors of induction outcomes in children.

Prognostic Factors of Post-remission Outcomes

Prognostic factors of specific post-remission outcomes, such as relapse, death during remission, and development of therapy-related myeloid neoplasms (t-MN) have been analyzed in only a marginal way in the majority of studies in APL. In addition, these events have generally been considered as a whole in a context of composite end points, such as EFS, DFS, and OS. However, the interpretation of composite end points with coexisting competing risks can reduce precision in estimating not only the probability of the occurrence of primary events [42], but also the prognostic factors involved in these adverse events. Therefore, in this chapter, we will review the prognostic factors implicated in the classical composite end points (EFS, DFS, OS), but also those found in the most important primary events (relapse, death during remission, t-MN).

Predictors of Composite End Points

Similar to induction response, the prognostic impact of WBC counts on the risk of relapse is universally accepted, regardless of the type of treatment used, with a higher risk for patients with WBC counts greater than 10 × 10^9/L at presentation. The prognostic value of WBC counts has a variable impact on composite end points in which relapse is one of the events directly considered, such as EFS, DFS, and RFS. Despite the indirect effect that relapse may have on OS, the impact of WBC counts on this end point may not appear evident due to the high antileukemic efficacy of salvage therapy in APL. In this regard, the score defined after a joint GIMEMA and PETHEMA study [43], based on the presenting WBC and platelet counts, has been regarded as the mainstay for risk stratification in most APL clinical trials, being so widely adopted because of its simplicity and reproducibility.

Other prognostic factors, such as male gender and morphologic classification, M3V, and classical M3 APL, have occasionally been associated with post-remission outcomes, but they lose their prognostic value when adjusted for the WBC or relapse risk score [44].

In general, prognostic factors different to WBC and relapse risk score have not been incorporated into decision-making, with the exception, to the best of our knowledge, of age and CD56 expression. Using a 20% cutoff point of leukemic promyelocytes expressing CD56 in three subsequent PETHEMA trials with AIDA-derived approaches (LPA96, LPA99, and LPA2005 trials), CD56 was found to be an independent prognostic factor not only for induction death, as previously mentioned, but also for relapse [28]. Subsequent to this study, PETHEMA trials have incorporated CD56 expression for refining risk stratification. In particular, in the context of risk-adapted consolidation therapy, patients classified according to relapse-risk score [43] are now upgraded one level when CD56 is positive. Thus, low- and intermediate-risk CD56-positive patients are treated for consolidation as intermediate- and high-risk patients, respectively.

It has been suggested that various molecular features could be useful to predict outcomes in APL, but most of these molecular predictors have still not been validated. In addition, logistic and technical issues have hampered a generalized use of these sophisticated tools so far.

The prognostic impact of FLT3 mutations has been widely analyzed in the context of ATRA plus chemotherapy with controversial results [45–55]. The methodological heterogeneity of these studies regarding the sample size, diversity of treatments, use or not of multivariable analysis, as well as the variables and end points analyzed, make it difficult to obtain reliable and definitive conclusions. The vast majority of these studies, however, have revealed a strong association between leukocytosis and FLT3 mutations. In this regard, the results reported in a large cohort by the PETHEMA-HOVON group [52] showed that FLT3-ITD status was removed from the regression equation when the WBC count was included in the multivariable analysis, suggesting that the adverse outcome of this mutation is attributable to its relationship with elevated WBC count. Furthermore, this study was unable to demonstrate the adverse prognostic impact that had previously been reported for the FLT3-D835 mutation [47] and the ratio and length of FLT3-ITD mutations [48].

The prognostic impact of FLT3 mutations has been less often studied in APL patients treated with ATO-based regimens. In this regard, neither the Australasian Leukaemia and Lymphoma Group [13] nor the North American Intergroup [35], both using ATRA, ATO, and chemotherapy, found differences in any post-remission outcome by FLT3 status. The Italian-German APL0406 randomized trial, using ATRA plus ATO without chemotherapy, but restricted to non-high risk patients, also failed to detect any impact of FLT3 status on outcome [55]. Finally, an elegant study carried out on 535 newly diagnosed APL patients treated with an ATRA/ATO-based protocol at Shanghai Institute of Hematology and affiliated centers [56] deserves special mention. This study showed that FLT3-ITD or FLT3-TKD, N-RAS, and WT1 mutations were the three most common additional gene mutations (15.8%, 4.5%, and 4.7%, respectively), but none of them had a significant impact on OS and DFS. In contrast, mutations of epigenetic modifier genes (EMG), such as DNMT3A (0.3%), TET2 (4.5%), IDH1 (0.4%), IDH2 (0.2%), and ASXL1 (1.6%), which together account for 6.5%, showed an independent prognostic value for DFS in multivariable analysis, together with the relapse risk score [43], whereas for OS this score was the only factor indicating poor prognosis.

In addition to mutations, the expression of several genes has also been explored as prognostic molecular markers in APL. Three subsequent studies of the German AML Cooperative Group (AMLCG) [57–59], carried out on relatively small cohorts of patients enrolled in two consecutive trials, showed that the expression levels of three different genes, BAALC [57], ERG [58], and WT1 [59] had an independent prognostic value for APL risk stratification. Based on these studies, a molecular risk score, which includes the expression level of the three genes, has been developed [60]. This integrative risk score was able to divide patients into two groups with statistically significant differences in OS, RFS, and CIR. The prognostic value of the expression of other genes has also been reported. A study carried out on patients enrolled in the International Consortium of APL trial showed that a low expression of KMT2E is associated with a shorter OS [61] and a higher DNp73/TAp73 RNA expression ratio with a lower OS and DFS, as well as higher risk of relapse in patients with APL. Finally, a Spanish group has reported that low PRAME expression defines a subgroup of APL patients with a short RFS [62].

Based on a large cohort of 187 PML/RARA-positive APL patients enrolled in three subsequent trials of the North American Leukemia Intergroup, it has been reported that telomere length (TL), in particular delta TL, defined as TL at remission minus TL at diagnosis, is a strong predictor of OS [63]. These findings, as well as those previously mentioned regarding mutations and gene expression, warrant prospective confirmation studies.

Several studies carried out on patients managed with state-of-the-art treatments were unable to demonstrate an independent prognostic impact of the presence of additional chromosomal abnormalities (ACA) on any post-remission outcome [32–35], with the exception of a recent study from the North American Intergroup [35]. In this study, the presence of a complex karyotype (≥2 ACAs) was strongly associated with an inferior OS independently of the post-remission treatment arm, even when ATO was given for consolidation therapy. This novel observation deserves further investigation in larger cohorts of patients treated with either chemotherapy-based or ATO-based state-of-the-art treatments.

Predictors of Specific Post-remission Events

The limitations of using composite end points for the analysis of prognostic factors have been widely discussed in the literature [42], but any discussion is outside the scope of this chapter. The precise estimate of post-remission events of primary interest, such as relapse and therapy-related adverse events, including death during remission and development t-MN, is affected by competing risks when analyzed using composite end points. Few studies have analyzed specifically these post-remission events taking into account competing risks.

Relapse

There is a general agreement that the impact of WBC count on prognosis of APL patients is not only restricted to induction response, mainly associated with induction deaths due to hemorrhages, but also is associated with the risk of relapse. Therefore, with EFS, DFS, and OS, the three meaningful composite end points in which relapse and death during remission have a considerable weight. Although some previous studies [18, 64, 65] have found a significantly higher incidence of relapse for patients with high WBC counts, the crucial prognostic value of this factor to predict relapse was definitively established in a joint GIMEMA and PETHEMA study [43]. In this study, multivariable analysis resulted in a simplified predictive model for relapse-free survival that has been widely adopted around the world. This model permits the identification of the following patient categories: (1) low-risk group, presenting WBC count below or equal to 10×10^9/L and platelet count above 40×10^9/L; (2) intermediate-risk group, presenting WBC and platelet counts below or equal to 10×10^9/L and 40×10^9/L, respectively; and (3) high-risk group, presenting WBC count greater than 10×10^9/L.

The expression of CD56 has also been defined as a predictor of relapse. This has been suggested in previous studies [27, 66, 67], and confirmed in a large study of the PETHEMA-HOVON group [28]. In addition to relapse risk score, the expression of CD56 using a 20% cutoff level is also an independent and accurate predictor for relapse in patients with APL treated with ATRA and anthracycline-based regimens. CD56-positive APL also showed a significantly higher risk of extramedullary relapse. Interestingly, CD56 positivity, with a prevalence of 11% of newly diagnosed patients, is correlated with the BCR3 isoform and the co-expression of other surface antigens, such as CD2, CD34, HLA-DR, and CD7 [28]. An increased body mass index at diagnosis has also been associated with a higher risk of disease relapse [38], but this finding has not yet been validated in larger series.

Several molecular markers have also been reported to be associated with relapse risk. This is the case of the expression of the gene PRAME, considered a good predictor of RFS [62], and an integrative risk score that includes the expression of three genes (BAALC, ERG, and WT1) [60], which are able to identify two groups with statistically significant differences in RFS and cumulative incidence of relapse.

Finally, in contrast to the lack of clinical value of molecular assessment of PML/RARA performed at the end of induction, it is widely accepted that patients with persistent or recurrent disease at the molecular level at any stage after completion of consolidation will invariably relapse, unless additional therapy is given. In contrast, continued persistent molecular negativity by RT-PCR or RQ-PCR is associated with a low relapse risk.

Central Nervous System Relapse

To the best of our knowledge, only two large studies [68, 69] have specifically analyzed the prognostic factors involved in extramedullary relapse, with particular reference to CNS relapse. In multivariable analysis, a study of the European APL group [68] found that only a high WBC count (cutoff point 10×10^9/L) is independently associated with CNS relapse, whereas a PETHEMA-HOVON study [69] found the occurrence of cerebral hemorrhage during induction and the relapse risk score, which is a composite of WBC and platelet counts [43], are the most valuable predictors of CNS relapse.

Regarding other potential risk factors for CNS relapse, some authors have suggested that FLT3-ITD mutations, which correlate with leukocytosis [47], and an increased expression of adhesion molecules, such as CD56, can promote leukemic infiltration in CNS and other extramedullary sites [28]. In fact, CD56 APL had a significantly higher risk of extramedullary relapse in a large series of patients included in several PETHEMA-HOVON trials [28].

Development of Therapy-Related Myeloid Neoplasms

Regarding risk factors of development of t-MN in APL, to our knowledge, only one study has addressed this issue [70]. The univariable analysis in this PETHEMA-HOVON study showed the following characteristics were associated with the development of t-MN: older age (cutoff 35 years), lower relapse risk score, and higher platelet count (cutoff 40 × 10^9/L). Multivariable analysis, however, only identified age and relapse risk score as independent prognostic factors for t-MN. There is no clear explanation for the apparent paradoxical finding of a higher risk of developing t-MN in patients with a lower risk of relapse, but it has been speculated that a greater frequency of competing events in patients with higher risk APL, particularly relapse and death in remission, decreases the chance of developing t-MN while in first CR [70].

Although a potential relationship between dose intensity of topoisomerase II inhibitors or intercalating agents and incidence of t-MN has been suggested, data from this PETHEMA-HOVON study [70] does not clearly support this hypothesis, since the increased risk of t-MN was observed in lower-risk APL patients, who overall were less heavily treated. Therefore, it is not clear whether anthracycline dose reduction, or even its replacement by arsenic trioxide, would be effective to decrease the incidence of t-MN.

Death During First Remission

Apart from the classical composite end points, such as OS, EFS, and DFS, in which death during first remission is one of the events considered, a precise estimate of this post-remission event of primary interest has hardly been analyzed. Nevertheless, it is generally accepted that death during first remission is mainly associated with age and comorbidities, along with dose intensity of post-remission therapy. It should be noted, however, that some deaths occur off-therapy due to causes not associated directly with therapy-related toxicity. The unquestionable impact of age on non-relapse mortality has led many groups to design age-adapted trials. In this regard, a recent report of the PETHEMA group [71] showed a significant improvement in long-term outcomes, which were mainly attributed to a decrease in hematologic toxicity and toxic death rates, using a less intensive frontline regimen with ATRA and anthracycline monochemotherapy in elderly patients with APL.

Whether non-relapse mortality can be reduced with age-adapted approaches, not only by decreasing dose intensity of chemotherapy in elderly patients, but also replacing chemotherapy by ATO, is still an open issue warranting further research.

Conclusions

The identification of prognostic factors has always been considered a matter of great interest in APL, since their recognition would allow the use of risk-adapted strategies aimed at optimizing the therapeutic efficacy and minimizing treatment-related toxicity, which in turn would translate into better outcomes. Early deaths during induction therapy and relapse are currently the most frequent events involved in therapeutic failures; however deaths in CR during post-remission therapy and even off-therapy, as well as the development of therapy-related neoplasms, are other important events with negative impact on outcome.

Several patient- and disease-related characteristics have been recognized as prognostic factors, but only age and WBC count, as well as a composite risk score including WBC and platelet counts to predict relapse and other surrogate end points, have been widely used for risk-adapted stratification in clinical trials. In addition to WBC count and the risk score, the expression of CD56 and the occurrence of cerebral hemorrhage during induction have been identified as independent and accurate predictors of hematologic and CNS relapse, respectively. Accordingly, patients included in the most recent risk-adapted PETHEMA trials are upgraded one level based on the relapse risk score when CD56 is positive, whereas those who develop a cerebral hemorrhage during induction are given systematic CNS prophylaxis. Other characteristics, such as an increased BMI, presence of additional chromosomal abnormalities, and mutational status and expression profiles of a variety of genes have also been recognized as independent prognostic factors. However, most of these predictors have not yet been validated in large and independent series.

It should be noted that the body of knowledge acquired over the last two decades on prognostic factors in APL has mainly been obtained in the context of ATRA plus chemotherapy-based regimens, while the impact of these factors after the incorporation of ATO in frontline therapy has not been established. Large studies with prolonged follow-up will be necessary to identify the best predictors of outcome in APL patients receiving ATO containing regimens, although it appears that age and WBC count will continue to play a key role.

References

1. Bernard J, Weil M, Boiron M, et al. Acute promyelocytic leukemia: results of treatment by daunorubicin. Blood. 1973;41:489–96.
2. Huang ME, Ye YC, Chen SR, et al. Use of all-trans retinoic acid in the treatment of acute promyelocytic leukemia. Blood. 1988;72:567–72.
3. Shen ZX, Chen GQ, Ni JH, et al. Use of arsenic trioxide (As2O3) in the treatment of acute promyelocytic leukemia (APL): II. Clinical efficacy and pharmacokinetics in relapsed patients. Blood. 1997;89:3354–60.
4. de la Serna J, Montesinos P, Vellenga E, et al. Causes and prognostic factors of remission induction failure in patients with acute promyelocytic leukemia treated with all-trans retinoic acid and idarubicin. Blood. 2008;111:3395–402. https://doi.org/10.1182/blood-2007-07-100669.
5. Adès L, Chevret S, Raffoux E, et al. Is cytarabine useful in the treatment of acute promyelocytic leukemia? Results of a randomized trial from the European Acute Promyelocytic Leukemia Group. J Clin Oncol. 2006;24:5703–10. https://doi.org/10.1200/JCO.2006.08.1596.
6. Asou N, Kishimoto Y, Kiyoi H, et al. A randomized study with or without intensified maintenance chemotherapy in patients with acute promyelocytic leukemia who have become negative for PML-RARalpha transcript after consolidation therapy: the Japan Adult Leukemia Study Group (JALSG) APL97 study. Blood. 2007;110:59–66. https://doi.org/10.1182/blood-2006-08-043992.
7. Lo-Coco F, Avvisati G, Vignetti M, et al. Front-line treatment of acute promyelocytic leukemia with AIDA induction followed by risk-adapted consolidation for adults younger than 61 years: results of the AIDA-2000 trial of the GIMEMA Group. Blood. 2010,116:3171–9. https://doi.org/10.1182/blood-2010-03-276196.
8. Sanz MA, Montesinos P, Rayón C, et al. Risk-adapted treatment of acute promyelocytic leukemia based on all-trans retinoic acid and anthracycline with addition of cytarabine in consolidation therapy for high-risk patients: further improvements in treatment outcome. Blood. 2010;115:5137–46. https://doi.org/10.1182/blood-2010-01-266007.
9. Burnett AK, Hills RK, Jovanovic JV, et al. Inclusion of chemotherapy in addition to anthracycline in the treatment of acute promyelocytic leukaemia does not improve outcomes: results of the MRC AML15 trial. Leukemia. 2013;27:843–51. https://doi.org/10.1038/leu.2012.360.
10. Hu J, Liu Y-F, Wu C-F, et al. Long-term efficacy and safety of all-trans retinoic acid/arsenic trioxide-based therapy in newly diagnosed acute promyelocytic leukemia. Proc Natl Acad Sci U S A. 2009;106:3342–7. https://doi.org/10.1073/pnas.0813280106.
11. Powell BL, Moser B, Stock W, et al. Arsenic trioxide improves event-free and overall survival for adults with acute promyelocytic leukemia: North American Leukemia Intergroup Study C9710. Blood. 2010;116:3751–7. https://doi.org/10.1182/blood-2010-02-269621.
12. Gore SD, Gojo I, Sekeres MA, et al. Single cycle of arsenic trioxide-based consolidation chemotherapy spares anthracycline exposure in the primary management of acute promyelocytic leukemia. J Clin Oncol. 2010;28:1047–53. https://doi.org/10.1200/JCO.2009.25.5158.
13. Iland HJ, Bradstock K, Supple SG, et al. All-trans-retinoic acid, idarubicin, and IV arsenic trioxide as initial therapy in acute promyelocytic leukemia (APML4). Blood. 2012;120:1570–80; quiz 1752. https://doi.org/10.1182/blood-2012-02-410746.

14. Iland HJ, Collins M, Bradstock K, et al. Use of arsenic trioxide in remission induction and consolidation therapy for acute promyelocytic leukaemia in the Australasian Leukaemia and Lymphoma Group (ALLG) APML4 study: a non-randomised phase 2 trial. Lancet Haematol. 2015;2:e357–66. https://doi.org/10.1016/S2352-3026(15)00115-5.
15. Zhu H-H, Wu D-P, Jin J, et al. Long-term survival of acute promyelocytic leukaemia patients treated with arsenic and retinoic acid. Br J Haematol. 2016;174:820–2. https://doi.org/10.1111/bjh.13809.
16. Lo-Coco F, Avvisati G, Vignetti M, et al. Retinoic acid and arsenic trioxide for acute promyelocytic leukemia. N Engl J Med. 2013;369:111–21. https://doi.org/10.1056/NEJMoa1300874.
17. Burnett AK, Russell NH, Hills RK, et al. Arsenic trioxide and all-trans retinoic acid treatment for acute promyelocytic leukaemia in all risk groups (AML17): results of a randomised, controlled, phase 3 trial. Lancet Oncol. 2015;16:1295–305. https://doi.org/10.1016/S1470-2045(15)00193-X.
18. Burnett AK, Grimwade D, Solomon E, et al. Presenting white blood cell count and kinetics of molecular remission predict prognosis in acute promyelocytic leukemia treated with all-trans retinoic acid: result of the Randomized MRC Trial. Blood. 1999;93:4131–43.
19. Di Bona E, Avvisati G, Castaman G, et al. Early haemorrhagic morbidity and mortality during remission induction with or without all-trans retinoic acid in acute promyelocytic leukaemia. Br J Haematol. 2000;108:689–95.
20. Schlenk RF, Germing U, Hartmann F, et al. High-dose cytarabine and mitoxantrone in consolidation therapy for acute promyelocytic leukemia. Leukemia. 2005;19:978–83. https://doi.org/10.1038/sj.leu.2403766.
21. Sanz MA, Martín G, González M, et al. Risk-adapted treatment of acute promyelocytic leukemia with all-trans-retinoic acid and anthracycline monochemotherapy: a multicenter study by the PETHEMA group. Blood. 2004;103:1237–43. https://doi.org/10.1182/blood-2003-07-2462.
22. Fenaux P, Chastang C, Chevret S, et al. A randomized comparison of all transretinoic acid (ATRA) followed by chemotherapy and ATRA plus chemotherapy and the role of maintenance therapy in newly diagnosed acute promyelocytic leukemia. The European APL Group. Blood. 1999;94:1192–200.
23. Lengfelder E, Haferlach C, Saussele S, et al. High dose ara-C in the treatment of newly diagnosed acute promyelocytic leukemia: long-term results of the German AMLCG. Leukemia. 2009;23:2248–58. https://doi.org/10.1038/leu.2009.183.
24. Rego EM, Kim HT, Ruiz-Argüelles GJ, et al. Improving acute promyelocytic leukemia (APL) outcome in developing countries through networking, results of the International Consortium on APL. Blood. 2013;121:1935–43. https://doi.org/10.1182/blood-2012-08-449918.
25. Ghavamzadeh A, Alimoghaddam K, Rostami S, et al. Phase II study of single-agent arsenic trioxide for the front-line therapy of acute promyelocytic leukemia. J Clin Oncol. 2011;29:2753–7. https://doi.org/10.1200/JCO.2010.32.2107.
26. Ravandi F, Estey E, Jones D, et al. Effective treatment of acute promyelocytic leukemia with all-trans-retinoic acid, arsenic trioxide, and gemtuzumab ozogamicin. J Clin Oncol. 2009;27:504–10. https://doi.org/10.1200/JCO.2008.18.6130.
27. Murray CK, Estey E, Paietta E, et al. CD56 expression in acute promyelocytic leukemia: a possible indicator of poor treatment outcome? J Clin Oncol. 1999;17:293–7. https://doi.org/10.1200/jco.1999.17.1.293.
28. Montesinos P, Rayón C, Vellenga E, et al. Clinical significance of CD56 expression in patients with acute promyelocytic leukemia treated with all-trans retinoic acid and anthracycline-based regimens. Blood. 2011;117:1799–805. https://doi.org/10.1182/blood-2010-04-277434.
29. Sunter NJ, Scott K, Hills R, et al. A functional variant in the core promoter of the CD95 cell death receptor gene predicts prognosis in acute promyelocytic leukemia. Blood. 2012;119:196–205. https://doi.org/10.1182/blood-2011-04-349803.
30. Slack JL, Arthur DC, Lawrence D, et al. Secondary cytogenetic changes in acute promyelocytic leukemia--prognostic importance in patients treated with chemotherapy alone and association with the intron 3 breakpoint of the PML gene: a Cancer and Leukemia Group B study. J Clin Oncol. 1997;15:1786–95. https://doi.org/10.1200/jco.1997.15.5.1786.
31. Hiorns LR, Swansbury GJ, Mehta J, et al. Additional chromosome abnormalities confer worse prognosis in acute promyelocytic leukaemia. Br J Haematol. 1997;96:314–21.
32. De Botton S, Chevret S, Sanz M, et al. Additional chromosomal abnormalities in patients with acute promyelocytic leukaemia (APL) do not confer poor prognosis: results of APL 93 trial. Br J Haematol. 2000;111:801–6.
33. Hernández JM, Martín G, Gutiérrez NC, et al. Additional cytogenetic changes do not influence the outcome of patients with newly diagnosed acute promyelocytic leukemia treated with an ATRA plus anthracyclin based protocol. A report of the Spanish group PETHEMA. Haematologica. 2001;86:807–13.
34. Cervera J, Montesinos P, Hernández-Rivas JM, et al. Additional chromosome abnormalities in patients with acute promyelocytic leukemia treated with all-trans retinoic acid and chemotherapy. Haematologica. 2010;95:424–31. https://doi.org/10.3324/haematol.2009.013243.
35. Poiré X, Moser BK, Gallagher RE, et al. Arsenic trioxide in front-line therapy of acute promyelocytic leukemia (C9710): prognostic significance of FLT3 mutations and complex karyotype. Leuk Lymphoma. 2014;55:1523–32. https://doi.org/10.3109/10428194.2013.842985.

36. De Botton S, Dombret H, Sanz M, et al. Incidence, clinical features, and outcome of all trans-retinoic acid syndrome in 413 cases of newly diagnosed acute promyelocytic leukemia. The European APL Group. Blood. 1998;92:2712–8.
37. Jeddi R, Ghédira H, Mnif S, et al. High body mass index is an independent predictor of differentiation syndrome in patients with acute promyelocytic leukemia. Leuk Res. 2010;34:545–7.
38. Breccia M, Mazzarella L, Bagnardi V, et al. Increased BMI correlates with higher risk of disease relapse and differentiation syndrome in patients with acute promyelocytic leukemia treated with the AIDA protocols. Blood. 2012;119:49–54.
39. Leblebjian H, Deangelo DJ, Skirvin JA, et al. Predictive factors for all-trans retinoic acid-related differentiation syndrome in patients with acute promyelocytic leukemia. Leuk Res. 2013;37:747–51. https://doi.org/10.1016/j.leukres.2013.04.011.
40. Norsworthy KJ, Altman JK. Optimal treatment strategies for high-risk acute promyelocytic leukemia. Curr Opin Hematol. 2016;23:127–36. https://doi.org/10.1097/MOH.0000000000000215.
41. Abla O, Ribeiro RC, Testi AM, et al. Predictors of thrombo-hemorrhagic early death in children and adolescents with t(15;17) positive acute promyelocytic leukemia treated with ATRA and chemotherapy. Ann Hematol. 2017;96(9):1449–56. https://doi.org/10.1007/s00277-017-3042-6.
42. Mell LK, Jeong J-H. Pitfalls of using composite primary end points in the presence of competing risks. J Clin Oncol. 2010,28.4297–9. https://doi.org/10.1200/JCO.2010.30.2802.
43. Sanz MA, Lo-Coco F, Martín G, et al. Definition of relapse risk and role of nonanthracycline drugs for consolidation in patients with acute promyelocytic leukemia: a joint study of the PETHEMA and GIMEMA cooperative groups. Blood. 2000;96:1247–53.
44. Tallman MS, Kim HT, Montesinos P, et al. Does microgranular variant morphology of acute promyelocytic leukemia independently predict a less favorable outcome compared with classical M3 APL? A joint study of the North American Intergroup and the PETHEMA Group. Blood. 2010;116:5650–9. https://doi.org/10.1182/blood-2010-06-288613.
45. Noguera NI, Breccia M, Divona M, et al. Alterations of the FLT3 gene in acute promyelocytic leukemia: association with diagnostic characteristics and analysis of clinical outcome in patients treated with the Italian AIDA protocol. Leukemia. 2002;16:2185–9. https://doi.org/10.1038/sj.leu.2402723.
46. Au WY, Fung A, Chim CS, et al. FLT-3 aberrations in acute promyelocytic leukaemia: clinicopathological associations and prognostic impact. Br J Haematol. 2004;125:463–9. https://doi.org/10.1111/j.1365-2141.2004.04935.x.
47. Gale RE, Hills R, Pizzey AR, et al. Relationship between FLT3 mutation status, biologic characteristics, and response to targeted therapy in acute promyelocytic leukemia. Blood. 2005;106:3768–76. https://doi.org/10.1182/blood-2005-04-1746.
48. Chillón MC, Santamaría C, García-Sanz R, et al. Long FLT3 internal tandem duplications and reduced PML-RARα expression at diagnosis characterize a high-risk subgroup of acute promyelocytic leukemia patients. Haematologica. 2010;95:745–51. https://doi.org/10.3324/haematol.2009.015073.
49. Beitinjaneh A, Jang S, Roukoz H, Majhail NS. Prognostic significance of FLT3 internal tandem duplication and tyrosine kinase domain mutations in acute promyelocytic leukemia: a systematic review. Leuk Res. 2010;34:831–6. https://doi.org/10.1016/j.leukres.2010.01.001.
50. Hong S-D, Kim Y-K, Kim H-N, et al. Treatment outcome of all-trans retinoic acid/anthracycline combination chemotherapy and the prognostic impact of FLT3/ITD mutation in acute promyelocytic leukemia patients. Korean J Hematol. 2011;46:24–30. https://doi.org/10.5045/kjh.2011.46.1.24.
51. Schnittger S, Bacher U, Haferlach C, et al. Clinical impact of FLT3 mutation load in acute promyelocytic leukemia with t(15;17)/PML-RARA. Haematologica. 2011;96:1799–807. https://doi.org/10.3324/haematol.2011.049007.
52. Barragán E, Montesinos P, Camos M, et al. Prognostic value of FLT3 mutations in patients with acute promyelocytic leukemia treated with all-trans retinoic acid and anthracycline monochemotherapy. Haematologica. 2011;96:1470–7. https://doi.org/10.3324/haematol.2011.044933.
53. Breccia M, Loglisci G, Loglisci MG, et al. FLT3-ITD confers poor prognosis in patients with acute promyelocytic leukemia treated with AIDA protocols: long-term follow-up analysis. Haematologica. 2013;98:e161–3. https://doi.org/10.3324/haematol.2013.095380.
54. Lucena-Araujo AR, Kim HT, Jacomo RH, et al. Internal tandem duplication of the FLT3 gene confers poor overall survival in patients with acute promyelocytic leukemia treated with all-trans retinoic acid and anthracycline-based chemotherapy: an International Consortium on Acute Promyelocytic Leukemia study. Ann Hematol. 2014;93:2001–10. https://doi.org/10.1007/s00277-014-2142-9.
55. Cicconi L, Divona M, Ciardi C, et al. PML-RARα kinetics and impact of FLT3-ITD mutations in newly diagnosed acute promyelocytic leukaemia treated with ATRA and ATO or ATRA and chemotherapy. Leukemia. 2016;30:1987–92. https://doi.org/10.1038/leu.2016.122.
56. Shen Y, Fu Y-K, Zhu Y-M, et al. Mutations of epigenetic modifier genes as a poor prognostic factor in acute promyelocytic leukemia under treatment with all-trans retinoic acid and arsenic trioxide. EBioMedicine. 2015;2:563–71. https://doi.org/10.1016/j.ebiom.2015.04.006.
57. Nolte F, Hecht A, Reinwald M, et al. In acute promyelocytic leukemia (APL) low BAALC gene expression identifies a patient group with favorable overall survival and improved relapse free survival.

Leuk Res. 2013;37:378–82. https://doi.org/10.1016/j.leukres.2012.11.018.
58. Hecht A, Nowak D, Nowak V, et al. High expression of the Ets-related gene (ERG) is an independent prognostic marker for relapse-free survival in patients with acute promyelocytic leukemia. Ann Hematol. 2013;92:443–9. https://doi.org/10.1007/s00277-012-1648-2.
59. Hecht A, Nolte F, Nowak D, et al. Prognostic importance of expression of the Wilms' tumor 1 gene in newly diagnosed acute promyelocytic leukemia. Leuk Lymphoma. 2015;56:2289–95. https://doi.org/10.3109/10428194.2014.990011.
60. Hecht A, Nowak D, Nowak V, et al. A molecular risk score integrating BAALC, ERG and WT1 expression levels for risk stratification in acute promyelocytic leukemia. Leuk Res. 2015;39:1172–7. https://doi.org/10.1016/j.leukres.2015.08.010.
61. Lucena-Araujo AR, Kim HT, Jacomo RH, et al. Prognostic impact of KMT2E transcript levels on outcome of patients with acute promyelocytic leukaemia treated with all-trans retinoic acid and anthracycline-based chemotherapy: an International Consortium on Acute Promyelocytic Leukaemia study. Br J Haematol. 2014;166:540–9. https://doi.org/10.1111/bjh.12921.
62. Santamaría C, Chillón MC, García-Sanz R, et al. The relevance of preferentially expressed antigen of melanoma (PRAME) as a marker of disease activity and prognosis in acute promyelocytic leukemia. Haematologica. 2008;93:1797–805. https://doi.org/10.3324/haematol.13214.
63. Baljevic M, Dumitriu B, Lee J-W, et al. Telomere length recovery: a strong predictor of overall survival in acute promyelocytic leukemia. Acta Haematol. 2016;136:210–8. https://doi.org/10.1159/000448160.
64. Mandelli F, Diverio D, Avvisati G, et al. Molecular remission in PML/RAR alpha-positive acute promyelocytic leukemia by combined all-trans retinoic acid and idarubicin (AIDA) therapy. Gruppo Italiano-Malattie Ematologiche Maligne dell'Adulto and Associazione Italiana di Ematologia ed Oncologia Pediatrica Cooperative Groups. Blood. 1997;90:1014–21.
65. Sanz MA, Martín G, Rayon C, et al. A modified AIDA protocol with anthracycline-based consolidation results in high antileukemic efficacy and reduced toxicity in newly diagnosed PML/RARalpha-positive acute promyelocytic leukemia. PETHEMA group. Blood. 1999;94:3015–21.
66. Ferrara F, Morabito F, Martino B, et al. CD56 expression is an indicator of poor clinical outcome in patients with acute promyelocytic leukemia treated with simultaneous all-trans-retinoic acid and chemotherapy. J Clin Oncol. 2000;18:1295–300. https://doi.org/10.1200/JCO.2000.18.6.1295.
67. Ito S, Ishida Y, Oyake T, et al. Clinical and biological significance of CD56 antigen expression in acute promyelocytic leukemia. Leuk Lymphoma. 2004;45:1783–9. https://doi.org/10.1080/10428190410001683624.
68. de Botton S, Sanz MA, Chevret S, et al. Extramedullary relapse in acute promyelocytic leukemia treated with all-trans retinoic acid and chemotherapy. Leukemia. 2005;20:35–41. https://doi.org/10.1038/sj.leu.2404006.
69. Montesinos P, Díaz-Mediavilla J, Debén G, et al. Central nervous system involvement at first relapse in patients with acute promyelocytic leukemia treated with all-trans retinoic acid and anthracycline monochemotherapy without intrathecal prophylaxis. Haematologica. 2009;94:1242–9. https://doi.org/10.3324/haematol.2009.007872.
70. Montesinos P, González JD, Gonzalez J, et al. Therapy-related myeloid neoplasms in patients with acute Promyelocytic leukemia treated with all-trans-retinoic acid and anthracycline-based chemotherapy. J Clin Oncol. 2010;28:3872–9. https://doi.org/10.1200/JCO.2010.29.2268.
71. Martínez-Cuadrón D, Montesinos P, Vellenga E, et al. Long-term outcome of elderly patients with newly diagnosed acute promyelocytic leukemia treated with ATRA plus anthracycline-based therapy. Leukemia accepted article preview 6 June 2017; doi: 10.1038/leu.2017.178.
72. Yanada M, Matsushita T, Asou N, et al. Severe hemorrhagic complications during remission induction therapy for acute promyelocytic leukemia: incidence, risk factors, and influence on outcome. Eur J Haematol. 2007;78:213–9. https://doi.org/10.1111/j.1600-0609.2006.00803.x.

8 First-Line Therapy for Acute Promyelocytic Leukemia: Chemotherapy-Based Approach

Aaron D. Goldberg and Martin S. Tallman

Introduction

The Role of Early ATRA

Patients with APL usually present with cytopenias with or without leukocytosis. Life-threatening coagulopathy also serves as one of the most concerning presentations of APL. In a patient with suspected acute leukemia, the presence of coagulopathy should prompt rapid evaluation of the peripheral smear for the possibility of APL. Even as this chapter focuses on chemotherapy, the paramount role of ATRA in APL must always be emphasized. Should APL be suspected, early treatment with ATRA must be initiated as soon as possible to induce APL blast differentiation and reverse or avert the development of the life-threatening coagulopathy. More than resistant disease, early death almost always from hemorrhage now represents the most important limitation to cure in APL [1–4]. Clinicians should not wait for the diagnostic confirmation of APL to initiate ATRA, as prompt administration of ATRA is likely critical to reduce the rate of early death [5].

A.D. Goldberg, M.D., Ph.D. • M.S. Tallman, M.D. (✉)
Leukemia Service, Memorial Sloan Kettering Cancer Center, Weill Cornell Medical College,
1275 York Avenue, New York, NY 10065, USA
e-mail: tallmanm@mskcc.org

Risk Stratification by White Blood Cell Count (WBC): Chemotherapy as a Component of Therapy for High-Risk APL

At diagnosis, patients with APL can be risk stratified for relapse into high-risk and low-risk disease, based on the presenting white blood cell count (WBC) [6–8]. Patients with high WBC (>10,000/μL) are considered to have high-risk disease, while patients with lower WBC (<10,000/μL) are considered to have low-risk disease. APL patients were previously risk stratified by WBC as well as platelet count into high-, intermediate-, and low-risk disease [7]. However, more recent data suggest that outcomes are similar in low- and intermediate-risk groups with contemporary therapies, thereby eliminating platelet count from risk stratification and enabling APL patients to be risk stratified only by WBC into high- and low-risk groups [8] (Fig. 8.1). Beyond blood counts, other factors including age greater than 60 years, male sex, and renal insufficiency with creatinine greater than 1.4 have been shown to be predictive of poor prognosis, largely due to death during induction [6–8]. Although data are mixed, some studies also suggest that APL patients with internal tandem duplication (ITD) of the FMS-like tyrosine kinase 3 gene (FLT3-ITD) may have an inferior prognosis, particularly patients treated with combined ATRA + idarubicin (AIDA) regimens [9–11].

O. Abla et al. (eds.), *Acute Promyelocytic Leukemia*, https://doi.org/10.1007/978-3-319-64257-4_8

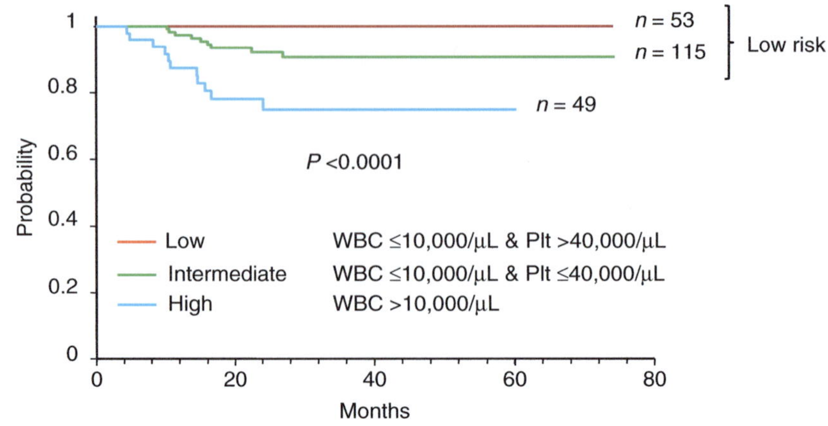

Fig. 8.1 Relapse-free survival by risk stratification in GIMEMA and PETHEMA trials. Kaplan-Meier product-limit estimate of relapse-free survival in the GIMEMA and PETHEMA trials according to risk groups defined by the predictive model. Figure is adapted from Sanz MA., et al., *Blood* 2000 [7]

Emerging data suggest this negative prognostic impact of FLT3-ITD in APL may be abrogated by the combined use of ATRA plus ATO [12]. However, at this time, despite the various prognostic factors noted above, only the presenting WBC is used to select the optimal choice of therapy.

The management of low-risk APL patients (WBC < 10,000/mcL) which accounts for approximately 75% of patients is addressed in other chapters. Notably, for patients with low-risk APL, recent studies have shown at least equivalent and apparently superior outcomes for ATRA plus ATO vs. ATRA plus chemotherapy [13, 14]. Therefore, in the modern management of APL, chemotherapy is generally not a component of standard therapy for low-risk disease. As this chapter highlights the role of first-line chemotherapy in APL, the remaining discussion focuses predominantly on patients with high-risk APL who would warrant combined chemotherapy + ATRA. Chemotherapy + ATRA also remains an option for low-risk patients unable to tolerate ATO. A detailed discussion of ATO-containing regimens will be provided in Chap. 9.

Tolerance of Anthracycline-Based Therapy

For patients with high-risk APL already started on treatment with ATRA, one of the first decision points is whether the patient can tolerate anthracycline-based chemotherapy. Given the potential cardiotoxicity of anthracyclines, cardiac evaluation with an echocardiogram or multiple-gated acquisition (MUGA) scan should be considered prior to anthracycline-based chemotherapy [8]. Delayed cardiomyopathy is a rare consequence of anthracycline-related toxicity in long-term disease-free survivors of APL [15]. Risk factors for anthracycline cardiotoxicity include cumulative anthracycline dose, rate of anthracycline administration, age, obesity, sex (with females at greater risk), and pre-existing cardiac risk factors [16].

Evolution of Chemotherapy and ATRA Regimens for APL

The current standard of care for newly diagnosed patients with high-risk APL remains ATRA- and anthracycline-based chemotherapy with or without ATO [17]. Prior to the introduction of ATRA, APL was treated with standard AML induction chemotherapy including anthracycline- and cytarabine-based chemotherapy. Anthracyclines have excellent activity as single agents in APL [18, 19]. One possible explanation for the high sensitivity of APL cells to anthracyclines involves reduced expression of the multidrug resistance (MDR1) gene product P-glycoprotein in APL in comparison to other leukemias [20, 21]. Even without the inclusion of modern therapies such as ATRA and arsenic, the majority of APL patients treated with anthracycline-based chemotherapy achieved complete remission (CR), with remission rates of 70–80% [22, 23]. However, with chemotherapy alone, early death from coagulopathy as well as relapse remained significant clinical barriers to cure for most APL patients [22–24]. Chemotherapy alone is also unlikely to lead to long-term cure in the absence of additional consolidation or maintenance therapy. In the North American Intergroup study I0129 (ECOG E2491), 5-year disease-free survival was 16% for APL patients randomized to induction and consolidation chemotherapy followed by observation without ATRA [25].

Therefore, the introduction of ATRA provided a powerful new tool in the treatment armamentarium for APL. ATRA targets the PML/RARa fusion protein, inducing differentiation of leukemic promyelocytes into mature cells [26–28]. During the 1980s and 1990s, single-agent ATRA was shown to have remarkable activity, with CR rates of 85% in APL [29].

The European APL91 trial and the North American Intergroup study I0129 (ECOG E2491) established that APL patients treated with ATRA had improved outcomes over those treated with chemotherapy alone [25, 30–32]. In the European APL91 trial, patients with newly diagnosed APL randomized to ATRA followed by chemotherapy had an improved survival and reduced relapse rate compared to patients randomized to chemotherapy alone [30, 31]. In the larger North American Intergroup study, single-agent ATRA was compared with daunorubicin and cytarabine in 401 patients with previously untreated APL. In this study, single-agent ATRA was shown to have equivalent rates of CR (70%) as induction chemotherapy with daunorubicin and cytarabine (73%) but markedly improved disease-free (69% vs. 29%) and overall survival (69% vs. 45%) at 5 years [25, 32]. These studies provided justification for the standard inclusion of ATRA in the treatment of APL. However, resistance and relapse are not uncommon for patients treated with single-agent ATRA, particularly if ATRA is only given as induction. The North American Intergroup study demonstrated a durable benefit for ATRA in both induction and maintenance therapy, as patients randomized to ATRA for both induction and maintenance had a 5-year DFS of 74%, in comparison to 55% for patients who received ATRA followed by observation. However, 35% of patients with high-risk APL failed to achieve a CR with ATRA alone, suggesting that there may be a role for additional chemotherapy for these high-risk patients [25]. In addition, differentiation syndrome remains a problem with ATRA monotherapy [33]. Multiple studies therefore tested combination therapies including ATRA and concurrent or sequential chemotherapy.

ATRA + Chemotherapy

Several large cooperative group studies demonstrated excellent outcomes with ATRA-based induction in combination with anthracycline-based chemotherapy, with greater than 90% of patients achieving CR [34, 35]. Although some of these patients relapsed with induction therapy alone, cure rates were increased to greater than 80% with the use of ATRA-based induction followed by consolidation with ATRA + anthracycline or cytarabine + anthracycline [34–36].

The European APL 93 trial demonstrated the superiority of concurrent ATRA + chemotherapy over sequential ATRA followed by chemotherapy. Chemotherapy in this study consisted of daunorubicin 60 mg/m^2/day for 3 days and cytarabine 200 mg/m^2/day for 7 days, starting on day 3 of ATRA for the concurrent group or after ATRA-induced CR for the sequential group. Chemotherapy was also added early to ATRA for increases in WBC. In this study of 413 newly diagnosed APL patients, the relapse rate at 2 years was 6% in the concurrent ATRA + chemotherapy group vs. 16% in the sequential ATRA followed by chemotherapy group [37].

The Italian GIMEMA 93 trial established the efficacy of the AIDA regimen (combined ATRA + idarubicin), consisting of induction chemotherapy with ATRA in combination with four 12 mg/m^2 doses of idarubicin given intravenously on days 2, 4, 6, and 8. With this regimen, 95% of patients achieved a hematologic remission [38, 39]. Patients then received three consolidation combination polychemotherapy regimens, with excellent event-free survival (EFS) of 79% at 2 years. The AIDA regimen provided the basis for further risk-adapted approaches that are still listed in NCCN Clinical Practice Guidelines in Oncology (NCCN Guidelines®) as appropriate first-line therapy for patients with high-risk APL [8, 35] (Fig. 8.2).

TREATMENT INDUCTION (HIGH RISK)		CONSOLIDATION THERAPY
Powell et al., Blood 2010. Intergroup C9710. **ATRA** 45mg/m^2 in divided doses until clinical remission + **daunorubicin** 50mg/m^2 x 4 days + **cytarabine** 200mg/m^2 x 7 days OR	→ At count recovery, LP and proceed with consolidation →	**Arsenic trioxide** 0.15mg/kg/day x 5 days for 5 weeks x 2 cycles, then **ATRA** 45mg/m^2 x 7 days + **daunorubicin** 50mg/m^2 x 3 days for 2 cycles
Iland et al., Blood 2012. APML4. **ATRA** 45mg/m^2 (days 1-36, divided) + age-adjusted **idarubicin** 6-12 mg/m^2 on days 2, 4, 6, 8 + **arsenic trioxide** 0.15 mg/kg (days 9-36 as 2h IV infusion) OR	→ At count recovery, LP and proceed with consolidation →	**ATRA** 45mg/m^2 x 28 days + **arsenic trioxide** 0.15mg/kg/day x 28 days x 1 cycle, then **ATRA** 45mg/m^2 x 7 d every 2 weeks x 3 + **arsenic trioxide** 0.15mg/kg/day x 5 days for 5 weeks x 1 cycle
Ades et al., Blood 2008. APL 2000. **ATRA** 45mg/m^2 in divided doses until clinical remission + **daunorubicin** 60mg/m^2 x 3 days + **cytarabine** 200mg/m^2 x 7 days OR	→ At count recovery, LP and proceed with consolidation →	**Daunorubicin** 60mg/m^2 x 3 days + **cytarabine** 200mg/m^2 x 7 days x 1 cycle, then **cytarabine** 2g/m^2 (age<50) or 1.5g/m2 (age 50-60) every 12 h x 5 days + **daunorubicin** 45mg/m^2 x 3 days x 1 cycle 5 doses of IT chemotherapy
Sanz et al., Blood 2010. PETHEMA LPA 2005 **ATRA** 45mg/m^2 in divided doses until clinical remission + **idarubicin** 12 mg/m^2 on days 2, 4, 6, 8 OR Clinical trial	→ At count recovery, LP and proceed with consolidation →	**ATRA** 45mg/m^2 x 15 days + **idarubicin** 5mg/m^2 and **cytarabine** 1g/m^2 x 4 days x 1 cycle, then **ATRA** x 15 days + **mitoxantrone** 10mg/m^2/day x 5 days x 1 cycle, then **ATRA** x 15 days + **idarubicin** 12mg/m^2 x 1 dose + **cytarabine** 150mg/m^2/8h x 4 days x 1 cycle

Fig. 8.2 Contemporary regimens for induction and consolidation therapy in high-risk APL. Highly effective induction and consolidation regimens supported by consensus guidelines for treatment of high-risk APL. ATRA, all-trans retinoic acid. Figure adapted with permission from the NCCN Clinical Practice Guidelines in Oncology (NCCN Guidelines®) for Acute Myeloid Leukemia V.3.2017. © 2017 National Comprehensive Cancer Network, Inc. All rights reserved. The NCCN Guidelines® and illustrations herein may not be reproduced in any form for any purpose without the express written permission of NCCN. To view the most recent and complete version of the NCCN Guidelines, go online to NCCN.org. The NCCN Guidelines are a work in progress that may be refined as often as new significant data becomes available. [8, 35, 41, 44, 49]. *ATRA all-trans* retinoic acid

The Spanish PETHEMA LPA 96 trial modified the AIDA regimen to reduce toxicity by omitting etoposide and cytarabine from consolidation [40]. In the PETHEMA LPA 96 trial, 51% of patients became PCR negative for *PML-RARA* after induction, and 93% were PCR negative after induction and consolidation. With this modified AIDA regimen, rates of 2-year OS were 82%, suggesting that cytarabine and etoposide may not be necessary for most APL patients.

Multivariate analysis of the GIMEMA 93 and PETHEMA LPA 96 trials demonstrated that the initial WBC and platelet counts in newly diagnosed APL patients provided robust independent prognostic value for patients who received AIDA-based therapies [7]. This analysis provided further evidence that the omission of non-intercalating drugs such as cytarabine and etoposide did not lead to inferior outcomes for most patients. However, APL patients with presenting WBC >10,000/mcL had inferior RFS with AIDA induction, providing justification for risk-adapted approaches based on WBC (Fig. 8.1). In the PETHEMA LPA99 risk-adapted study by Sanz and colleagues, all patients received AIDA induction followed by consolidation chemotherapy, with ATRA added to consolidation cycles 1 and 3 in all but low-risk patients (WBC < 10,000/mcL and platelets > 40,000/mcL) [6]. The LPA99 study demonstrated that ATRA in consolidation therapy significantly reduced rates of relapse from 20.1 to 8.7%. This benefit of ATRA in consolidation was most notable in intermediate-risk patients, where relapse rates decreased from 14 to 2.5% [6].

Role of Cytarabine in High-Risk APL

Given the excellent outcomes of the modified AIDA regimen which eliminated cytarabine, the role of cytarabine in APL induction and consolidation chemotherapy remains controversial. Comparison of the French APL 2000 trial and the PETHEMA LPA 99 trials provides some insight into the role of cytarabine [41, 42]. Both the APL 2000 and the PETHEMA LPA 99 trials used ATRA in combination with chemotherapy for induction. The European APL 2000 trial combined ATRA with 7 + 3 (cytarabine 200 mg/m^2/day × 7 days and daunorubicin 60 mg/m^2/day × 3 days), while the PETHEMA LPA 99 study used an AIDA induction regimen. APL 2000 and PETHEMA LPA 99 also provided different consolidation approaches that were risk stratified based on the presenting WBC. No PETHEMA LPA 99 patients received cytarabine. However, all high-risk APL 2000 patients received cytarabine during induction as well as consolidation in combination with ATRA and daunorubicin. For high-risk patients, rates of CR (95.1% vs. 83.6%, $P = 0.018$) and 3-year OS (91.5% vs. 80.8%, $P = 0.026$) were significantly higher in the cytarabine-containing APL 2000 vs. LPA 99 trial. In an initial analysis of 104 high-risk patients in the LPA 99 trial, there was also a trend toward a lower 3-year incidence of relapse in the APL 2000 trial (9.9% in APL 2000 vs. 18.5% in LPA 99, $P = 0.12$), further suggesting a potential role for cytarabine in high-risk patients. In the final analysis of a total of 140 high-risk patients in the cytarabine-free LPA 99 trial, the 3-year cumulative incidence of relapse (CIR) was even higher at 26% [35]. In contrast, for patients with WBC < 10,000/mcL, CR rates and 3-year OS were similar, but rates of relapse were higher in the APL 2000 trial vs. the LPA 99 trial (14.3% vs. 4.2%), indicating that this non-cytarabine containing AIDA-based regimen is appropriate for low-risk patients. Based on these data, the APL 2000 induction and consolidation regimen using ATRA + chemotherapy including both daunorubicin and cytarabine represents one standard approach for treatment of high-risk APL [8, 41] (Fig. 8.2).

Although cytarabine may be reasonably excluded from AIDA-based therapy for low-risk APL, recent data indicate that cytarabine should not be excluded from regimens using daunorubicin [43]. Longer-term follow-up from the APL 2000 trial demonstrated unacceptably high rates of relapse for patients treated without cytarabine. Even in low-risk APL patients with WBC < 10,000/mcL, those who received daunorubicin without cytarabine had a 7-year CIR of 28.6% vs. 12.9% for those who received daunorubicin and cytarabine. This study therefore suggests that if daunorubicin is used as the anthracycline for APL induction and consolidation, cytarabine may not be dispensable for patients in any risk group [43].

Cytarabine has also been studied in combination with ATRA and idarubicin during consolidation therapy following AIDA-based induction for high-risk APL patients younger than 60 in the PETHEMA LPA 2005 trial [35]. The LPA 2005 trial followed the excellent results of the risk-adapted PETHEMA LPA 99 trial and was designed with the goal of further improving outcomes for younger high-risk APL patients. In the LPA 2005 trial, for high-risk patients younger than 60 years, cytarabine was added to the combination of ATRA and idarubicin during cycles 1 and 3 of consolidation therapy. Low- and intermediate-risk patients received a reduced course of mitoxantrone for the second consolidation course and did not receive cytarabine. For high-risk patients in the LPA 2005 trial, the 3-year relapse rate was 11%, significantly lower ($P = 0.03$) than the 3-year relapse rate of 26% in the LPA 99 trial. The 3-year DFS rates were 92% for the entire LPA 2005 study, with excellent 3-year DFS of 82% for high-risk patients. Therefore, the LPA2005 trial regimen using AIDA-based induction followed by ATRA + idarubicin + cytarabine for cycles 1 and 3 of consolidation and ATRA + mitoxantrone for cycle 2 of consolidation now represents another standard approach for treatment of high-risk APL [8, 35]. The APL 2000 and LPA 2005 regimens have never been directly compared, and they both represent highly effective approaches for induction and consolidation therapy for high-risk APL patients (Fig. 8.2).

In the modern era, following the demonstration of arsenic trioxide (ATO) as the most active single agent in APL, multiple studies have also tested combinations of ATRA, ATO, and chemotherapy. In particular, the APML4 regimen including combination ATRA + ATO + idarubicin for induction represents a highly efficacious option for treatment of high-risk APL patients [8, 44–46]. Please see Chaps. 9 and 10 for details regarding the use of ATO with and without ATRA and chemotherapy.

Bone Marrow Evaluation After Induction Therapy

The timing of bone marrow evaluation after induction therapy for APL differs from evaluation in the setting of other subtypes of AML. With modern regimens, much of the efficacy of APL induction therapy results from prolonged ATRA-induced differentiation of APL promyelocytes, in addition to the more rapid cytotoxic effects of chemotherapy and the induction of apoptosis caused by ATO [26–28, 47, 48]. Therefore, an initial bone marrow evaluation on day 14 is too early to adequately evaluate the effects of APL induction therapy. Contemporary consensus guidelines recommend marrow evaluation in APL after recovery of blood counts, often 4–6 weeks after induction therapy. While cytogenetic evaluation may no longer detect the t(15;17) translocation after modern induction therapy, PCR for molecular detection of PML-RARa may remain positive. Therefore, additional therapy for APL in the form of consolidation is required before assessment of molecular remission [8].

Consolidation Regimens

Following the use of induction therapy, the goal of additional consolidation therapy is to eliminate residual APL cells to achieve a durable molecular remission and prevent relapse [8, 17]. As noted above, various trials including the North American Intergroup study E2491 have shown that outcomes for APL patients who underwent induction therapy but failed to undergo further therapy had higher rates of relapse than patients who received further therapy with consolidation or maintenance [25].

For high-risk APL patients, chemotherapy is included in consolidation regimens for all modern standard therapies with the exception of the APML4 trial, which uses ATRA and ATO during consolidation and includes chemotherapy only during induction and maintenance [44, 45]. Anthracyclines, such as daunorubicin and idarubicin, and the related anthraquinone, mitoxantrone represent key components of consolidation for contemporary regimens including the Intergroup C9710, APL 2000, and PETHEMA LPA 2005 trials [35, 41, 49] (Fig. 8.2). As these consolidation regimens may include high cumulative doses of cardiotoxic medications, repeat cardiac evaluation is important prior to initiating each cycle of consolidation chemotherapy containing anthracyclines or mitoxantrone [8]. The pyrimidine analog cytarabine is also a component of consolidation therapy in the APL 2000 and LPA 2005 trials, and clinicians following these protocols may need to dose adjust for age or renal dysfunction [35, 41].

Differentiation or apoptosis-inducing therapies such as ATRA ± ATO also serve as critically important components of contemporary consolidation regimens for high-risk APL. As described above, the inclusion of these agents during consolidation is based upon multiple studies showing improvements in DFS and OS with the use of ATRA and ATO [6, 35, 41, 44, 45, 49]. For example, the LPA99 study demonstrated that adding ATRA to consolidation therapy significantly reduced rates of relapse [6]. This finding was confirmed by the GIMEMA AIDA-2000 trial, which demonstrated that the inclusion of ATRA in consolidation particularly improved outcomes for high-risk patients [36]. The Intergroup C9710 study demonstrated that adding two cycles of ATO consolidation prior to two cycles of ATRA + daunorubicin consolidation improved outcomes including DFS and OS across APL risk groups [49]. Even in the ATRA and ATO era, chemotherapy likely plays an important role for patients with high-risk APL, as evidenced by the poor outcomes for high-risk APL patients with ATRA or ATO monotherapy [32, 50].

Contemporary protocols therefore still include chemotherapy during consolidation or maintenance for patients with high-risk APL. Both the Intergroup C9710 and PETHEMA LPA 2005 protocols use ATRA in combination with chemotherapy during consolidation therapy for high-risk APL, while the APML4 trial uses ATRA + ATO without chemotherapy for consolidation and reintroduces low-dose chemotherapy + ATRA during maintenance (Figs. 8.2 and 8.3) [44, 45, 49]. Despite the omission of chemotherapy during consolidation, the APML4 trial using only ATRA + ATO consolidation has excellent 5-year OS rates of 87% and DFS rates of 95% for high-risk patients [44, 45] (Table 8.1). The European APL 2000 study uses

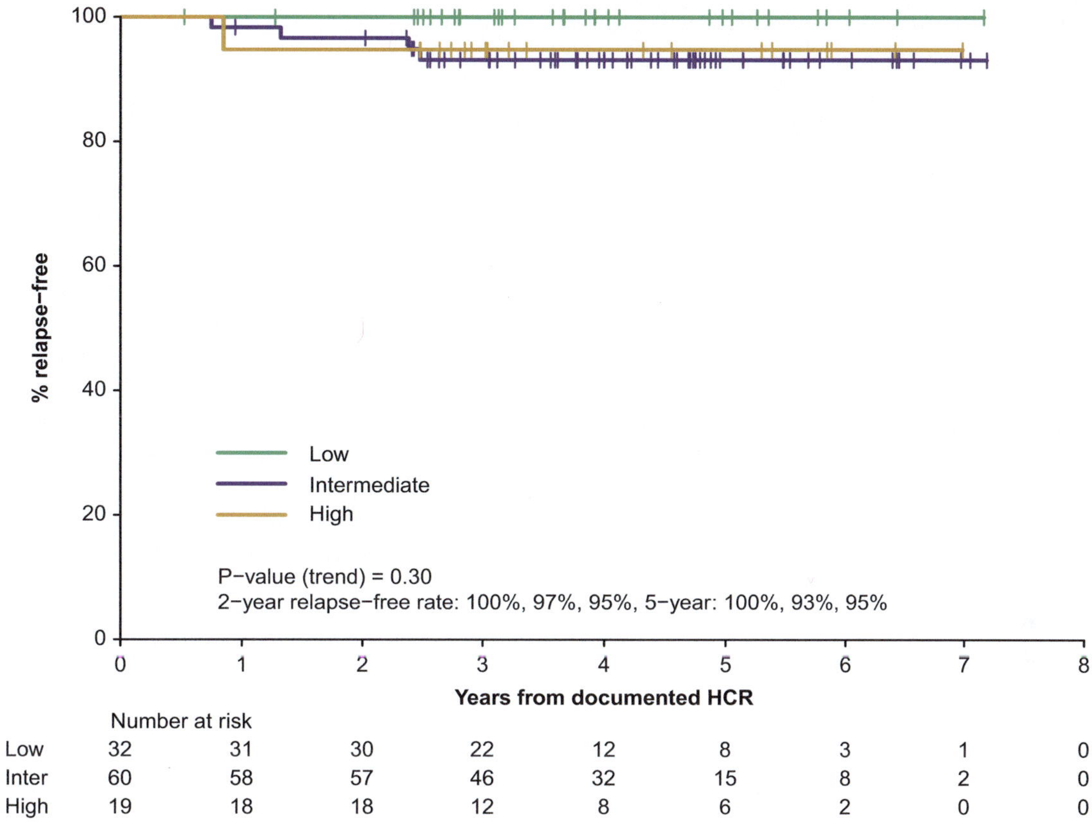

Fig. 8.3 Relapse-free survival by risk stratification in APML4. Kaplan-Meier curves for relapse-free survival following achievement of documented hematologic complete remission (HCR) in the APML4 trial, stratified by Sanz risk groups. Figure from Collins M, Di Iulio J, Beresford J. Australasian Leukaemia & Lymphoma Group APML4 Statistical Report, June 2013, courtesy of H Iland (APML4 principal investigator) [46]

Table 8.1 Outcomes for selected trials of ATRA + risk-adapted chemotherapy vs. APML4 in high-risk APL

	Number	Median follow-up (months)	IDA equivalent (mg/m^2)	Ara-C (g/m^2)	DFS (%)	CIR (%)	OS (%)
ALLG APML4 [44, 45]	23	50	48	0	95	5	87
European APL2000 [43]	74	103	99	22.8	–	7	88
PETHEMA LPA2005 [35]	118	28	122	5.8	82	14	79
GIMEMA AIDA2000 [36]	129	59	122	6.3	85	9	83

only chemotherapy for consolidation, but these cycles of consolidation chemotherapy are sandwiched between ATRA + chemotherapy during induction and maintenance [41].

In choosing consolidation and maintenance therapies following induction for high-risk disease, clinicians should follow the specific consolidation and maintenance regimen for the protocol used for induction therapy [8]. With the participation of hundreds of APL patients in numerous clinical trials as described above, treatment outcomes have continued to improve over the last several decades, transforming APL into a largely curable disease. However, realization of this success for individual patients depends upon rigorous adherence to established protocols. Although the outstanding outcomes of protocols such as APML4 might tempt clinicians to use ATRA + ATO consolidation following any induction regimen, mixing and matching regimens should be strongly discouraged outside of the context of a clinical trial. One exceptional circumstance involves consolidation therapy for a high-risk APL patient with cardiotoxicity or for whom an anthracycline is otherwise contraindicated. In that setting, consensus guidelines suggest the use of consolidation with combination ATRA and ATO as recently described for low-risk APL [8, 13].

Maintenance Therapy

The goal of maintenance therapy is to maintain molecular remission, decrease rates of relapse, and ideally to increase rates of cure. Given the high efficacy of treatment strategies in the modern era of ATRA + ATO, the role of maintenance therapy in contemporary APL treatment is controversial and may not be necessary for patients who achieve a molecular CR [51–53]. In addition, the use of chemotherapy in maintenance has the potential to harm some patients who might already be cured with induction and consolidation therapy [17]. Maintenance is therefore no longer a component of therapy for low-risk APL patients treated with ATRA + ATO induction and consolidation [13]. However, based upon evidence from previous clinical trials discussed below, the use of maintenance therapy still represents the standard of care for patients with high-risk APL [8, 17].

Agents used in maintenance regimens for APL include ATRA, the folate antimetabolite methotrexate (MTX), and the purine antagonist 6-mercaptopurine (6-MP). The North American Intergroup E2491 study showed superior 5-year DFS with maintenance ATRA over observation (61% vs. 36%, $P < 0.0001$) [25, 32]. The European APL93 trial tested four different maintenance strategies: no maintenance, intermittent ATRA, continuous chemotherapy with 6-MP and MTX, and combination ATRA + 6-MP + MTX [34, 37]. In this study, the 10-year CIR was significantly decreased from 43.2% to 33%, 23.4%, and 13.4%, respectively, with the regimens above, with the lowest incidence of relapse seen with ATRA in combination with chemotherapy ($P < 0.001$). The greatest benefit of maintenance therapy was seen in patients with WBC > 5000/μL, with a decrease in CIR from 68.4% to 53.1%, 32.8%, and 20.6% ($P < 0.001$). However, this decrease in relapse from maintenance therapy came at the price of increased toxicity, particularly in older patients, with a marked 21.7% 10-year cumulative incidence of death in CR for patients older than 65 years, primarily from myelosuppression [34, 37].

A recent Cochrane review conducted a meta-analysis to evaluate the role of maintenance therapy for APL in CR1 [51]. In this meta-analysis of ten randomized controlled trials in APL, maintenance therapy had no statistically significant effect on OS but did improve DFS. Studies including the Japanese APL 97 study and the AIDA 0493 trial have suggested that there are no long-term benefits to maintenance therapy [54, 55]. The SWOG 0521 trial randomized low-risk patients in molecular CR after standard induction and consolidation including ATO to maintenance ATRA + 6-MP + MTX vs. observation. Although enrollment was stopped early because of slow accrual, no relapses were seen in the 68 patients randomized to either arm with a median follow-up of 36 months. This study therefore suggests that if an intensive post-remission consolidation regimen including ATO is used to achieve molecular CR, further maintenance may not be necessary for low-risk patients [52]. However, the best long-term outcomes for high-risk patients have all been achieved using protocols that use maintenance therapy, including the APL

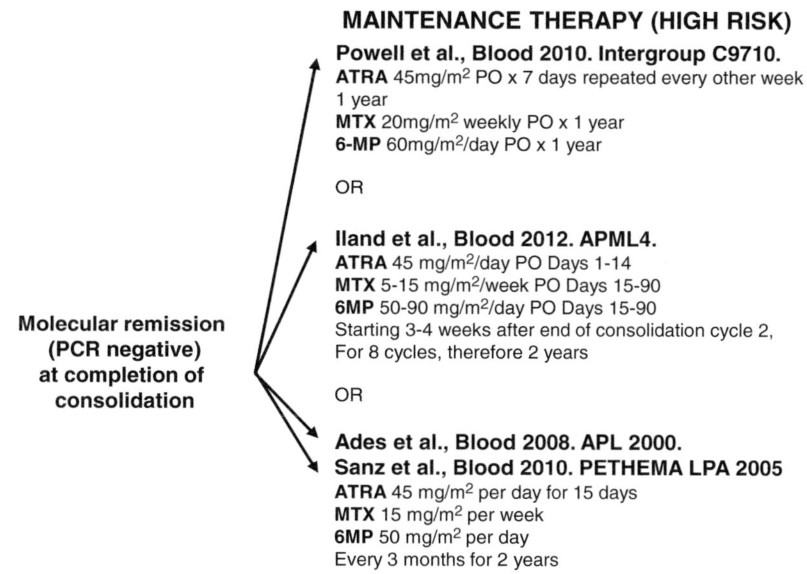

Fig. 8.4 Maintenance therapy in high-risk APL. Regimens for maintenance therapy in high-risk APL patients, following achievement of molecular remission at completion of consolidation [35, 41, 44, 49]. *ATRA all-trans* retinoic acid, *MTX* methotrexate, *6MP* 6-mercaptopurine

2000, LPA 2005, APML4, and Intergroup C9710 [35, 41, 44, 45, 49]. Improvements in outcomes for high-risk APL patients over time are likely due to a variety of factors, but combined ATRA + chemotherapy maintenance has been suggested as a factor leading to reduced rates of relapse in European clinical trials [56].

Following the completion of consolidation therapy, APL patients should be assessed for molecular remission using RT-PCR on bone marrow samples. Patients who are PCR positive and remain so on a repeat bone marrow PCR in 2–4 weeks should be treated as relapsed APL [8] (see Chap. 13). High-risk APL patients who are PCR negative following consolidation should be treated with maintenance therapy per the initial treatment protocol (Fig. 8.4). The importance of not mixing and matching treatment regimens applies to maintenance strategies as well as consolidation as discussed above, although most modern maintenance approaches are nearly identical. In contemporary treatment of APL, the APL 2000 and PETHEMA LPA 2005 protocols include the same regimen of maintenance as the LPA 99 trial: 2 years of 6-mercaptopurine (50 mg/m^2/day), methotrexate (15 mg/m^2/week), and intermittent ATRA (45 mg/m^2/day) for 15 days every 3 months [6, 35, 41]. The APML4 trial also uses a nearly identical regimen for 2 years of maintenance therapy starting 3–4 weeks following the end of consolidation cycle 2 [44, 45]. The North American Intergroup C9710 attempted to evaluate the role of maintenance ATRA vs. ATRA + chemotherapy but was underpowered to detect a difference. For those patients who received ATRA + chemotherapy maintenance, the regimen was a similar combination of ATRA, MTX, and 6-MP, although only given for 1 year [49] (Fig. 8.4). As it is advisable to follow an established protocol from induction through consolidation and maintenance, foregoing maintenance therapy for high-risk APL patients should not be undertaken outside of a clinical trial.

CNS Relapse and the Role of Prophylactic Intrathecal Chemotherapy

The role of prophylactic intrathecal (IT) chemotherapy to prevent CNS relapse remains controversial. However, several lines of evidence suggest that prophylactic IT chemotherapy may be important for preventing CNS relapse, particularly in high-risk APL patients. Although ATRA and ATO cross the blood-brain barrier, CSF concentrations may vary significantly from patient to patient and may not be adequate for significant antileukemic activity [57]. As treatment of systemic disease improved over time with the use of ATRA, relapsed CNS disease was increasingly reported in APL patients who presented with high WBC [58]. In the European experience, trials with prophylactic IT chemotherapy for high-risk APL patients demonstrated decreased rates of relapse. Patients with high-risk APL had a 4% incidence of CNS relapse in the APL 93 trial, while the APL 2000 trial had no CNS relapses at 5 years [56]. This decreased rate of relapse may have been due to the use of five doses of IT chemotherapy in high-risk APL patients in APL 2000, as well as the use of higher doses of cytarabine during consolidation [56]. Longer-term 7-year follow-up from the APL 2000 trial did reveal one CNS relapse, although this occurred in a patient with low-risk APL treated without cytarabine and without prophylactic IT chemotherapy [43]. For patients with high-risk APL, lumbar puncture should therefore be considered at count recovery prior to consolidation therapy as the CNS can serve as a sanctuary site for residual APL cells [8, 58]. Consensus guidelines support the use of four to six doses of IT chemotherapy with MTX or liposomal cytarabine combined with corticosteroids to be given during consolidation for patients with high-risk APL [8].

Aggressive Supportive Care for Thrombocytopenia in the Setting of Chemotherapy and Coagulopathy

Life-threatening coagulopathy represents a potentially catastrophic complication of APL and is discussed in detail elsewhere (see Chap. 5). With the advent of remarkably effective therapies in the modern era of treatment for APL, early death from coagulopathy has emerged as the single most important barrier to cure [1–4, 59–62]. The prompt use of ATRA is likely critical to prevent early death from hemorrhage [59, 61, 63]. From the perspective of induction chemotherapy for high-risk APL, cytotoxic chemotherapy including anthracyclines and cytarabine has the potential to exacerbate thrombocytopenia. In addition to vigilant monitoring of coagulation parameters and repletion of fibrinogen with cryoprecipitate, meticulous monitoring of the CBC and frequent transfusions of platelets are often needed to prevent death from hemorrhage. Platelet counts should be maintained above 30,000–50,000/μL and fibrinogen above 100–150 mg/dL [5].

Differentiation Syndrome and the Role of Prophylactic Steroids and Early Chemotherapy for High-Risk APL

Differentiation syndrome represents a unique complication of APL therapy (see Chap. 17). Upon treatment of APL blasts with ATRA, the block to lineage differentiation induced by PML/RARα is reversed, and the resulting surge of differentiated myeloid cells can result in pleural and pericardial effusions, pulmonary infiltrates, dyspnea, hypotension, and renal failure [64, 65]. Prophylactic steroids with either prednisone or dexamethasone are recommended for patients with high WBC count to prevent differentiation syndrome [8, 66]. As the risk of differentiation syndrome is increased in patients with high WBC [67], early introduction of chemotherapy is recommended for high-risk disease. For APL patients with WBC > 10,000/μL, some expert guidelines recommend initiation of chemotherapy as early as day 1 within a few hours of the first dose of ATRA, both to reduce the risk of differentiation syndrome and to achieve better control of coagulopathy [5, 64].

Alternate Role of Chemotherapy: Patients Unable to Tolerate Arsenic Trioxide

Current standard treatment for APL utilizes chemotherapy mostly in the setting of high-risk disease. However, unusual circumstances may also warrant the use of chemotherapy in low-risk APL to increase rates of cure. Rarely, a low-risk APL patient on ATRA + ATO may experience a complication from ATO such as pancreatitis or a prolonged QT interval leading to significant arrhythmia. ATO is commonly associated with QT interval prolongation (24–32%), but clinically significant arrhythmias are rare and can generally be avoided with appropriate precautions including careful monitoring and electrolyte repletion [68]. In cases of unusual complications precluding further ATO, switching to a non-ATO chemotherapy-based approach such as APL 2000 or LPA 2005 is reasonable, as combined ATRA + chemotherapy improves rates of cure over ATRA alone [25, 32].

Conclusion

Despite the development of highly effective disease-directed agents such as ATRA and ATO, cytotoxic chemotherapy still plays an important role in contemporary treatment of APL. Although recent data demonstrate that chemotherapy is not required for patients with low-risk APL [13, 69, 70], chemotherapy remains an important component of curative therapy for high-risk disease. Several ATRA + chemotherapy combination approaches are appropriate for standard induction therapy, and ATRA + ATO + idarubicin induction results in particularly excellent outcomes [35, 41, 44, 45, 49]. Early ATRA and aggressive supportive care remain critical for preventing early death from coagulopathy and hemorrhage [5, 59, 61, 63]. Early chemotherapy following ATRA is also important to reduce the risk of differentiation syndrome and for controlling coagulopathy in high-risk patients [5, 64]. Prophylactic steroids are recommended to reduce the risk of differentiation syndrome in this patient population [8, 66].

Various agents are used for consolidation and maintenance therapies, including ATRA, ATO, anthracyclines, and cytarabine during consolidation, as well as ATRA, 6-MP, and MTX for maintenance. However, mixing and matching induction, consolidation, and maintenance regimens should be strongly discouraged. Following induction, consolidation and maintenance therapy for patients with high-risk APL should be given according to the initial protocol. Although controversial, prophylactic intrathecal chemotherapy during consolidation is advisable to prevent CNS relapse in high-risk APL patients [8]. Some APL patients experience long-term complications including therapy-related myeloid neoplasms as well as cardiomyopathy [15, 70]. Although APL has been transformed over the last several decades into a largely curable disease, future studies are needed to reduce rates of early death and increase rates of cure and to minimize the use of chemotherapy where possible.

References

1. Lehmann S, Ravn A, Carlsson L, Antunovic P, Deneberg S, Mollgard L, et al. Continuing high early death rate in acute promyelocytic leukemia: a population-based report from the Swedish Adult Acute Leukemia Registry. Leukemia. 2011;25(7):1128–34.
2. Paulson K, Serebrin A, Lambert P, Bergeron J, Everett J, Kew A, et al. Acute promyelocytic leukaemia is characterized by stable incidence and improved survival that is restricted to patients managed in leukaemia referral centres: a pan-Canadian epidemiological study. Br J Haematol. 2014;166(5):660–6.
3. Rahme R, Thomas X, Recher C, Vey N, Delaunay J, Deconinck E, et al. Early death in acute promyelocytic leukemia (APL) in French centers: a multicenter study in 399 patients. Leukemia. 2014;28(12):2422–4.
4. Altman JK, Rademaker A, Cull E, Weitner BB, Ofran Y, Rosenblat TL, et al. Administration of ATRA to newly diagnosed patients with acute promyelocytic leukemia is delayed contributing to early hemorrhagic death. Leuk Res. 2013;37(9):1004–9.
5. Sanz MA, Grimwade D, Tallman MS, Lowenberg B, Fenaux P, Estey EH, et al. Management of acute promyelocytic leukemia: recommendations from an expert panel on behalf of the European LeukemiaNet. Blood. 2009;113(9):1875–91.
6. Sanz MA, Martin G, Gonzalez M, Leon A, Rayon C, Rivas C, et al. Risk-adapted treatment of acute promyelocytic leukemia with all-trans-retinoic acid and anthracycline monochemotherapy: a multicenter study by the PETHEMA group. Blood. 2004;103(4):1237–43.
7. Sanz MA, Lo Coco F, Martin G, Avvisati G, Rayon C, Barbui T, et al. Definition of relapse risk and role of nonanthracycline drugs for consolidation in patients with acute promyelocytic leukemia: a joint study of the PETHEMA and GIMEMA cooperative groups. Blood. 2000;96(4):1247–53.
8. Referenced with permission from the NCCN Clinical Practice Guidelines in Oncology (NCCN Guidelines®) for Acute Myeloid Leukemia V.3.2017. © National Comprehensive Cancer Network, Inc. 2017. All rights reserved. Accessed August 21, 2017. To view the most recent and complete version of the guideline, go online to NCCN.org. NCCN makes no warranties of any kind whatsoever regarding their content, use or application and disclaims any responsibility for their application or use in any way. [Internet].

9. Molica M, Breccia M. FLT3-ITD in acute promyelocytic leukemia: clinical distinct profile but still controversial prognosis. Leuk Res. 2015;39(4):397–9.
10. Breccia M, Loglisci G, Loglisci MG, Ricci R, Diverio D, Latagliata R, et al. FLT3-ITD confers poor prognosis in patients with acute promyelocytic leukemia treated with AIDA protocols: long-term follow-up analysis. Haematologica. 2013;98(12):e161–3.
11. Schnittger S, Bacher U, Haferlach C, Kern W, Alpermann T, Haferlach T. Clinical impact of FLT3 mutation load in acute promyelocytic leukemia with t(15;17)/PML-RARA. Haematologica. 2011;96(12):1799–807.
12. Cicconi L, Divona M, Ciardi C, Ottone T, Ferrantini A, Lavorgna S, et al. PML-RARalpha kinetics and impact of FLT3-ITD mutations in newly diagnosed acute promyelocytic leukaemia treated with ATRA and ATO or ATRA and chemotherapy. Leukemia. 2016;30(10):1987–92.
13. Lo-Coco F, Avvisati G, Vignetti M, Thiede C, Orlando SM, Iacobelli S, et al. Retinoic acid and arsenic trioxide for acute promyelocytic leukemia. N Engl J Med. 2013;369(2):111–21.
14. Lo-Coco F, Orlando SM, Platzbecker U. Treatment of acute promyelocytic leukemia. N Engl J Med. 2013;369(15):1472.
15. Thomas X, Le QH, Fiere D. Anthracycline-related toxicity requiring cardiac transplantation in long-term disease-free survivors with acute promyelocytic leukemia. Ann Hematol. 2002;81(9):504–7.
16. Raj S, Franco VI, Lipshultz SE. Anthracycline-induced cardiotoxicity: a review of pathophysiology, diagnosis, and treatment. Curr Treat Options Cardiovasc Med. 2014;16(6):315.
17. Watts JM, Tallman MS. Acute promyelocytic leukemia: what is the new standard of care? Blood Rev. 2014;28(5):205–12.
18. Avvisati G, Mandelli F, Petti MC, Vegna ML, Spadea A, Liso V, et al. Idarubicin (4-demethoxydaunorubicin) as single agent for remission induction of previously untreated acute promyelocytic leukemia: a pilot study of the Italian cooperative group GIMEMA. Eur J Haematol. 1990;44(4):257–60.
19. Bernard J, Weil M, Boiron M, Jacquillat C, Flandrin G, Gemon MF. Acute promyelocytic leukemia: results of treatment by daunorubicin. Blood. 1973;41(4):489–96.
20. Paietta E, Andersen J, Racevskis J, Gallagher R, Bennett J, Yunis J, et al. Significantly lower P-glycoprotein expression in acute promyelocytic leukemia than in other types of acute myeloid leukemia: immunological, molecular and functional analyses. Leukemia. 1994;8(6):968–73.
21. Michieli M, Damiani D, Ermacora A, Geromin A, Michelutti A, Masolini P, et al. P-glycoprotein (PGP), lung resistance-related protein (LRP) and multidrug resistance-associated protein (MRP) expression in acute promyelocytic leukaemia. Br J Haematol. 2000;108(4):703–9.
22. Cunningham I, Gee TS, Reich LM, Kempin SJ, Naval AN, Clarkson BD. Acute promyelocytic leukemia: treatment results during a decade at Memorial Hospital. Blood. 1989;73(5):1116–22.
23. Head DR, Kopecky KJ, Willman C, Appelbaum FR. Treatment outcome with chemotherapy in acute promyelocytic leukemia: the Southwest Oncology Group (SWOG) experience. Leukemia. 1994;8(Suppl 2):S38–41.
24. Rodeghiero F, Avvisati G, Castaman G, Barbui T, Mandelli F. Early deaths and anti-hemorrhagic treatments in acute promyelocytic leukemia. A GIMEMA retrospective study in 268 consecutive patients. Blood. 1990;75(11):2112–7.
25. Tallman MS. All-trans retinoic acid in acute promyelocytic leukemia: long-term outcome and prognostic factor analysis from the North American Intergroup protocol. Blood. 2002;100(13):4298–302.
26. Castaigne S, Chomienne C, Daniel MT, Ballerini P, Berger R, Fenaux P, et al. All-trans retinoic acid as a differentiation therapy for acute promyelocytic leukemia. I. Clinical results. Blood. 1990;76(9):1704–9.
27. Chomienne C, Ballerini P, Balitrand N, Daniel MT, Fenaux P, Castaigne S, et al. All-trans retinoic acid in acute promyelocytic leukemias. II. In vitro studies: structure-function relationship. Blood. 1990;76(9):1710–7.
28. Warrell RP Jr, Frankel SR, Miller WH Jr, Scheinberg DA, Itri LM, Hittelman WN, et al. Differentiation therapy of acute promyelocytic leukemia with tretinoin (all-trans-retinoic acid). N Engl J Med. 1991;324(20):1385–93.
29. Huang ME, Ye YC, Chen SR, Chai JR, Lu JX, Zhoa L, et al. Use of all-trans retinoic acid in the treatment of acute promyelocytic leukemia. Blood. 1988;72(2):567–72.
30. Fenaux P, Le Deley MC, Castaigne S, Archimbaud E, Chomienne C, Link H, et al. Effect of all transretinoic acid in newly diagnosed acute promyelocytic leukemia. Results of a multicenter randomized trial. European APL 91 Group. Blood. 1993;82(11):3241–9.
31. Fenaux P, Chastang C, Chomienne C, Degos L. Tretinoin with chemotherapy in newly diagnosed acute promyelocytic leukaemia. European APL Group. Lancet. 1994;343(8904):1033.
32. Tallman MS, Andersen JW, Schiffer CA, Appelbaum FR, Feusner JH, Ogden A, et al. All-trans-retinoic acid in acute promyelocytic leukemia. N Engl J Med. 1997;337(15):1021–8.
33. Tallman MS, Andersen JW, Schiffer CA, Appelbaum FR, Feusner JH, Ogden A, et al. Clinical description of 44 patients with acute promyelocytic leukemia who developed the retinoic acid syndrome. Blood. 2000;95(1):90–5.
34. Ades L, Guerci A, Raffoux E, Sanz M, Chevallier P, Lapusan S, et al. Very long-term outcome of acute promyelocytic leukemia after treatment with all-trans retinoic acid and chemotherapy: the European APL Group experience. Blood. 2010;115(9):1690–6.
35. Sanz MA, Montesinos P, Rayon C, Holowiecka A, de la Serna J, Milone G, et al. Risk-adapted treatment of acute promyelocytic leukemia based on all-trans retinoic acid and anthracycline with addition of cytarabine in consolidation therapy for high-risk patients:

further improvements in treatment outcome. Blood. 2010;115(25):5137–46.

36. Lo-Coco F, Avvisati G, Vignetti M, Breccia M, Gallo E, Rambaldi A, et al. Front-line treatment of acute promyelocytic leukemia with AIDA induction followed by risk-adapted consolidation for adults younger than 61 years: results of the AIDA-2000 trial of the GIMEMA Group. Blood. 2010;116(17):3171–9.
37. Fenaux P, Chastang C, Chevret S, Sanz M, Dombret H, Archimbaud E, et al. A randomized comparison of all transretinoic acid (ATRA) followed by chemotherapy and ATRA plus chemotherapy and the role of maintenance therapy in newly diagnosed acute promyelocytic leukemia. The European APL Group. Blood. 1999;94(4):1192–200.
38. Mandelli F, Diverio D, Avvisati G, Luciano A, Barbui T, Bernasconi C, et al. Molecular remission in PML/RAR alpha-positive acute promyelocytic leukemia by combined all-trans retinoic acid and idarubicin (AIDA) therapy. Gruppo Italiano-Malattie Ematologiche Maligne dell'Adulto and Associazione Italiana di Ematologia ed Oncologia Pediatrica Cooperative Groups. Blood. 1997;90(3):1014–21.
39. Avvisati G, Lo Coco F, Diverio D, Falda M, Ferrara F, Lazzarino M, et al. AIDA (all-trans retinoic acid + idarubicin) in newly diagnosed acute promyelocytic leukemia: a Gruppo Italiano Malattie Ematologiche Maligne dell'Adulto (GIMEMA) pilot study. Blood. 1996;88(4):1390–8.
40. Sanz MA, Martin G, Rayon C, Esteve J, Gonzalez M, Diaz-Mediavilla J, et al. A modified AIDA protocol with anthracycline-based consolidation results in high antileukemic efficacy and reduced toxicity in newly diagnosed PML/RARalpha-positive acute promyelocytic leukemia. PETHEMA group. Blood. 1999;94(9):3015–21.
41. Ades L, Sanz MA, Chevret S, Montesinos P, Chevallier P, Raffoux E, et al. Treatment of newly diagnosed acute promyelocytic leukemia (APL): a comparison of French-Belgian-Swiss and PETHEMA results. Blood. 2008;111(3):1078–84.
42. Ades L, Chevret S, Raffoux E, de Botton S, Guerci A, Pigneux A, et al. Is cytarabine useful in the treatment of acute promyelocytic leukemia? Results of a randomized trial from the European Acute Promyelocytic Leukemia Group. J Clin Oncol. 2006;24(36):5703–10.
43. Ades L, Chevret S, Raffoux E, Guerci-Bresler A, Pigneux A, Vey N, et al. Long-term follow-up of European APL 2000 trial, evaluating the role of cytarabine combined with ATRA and Daunorubicin in the treatment of nonelderly APL patients. Am J Hematol. 2013;88(7):556–9.
44. Iland HJ, Bradstock K, Supple SG, Catalano A, Collins M, Hertzberg M, et al. All-trans-retinoic acid, idarubicin, and IV arsenic trioxide as initial therapy in acute promyelocytic leukemia (APML4). Blood. 2012;120(8):1570–80; quiz 752.
45. Iland HJ, Collins M, Bradstock K, Supple SG, Catalano A, Hertzberg M, et al. Use of arsenic trioxide in remission induction and consolidation therapy for acute promyelocytic leukaemia in the Australasian Leukaemia and Lymphoma Group (ALLG) APML4 study: a non-randomised phase 2 trial. Lancet Haematol. 2015;2(9):e357–66.
46. Collins M, Di Iulio J, Beresford J. Australasian Leukaemia & Lymphoma Group APML4 Statistical Report. 2013.
47. Lallemand-Breitenbach V, Jeanne M, Benhenda S, Nasr R, Lei M, Peres L, et al. Arsenic degrades PML or PML–RARα through a SUMO-triggered RNF4/ubiquitin-mediated pathway. Nat Cell Biol. 2008;10(5):547–55.
48. Zhang XW, Yan XJ, Zhou ZR, Yang FF, Wu ZY, Sun HB, et al. Arsenic trioxide controls the fate of the PML-RAR oncoprotein by directly binding PML. Science. 2010;328(5975):240–3.
49. Powell BL, Moser B, Stock W, Gallagher RE, Willman CL, Stone RM, et al. Arsenic trioxide improves event-free and overall survival for adults with acute promyelocytic leukemia: North American Leukemia Intergroup Study C9710. Blood. 2010;116(19):3751–7.
50. Mathews V, George B, Chendamarai E, Lakshmi KM, Desire S, Balasubramanian P, et al. Single-agent arsenic trioxide in the treatment of newly diagnosed acute promyelocytic leukemia: long-term follow-up data. J Clin Oncol. 2010;28(24):3866–71.
51. Muchtar E, Vidal L, Ram R, Gafter-Gvili A, Shpilberg O, Raanani P. The role of maintenance therapy in acute promyelocytic leukemia in the first complete remission. Cochrane Database Syst Rev. 2013;(3):CD009594.
52. Coutre SE, Othus M, Powell B, Willman CL, Stock W, Paietta E, et al. Arsenic trioxide during consolidation for patients with previously untreated low/intermediate risk acute promyelocytic leukaemia may eliminate the need for maintenance therapy. Br J Haematol. 2014;165(4):497–503.
53. Coombs CC, Tavakkoli M, Tallman MS. Acute promyelocytic leukemia: where did we start, where are we now, and the future. Blood Cancer J. 2015;5:e304.
54. Asou N, Kishimoto Y, Kiyoi H, Okada M, Kawai Y, Tsuzuki M, et al. A randomized study with or without intensified maintenance chemotherapy in patients with acute promyelocytic leukemia who have become negative for PML-RAR transcript after consolidation therapy: the Japan Adult Leukemia Study Group (JALSG) APL97 study. Blood. 2007;110(1):59–66.
55. Avvisati G, Lo-Coco F, Paoloni FP, Petti MC, Diverio D, Vignetti M, et al. AIDA 0493 protocol for newly diagnosed acute promyelocytic leukemia: very long-term results and role of maintenance. Blood. 2011;117(18):4716–25.
56. Kelaidi C, Chevret S, De Botton S, Raffoux E, Guerci A, Thomas X, et al. Improved outcome of acute promyelocytic leukemia with high WBC counts over the last 15 years: the European APL Group Experience. J Clin Oncol. 2009;27(16):2668–76.
57. Au WY, Tam S, Fong BM, Kwong YL. Determinants of cerebrospinal fluid arsenic concentration in patients with acute promyelocytic leukemia on oral arsenic trioxide therapy. Blood. 2008;112(9):3587–90.

58. Breccia M, Carmosino I, Diverio D, De Santis S, De Propris MS, Romano A, et al. Early detection of meningeal localization in acute promyelocytic leukaemia patients with high presenting leucocyte count. Br J Haematol. 2003;120(2):266–70.
59. Breccia M, Lo CF. Thrombo-hemorrhagic deaths in acute promyelocytic leukemia. Thromb Res. 2014;133(Suppl 2):S112–6.
60. McClellan JS, Kohrt HE, Coutre S, Gotlib JR, Majeti R, Alizadeh AA, et al. Treatment advances have not improved the early death rate in acute promyelocytic leukemia. Haematologica. 2012;97(1):133–6.
61. Tallman M, Lo-Coco F, Kwaan H, Sanz M, Gore S. Clinical roundtable monograph. Early death in patients with acute promyelocytic leukemia. Clin Adv Hematol Oncol. 2011;9(2):1–16.
62. Park JH, Qiao B, Panageas KS, Schymura MJ, Jurcic JG, Rosenblat TL, et al. Early death rate in acute promyelocytic leukemia remains high despite all-trans retinoic acid. Blood. 2011;118(5):1248–54.
63. Mantha S, Tallman MS, Soff GA. What's new in the pathogenesis of the coagulopathy in acute promyelocytic leukemia? Curr Opin Hematol. 2016;23(2):121–6.
64. Sanz MA, Montesinos P. How we prevent and treat differentiation syndrome in patients with acute promyelocytic leukemia. Blood. 2014;123(18):2777–82.
65. Montesinos P, Bergua JM, Vellenga E, Rayon C, Parody R, de la Serna J, et al. Differentiation syndrome in patients with acute promyelocytic leukemia treated with all-trans retinoic acid and anthracycline chemotherapy: characteristics, outcome, and prognostic factors. Blood. 2009;113(4):775–83.
66. Wiley JS, Firkin FC. Reduction of pulmonary toxicity by prednisolone prophylaxis during all-trans retinoic acid treatment of acute promyelocytic leukemia. Australian Leukaemia Study Group. Leukemia. 1995;9(5):774–8.
67. Camacho LH, Soignet SL, Chanel S, Ho R, Heller G, Scheinberg DA, et al. Leukocytosis and the retinoic acid syndrome in patients with acute promyelocytic leukemia treated with arsenic trioxide. J Clin Oncol. 2000;18(13):2620–5.
68. Roboz GJ, Ritchie EK, Carlin RF, Samuel M, Gale L, Provenzano-Gober JL, et al. Prevalence, management, and clinical consequences of QT interval prolongation during treatment with arsenic trioxide. J Clin Oncol. 2014;32(33):3723–8.
69. Lo-Coco F, Cicconi L, Breccia M. Current standard treatment of adult acute promyelocytic leukaemia. Br J Haematol. 2016;172(6):841–54.
70. Burnett AK, Russell NH, Hills RK, Bowen D, Kell J, Knapper S, et al. Arsenic trioxide and all-trans retinoic acid treatment for acute promyelocytic leukaemia in all risk groups (AML17): results of a randomised, controlled, phase 3 trial. Lancet Oncol. 2015;16(13):1295–305.

9 First-Line Therapy: ATRA-ATO/ Reduced Chemotherapy Approach

Harry Iland

Introduction

As our understanding of the genetic events that initiate APL has increased, the treatment paradigms that have proven successful have diverged from standard acute myeloid leukemia (AML) chemotherapy protocols. This divergence has sequentially involved the addition of ATRA to chemotherapy, greater reliance on anthracyclines, intensification of chemotherapy with cytarabine for Sanz high-risk patients [1], the incorporation of ATO, and the subsequent elimination of chemotherapy for patients with standard (low and intermediate)-risk disease. One of the major challenges that remains is how to balance the combined use of ATRA, ATO, and reduced doses of chemotherapy for the subset of patients at greatest risk of failure [2] in order to maximize efficacy while reducing both short-term and long-term toxicity.

H. Iland, M.B.B.S., F.R.A.C.P., F.R.C.P.A.
Institute of Haematology, Royal Prince Alfred Hospital, Missenden Road, Camperdown, NSW 2050, Australia
e-mail: harryiland@gmail.com

Chemotherapy-Associated Problems

Improved outcomes for patients with APL have unfortunately been accompanied by the emergence of several major complications, particularly in the context of risk-adapted chemotherapy intensification during consolidation. The most important of these are increased deaths in complete remission (CR) resulting from excessive myelosuppression, therapy-related myeloid neoplasms (t-MN) including myelodysplasia (MDS) and AML, and anthracycline-related cardiomyopathy.

Deaths in CR

Virtually all patients who survive induction achieve morphological CR. In order to maximize their chances of cure, not only must relapse be prevented, but death due to post-remission therapy must also be avoided. The vast majority of ATRA + chemotherapy protocols have consistently been associated with a low but not insignificant incidence of death in CR (Table 9.1). In general, the probability of death in CR is greater in those protocols where large doses of cytarabine and/or anthracycline have been incorporated during consolidation, despite the fact that these protocols are usually age-restricted.

O. Abla et al. (eds.), *Acute Promyelocytic Leukemia*, https://doi.org/10.1007/978-3-319-64257-4_9

Table 9.1 Representative trials showing reported deaths in CR and their association with consolidation components

Reference — trial	Cumulative[a] idarubicin-equivalent dose (mg/m^2) in consolidation[b]	Cumulative cytarabine dose (g/m^2) in consolidation	Other drugs used in consolidation[c]	Number of deaths in CR (%)			Age restriction (years)
				All patients	Standard-risk	High risk	
Non-risk-adapted consolidation							
Iland, 2012 [67] ALLG APML3	48.0	0	ATRA	2/91 (2.2%)	ns[d]	ns	–
Sanz, 2004 [70] PETHEMA LPA96	73.7	0	–	3/157 (1.9%)	ns	ns	–
Lo-Coco, 2010 [110] GIMEMA AIDA0493	73.7	6.25	VP16, 6TG	3/592 (0.5%)	ns	ns	≤61
Burnett, 2013 [111] MRC AML15 (MRC arm)	71.7	8.6	ATRA, VP16, AMSA, ±GO	13/132 (9.8%)	ns	ns	–
Lengfelder, 2009 [91] German AMLCG	72.0–97.0	37.5–55.4	6TG, CPX	11/131 (8.4%)	9/100 (9.0%)	2/31 (6.5%)	≤60
Risk-adapted consolidation							
Adès and Sanz, 2008 [112] PETHEMA LPA99	73.7–93.7	0	ATRA	5/381 (1.3%)	4/294 (1.4%)	1/87 (1.1%)	<65
Adès and Sanz, 2008 [112] French-Belgian-Swiss APL2000	63.0	9.4–21.4	–	5/173 (2.9%)	2/95 (2.1%)	3/78 (3.8%)	<65
Sanz, 2010 [113] LPA2005	57.0–77.0	0–5.8	ATRA	4/372 (1.1%)	1/270 (0.4%)	3/98 (3.1%)	–
Lo-Coco, 2010 [110] GIMEMA AIDA2000	73.7	0–6.25	VP16, 6TG, ATRA	8/395 (2.0%)	3/297 (1.0%)	5/9 (5.1%)	≤61
Trials with only ATRA + ATO in consolidation							
Ravandi, 2009 [73] MD Anderson	0	0	ATRA, ATO	1/75 (1.3%)[e]	ns	ns	–

Iland, 2015 [71] ALLG APML4	0	0	ATRA, ATO	0/112 (0%)	0/93 (0%)	0/19 (0%)	–
Burnett, 2015 [76] NCRI AML17 (ATRA + ATO arm)	0	0	ATRA, ATO	Cumulative incidence 2%	ns	ns	–
Platzbecker, 2016 [75] GIMEMA-AMLSG-SAL APL0406 (ATRA + ATO arm)	0	0	ATRA, ATO	1/127 (0.8%)	1/127 (0.8%)	na[f]	≤71

[a]Cumulative dose for idarubicin (or equivalent) and for cytarabine includes all exposure during consolidation only
[b]Idarubicin equivalence calculated as 10 mg idarubicin = 12 mg mitoxantrone = 50 mg daunorubicin [3, 114]
[c]*AMSA* amsacrine, *ATO* arsenic trioxide, *ATRA* all-*trans* retinoic acid, *CPX* cyclophosphamide, *GO* gemtuzumab ozogamicin, *6TG* 6-thioguanine, *VP16* etoposide
[d]Not stated in the original publication
[e]There were actually 4/75 (5.3%) deaths in CR, but 3 deaths were attributable to pre-existing malignancy
[f]Not applicable as APL0406 was restricted to standard-risk patients only

Therapy-Related Myeloid Neoplasms

The anthracycline-enhanced regimens used for the treatment of APL by several cooperative groups have included cumulative idarubicin or idarubicin-equivalent [3] doses ranging from 100 to 140 mg/m^2. It is well established that higher cumulative doses and increasing dose intensity of many cytotoxic agents, including anthracyclines, alkylating agents, and epipodophyllotoxins, are associated with a corresponding increased risk of t-MN after treatment of solid tumors [4, 5]. t-MN have also been documented after treatment of APL with chemotherapy-based regimens [6–14], and the reported incidence ranges from 1 to 10% [15–18].

The spectrum of cytogenetic abnormalities seen in t-MN after the treatment of APL includes those associated with topoisomerase II inhibitors (such as anthracyclines and etoposide) and also those typically seen following alkylating agents, despite the fact that alkylating agents are rarely used to treat APL. Rearrangements involving 11q23 (*MLL*) and 22q11 (*RUNX1*), abnormalities of chromosomes 5 and/or 7, and disruption of *TP53* have all been described [9, 19–24].

Cardiotoxicity

Despite the emphasis on anthracyclines in APL regimens and the well-established risk of anthracycline-induced cardiotoxicity [25], there has been little in the way of comprehensive evaluation of long-term cardiotoxicity in APL patients. Nevertheless, in a study of 34 APL patients treated with idarubicin and mitoxantrone, echocardiography demonstrated frequent regional wall motion abnormalities and subclinical diastolic dysfunction when compared with 47 well-matched controls [26]. Fatal anthracycline cardiotoxicity has also been reported by the Japanese Children's Cancer and Leukemia Study Group in 3 of 40 children with APL [27].

Occurrences of death in CR, t-MN, and anthracycline-induced cardiomyopathy in patients who have a high probability of cure of their original APL are of considerable concern and provide a compelling argument to devise treatment strategies that minimize exposure to anthracyclines and large doses of cytarabine.

Therapeutic Arsenic: Historical Aspects

Natural sources of arsenic include rocks, soil, water, air, and biota [28] where it is found in both inorganic and organic forms. Arsenic exists in multiple valence states, primarily +V (arsenate), +III (arsenite), +I (arsonium metal), 0 (arsenic), and –III (arsine). The major inorganic forms of arsenic are red arsenic (As_4S_4, also known as realgar), yellow arsenic (As_2S_3, also known as orpiment), and white arsenic (As_2O_3, ATO). The metabolism of arsenic species involves repeated sequential reduction from the pentavalent to the trivalent state, followed by coupled oxidation and methylation [29]. Thus $As^V \rightarrow As^{III} \rightarrow$ monomethylarsonic acid^V (MMA^V) $\rightarrow$ monomethylarsenous acid^{III} (MMA^{III}) $\rightarrow$ dimethylarsinic acid^V (DMA^V) $\rightarrow$ dimethylarsinous acid^{III} (DMA^{III}).

The origins of inorganic arsenic therapy in traditional Chinese medicine more than 2000 years ago, and subsequently in Western medicine at least 250 years ago, have been eloquently reviewed [30, 31]. The use of both realgar and ATO was documented in the Shennong Materia Medica as far back as the Han dynasty around 200BC, but therapeutic arsenic did not appear in the Western literature until the latter part of the eighteenth century. The first published report of its use in leukemia dates back to 1865 when potassium arsenite (Fowler's solution) was administered to a woman with chronic myeloid leukemia (CML), and in 1931, it was shown to have clinically relevant activity in CML with substantial improvements in blood counts and reduction of splenomegaly [32].

Introduction of Arsenic Trioxide into the APL Armamentarium

The earliest recognition that arsenic was active against APL emerged from a series of experiments performed in 1973 by Dr. TD Zhang using several combinations of ATO, mercuric oxide, and toad extracts against various leukemias. He identified ATO as the active antileukemic agent and subsequently reported the use of 1% ATO with a trace of mercury chloride (Ai-Lin I) given intravenously to 73 patients with APL [33]. The same group from Harbin Medical University subsequently reported over 100 cases of previously untreated and relapsed patients treated with Ai-Lin I who achieved CR rates ranging from 52 to 73% [34, 35].

The first report of ATO use in APL appeared in the Western literature in 1997; investigators from Shanghai and Harbin documented the outcome of ATO therapy in 15 patients that had relapsed after ATRA induction and chemotherapy consolidation [36]. CR was achieved in 9 of 10 patients treated only with intravenous ATO 10 mg/day and in all 5 of those treated with ATO and either low-dose chemotherapy or ATRA. The overall CR rate was 93% and was reached after a median of 38 days of ATO therapy (range 28–54). Five patients exhibited transient leukocytosis (peak WBC count 12.5–167 × 10^9/L), similar to ATRA-induced hyperleukocytosis, and significant myelosuppression was not seen. Fibrin degradation products and D-dimers fell rapidly after commencement of ATO. The most frequent side effects involved the skin (dryness, itching, erythema), the gastrointestinal tract (anorexia, nausea, vomiting), and elevation of liver enzymes, but no patients discontinued arsenic because of toxicity. These investigators extended their results with additional relapsed and previously untreated patients [37]. The CR rates were 85% and 73%, respectively. Molecular CR was infrequently seen in both subgroups at the time hematological CR was achieved but was documented in some patients after maintenance chemotherapy and/or ATO. Whereas hepatic toxicity in relapsed patients was mild, significant hepatic toxicity occurred in 7 of the 11 previously untreated patients and was regarded as a contributory factor in the deaths of 2. The first experience with ATO in Australia for relapsed APL was also reported around that time, with two cases showing different outcomes. One patient responded promptly to Ai-Lin I after failing reinduction with ATRA + chemotherapy, whereas the second was overtly refractory to Ai-Lin I [38].

Arsenic Trioxide as Standard Therapy for Relapsed APL

The impressive results reported from China were promptly reproduced in a pilot study in New York [39], and the success of the pilot study paved the way for a subsequent US multicenter study of 40 patients with APL in first or second relapse who had previously received ATRA and anthracycline-based chemotherapy [40]. They were treated with intravenous ATO for up to 60 days, and patients who achieved CR were eligible for consolidation with ATO for 25 days and up to four similar maintenance cycles. The CR rate was 85%, and 86% of those tested after consolidation achieved molecular remission. Overall survival (OS) at 18 months was 66%, and disease-free survival (DFS) was 56%, although these results were not censored for patients who underwent transplantation. There were no treatment-related deaths. Frequent adverse events included hypokalemia, hyperglycemia, neutropenia, prolongation of the corrected QT interval (QTc), transient elevation of liver function tests, and neuropathic symptoms which were predominantly mild and reversible. Coagulopathy resolved a median of 11 days from the start of ATO. Hyperleukocytosis and other features consistent with APL DS were also common.

Despite the small sample size, these data secured regulatory approval for ATO in the treatment of relapsed/refractory APL in the USA, Europe, and Australia, and the effectiveness of ATO in the treatment of relapsed APL was subsequently demonstrated in reports from centers around the world [41–49]. In the majority of these reports, the daily dose of ATO was either 10 mg or 0.15–0.16 mg/kg. Of note, a study from Shanghai described comparable results with less toxicity in 20 patients treated with approximately half-dose ATO (0.08 mg/kg) [50]. As a result, when ATO dose reduction rather than cessation is deemed appropriate because of moderate toxicity, 0.08 mg/kg/day is generally chosen as this represents the lowest dose with proven efficacy.

Incorporating ATO into Initial Therapy

Although ATO achieved recognition as the treatment of choice for relapsed APL following failure of ATRA and chemotherapy, concern about its use as initial therapy lingered for some time, based on higher than expected fatal toxicity in some reports [37, 51]. An important study from Shanghai [52] did much to dispel these concerns, and also rebutted *in vitro* data that had suggested ATO and ATRA were antagonistic when used concurrently [53]. In the Shanghai study, 61 patients were randomized to induction with ATRA ($n = 20$), ATO ($n = 21$), or the combination ($n = 20$). The CR rates were comparable (95%, 90%, and 95%, respectively), but the median time to achieve CR was significantly shorter with ATO than with ATRA (31 vs. 40.5 days, $P = 0.0233$) and occurred even more rapidly with the combination (median 25.5 days, $P = 0.0003$). Synergism was also shown by the fact that *PML-RARA* transcripts were reduced by a significantly greater extent after induction with combination therapy (118.9-fold reduction) than with ATRA (6.7-fold, $P = 0.0001$) or ATO (32.1-fold, $P = 0.0079$) monotherapy. These findings translated into a reduced relapse rate and improved DFS in the group induced with combination therapy. Liver dysfunction was more common in the two cohorts that received ATO compared with the ATRA monotherapy group, but all patients had recovery of liver function within 2 weeks.

In 2009 the Shanghai group updated their experience with 85 patients treated with the combined ATRA + ATO induction regimen [54] and subsequently reported the long-term experience with this regimen in 217 patients [55]. The CR rate was 91.7% with 7.4% early deaths (ED) and 0.9% failure to respond. The 10-year DFS for standard-risk patients was 91% but was only 73% for patients with high-risk APL. The difference was primarily attributable to a significantly higher cumulative incidence of relapse (CIR) in high-risk patients (26.9% vs. 8% for standard-risk, $P = 0.003$). Although the Shanghai protocol is appropriately acknowledged as the originator of ATRA + ATO combination therapy, high-risk patients also received idarubicin during induction, and 61.6% of standard-risk patients required idarubicin or hydroxyurea to control treatment-induced leukocytosis. Furthermore, combinations of daunorubicin or idarubicin, conventional- and intermediate-dose cytarabine, and homoharringtonine were utilized in three cycles of consolidation, followed by five cycles of maintenance therapy each involving monthly rotations through ATRA, ATO, 6-mercaptopurine (6MP), and methotrexate (MTX). Two other Chinese groups have also published data attesting to the superiority of ATRA combined with ATO during induction for previously untreated APL [56, 57]. Collectively, these studies provide a convincing argument for the use of combination ATRA + ATO during induction rather than either used alone.

In North America, incorporation of ATO into frontline therapy has predominantly focused on its use in consolidation. In the North American Leukemia Intergroup Study C9710 [58], induction with ATRA, 7 days of infusional cytarabine, and four doses of daunorubicin were followed by consolidation with two cycles of ATRA and daunorubicin. The investigational arm involved the same induction and consolidation but also included two cycles of ATO (0.15 mg/kg/day, 5 days per week for 4 weeks per cycle) sandwiched between induction and consolidation. Event-free survival (EFS), the primary end point, was significantly better at 3 years in the ATO arm (80% vs. 63%, $P < 0.0001$), and the benefit was evident in both high-risk and standard-risk patients. ATO was also associated with superior DFS in both risk categories, but the improvement in OS with ATO did not quite reach statistical significance. ATO was also used in consolidation in an American single-arm study with the aim of reducing anthracycline exposure [59, 60]. The results (OS 93%, EFS 89%, and DFS 92%) were comparable with the ATO arm of C9710, despite a 28% reduction in daunorubicin. These North American data clearly demonstrated that one or two cycles of ATO could be safely added to a protocol that was predominantly based around ATRA + chemotherapy and could effectively facilitate a reduction in chemotherapy intensity.

In some countries, the high cost of ATRA and chemotherapy, combined with the relatively low cost of ATO in the absence of patent protection, has encouraged the use of ATO monotherapy for induction and consolidation ± maintenance, despite the fact that the combination of ATRA + ATO is superior [52, 56, 57]. Studies from Vellore (India) [61] and Tehran (Iran) [62] have both reported a CR rate of 86% with ATO monotherapy, although both protocols employed hydroxyurea for patients with high initial WBC counts, and limited anthracycline was used in a minority of patients in Vellore. Mature survival data show 5-year DFS, and OS in Vellore [63] was 80% and 74%, respectively, compared with 67% and 64% in Tehran [64], and the better outcomes observed in Vellore most likely reflect differences in ATO scheduling. In both studies, high-risk patients had inferior outcomes. Accordingly, in countries where ATO monotherapy is more affordable than ATRA + chemotherapy, it provides a reasonable option for patients who have standard-risk disease but is clearly inadequate for high-risk patients.

Optimizing Outcomes by Combining ATRA, ATO, and Chemotherapy

Following the pivotal studies from Shanghai which utilized ATRA + ATO in induction and maintenance, with intensive chemotherapy as consolidation, other Chinese investigators have demonstrated the ability to successfully combine ATRA, ATO, and chemotherapy for previously untreated patients with APL [65]. As with the Shanghai approach, additional limited chemotherapy was combined with ATRA and ATO during induction for high-risk patients. Post-remission therapy was based on multiple cycles of chemotherapy for consolidation and maintenance together with additional ATRA and ATO given sequentially over a 3-year period [65].

The Australasian Leukaemia and Lymphoma Group (ALLG) adopted a different approach to the combination of ATRA, ATO, and chemotherapy. Their rationale was based on a desire to maximize antileukemic efficacy by combining the three most active agents (ATRA, ATO, and idarubicin) while simultaneously minimizing overall anthracycline exposure. In their APML4 protocol [66], the ALLG used an AIDA backbone in induction (ATRA days 1–36 with idarubicin days 2, 4, 6, 8) and added ATO 0.15 mg/kg from days 9 to 36. The ability to successfully deliver ATRA, ATO, and idarubicin concurrently was confirmed in an analysis of the proportion of patients who received the protocol-specified maximum and minimum cumulative doses of each drug during induction [66]. The synergism of ATRA and ATO was further exploited in two chemotherapy-free cycles of consolidation. Two years of maintenance (ATRA, 6MP, and MTX) were also included, as this had proven effective in the ALLG's previous AIDA-based APML3 protocol [67]. Despite controversy over the value of prophylactic corticosteroids [68–70], all patients received prednisone for at least the first 10 days of induction as prophylaxis against DS, as well as protocol-specified hemostatic support.

The results were initially published in 2012 with a median follow-up of 2 years [66] and were updated in 2015 with extended follow-up (median 4.2 years) [71]. Hematological CR was documented in 118 of 124 (95%) patients after induction. The ED rate was 3.2%, and none were due to DS. The only pre-treatment variable significantly associated with ED was age > 70. One hundred and twelve patients commenced consolidation; the first cycle comprised ATRA and ATO given daily for 28 days, and the second cycle utilized intermittent therapy (ATO 5 days per week for 5 weeks and ATRA daily on weeks 1, 3, and 5). All 112 patients completed both consolidation cycles, and all achieved molecular CR. The outcomes were durable with extended follow-up, as shown by the 5-year figures for CIR (5%), DFS (95%), EFS (90%), and OS (94%) [71]. The results were particularly gratifying in the high-risk subgroup ($n = 23$), since the 5-year CIR and DFS were virtually identical in high-risk patients (5%, 95%, respectively) with the results in standard-risk patients (5%, 96%, respectively, Fig. 9.1a). The only statistically significant association with DFS in multivariate analysis was the presence or absence of a complex karyotype, defined as two or more cytogenetic abnormalities in addition to t(15;17) or *PML-RARA* positivity (Fig. 9.1b).

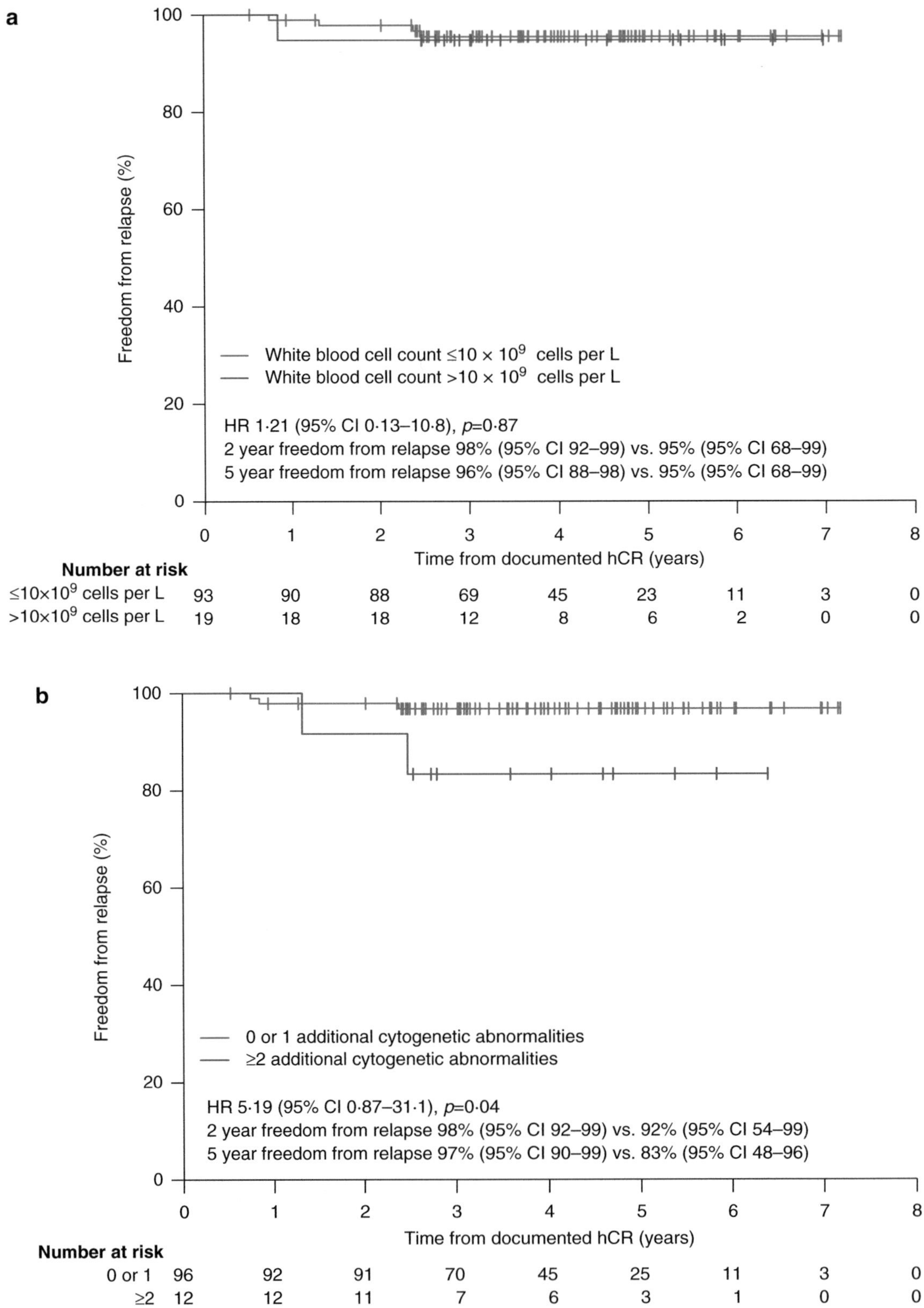

Fig. 9.1 Kaplan-Meier curves of freedom from relapse (and DFS) with APML4 therapy stratified by (**a**) white blood cell count and (**b**) karyotype. *HR* hazard ratio, *hCR* hematological complete remission. Originally published in Iland et al., The Lancet Haematology. 2015;2(9):e357–e66 [71]

The APML4 outcomes were compared with the results of the ALLG's previous APML3 trial [67], which involved AIDA induction followed by a second cycle of idarubicin and three blocks of ATRA in consolidation. Maintenance was not part of the original APML3 protocol but was added in an amendment after an unacceptably high relapse rate was noted and proved to be the only factor that significantly influenced DFS in multivariate analysis. The use of APML3 as a historical control for APML4 was restricted to the 70 patients who were registered after the maintenance amendment to eliminate confounding effects of differences in post-consolidation therapy. There was no significant difference in the rates of CR (APML4 95%, APML3 90%) or ED (APML4 3.2%, APML3 7.1%). In contrast, highly significant differences in freedom from relapse (FFR), DFS, and EFS favoring APML4 were already apparent at the time of the initial analysis [66], and these endpoint differences were even more pronounced in 5-year data at the final analysis (FFR 95% vs. 80%, $P = 0.002$, Fig. 9.2a; DFS 95% vs. 79%, $P = 0.001$, Fig. 9.2b; EFS 90% vs. 72%, $P = 0.002$, Fig. 9.2c). The extended follow-up also revealed a statistically significant 5-year OS advantage for the ATO-based APML4 protocol (94% vs. 83%, $P = 0.02$, Fig. 9.2d), despite the availability of ATO as salvage therapy for APML3 patients who had experienced relapse. Whereas the presence of *FLT3* internal tandem duplications (ITD) or kinase domain (KD)

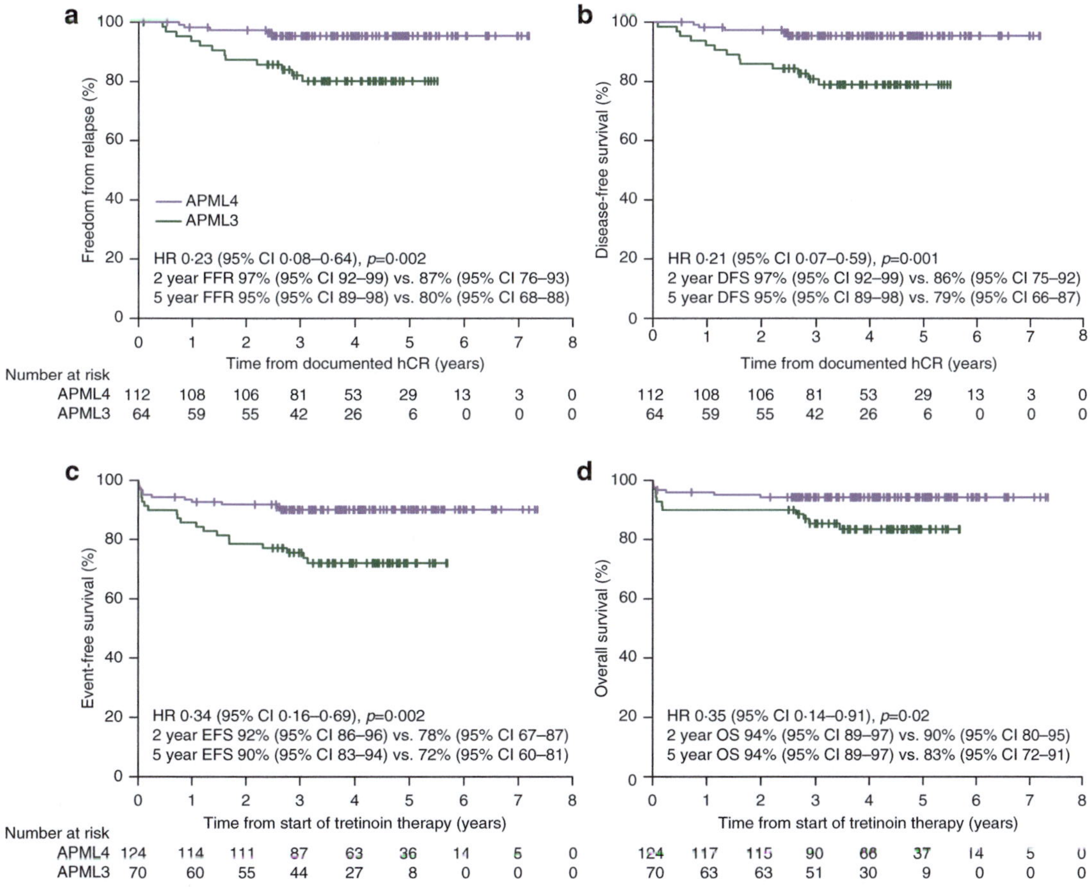

Fig. 9.2 Kaplan-Meier survival curves for APML4 and APML3 treatment protocols. (**a**) Freedom from relapse. (**b**) Disease-free survival. (**c**) Event-free survival. (**d**) Overall survival. *HR* hazard ratio, *FFR* freedom from relapse, *DFS* disease-free survival, *EFS* event-free survival, *OS* overall survival, *hCR* hematological complete remission. Originally published in Iland et al., The Lancet Haematology. 2015;2(9):e357–e66 [71]

point mutations was the single most important determinant of OS in the APML3 trial [67], ATO-based therapy in the APML4 trial completely abrogated the adverse effect of *FLT3* mutations [71]. The overwhelming superiority of APML4 over APML3 was clearly a consequence of incorporating ATO, since the total idarubicin content had contemporaneously been reduced by 50% (48 mg/m^2 in APML4 vs. 96 mg/m^2 in APML3). Although APML4 was not specifically powered for subgroup comparisons with APML3, a post-hoc subgroup analysis, stratified by risk category, showed high-risk APML4 patients had significantly better FFR ($P = 0.024$) and DFS ($P = 0.011$) than high-risk APML3 patients, thereby confirming the benefit of ATRA + ATO + reduced chemotherapy in the high-risk context.

Eliminating Chemotherapy from Frontline Treatment

Given the data supporting synergism between ATRA and ATO in induction and given the short- and long-term toxicity concerns related to intensive chemotherapy, an obvious question that arises is whether there still exists a role for any chemotherapy in the initial management of APL? In the following chapter, the use of chemotherapy-free protocols is reviewed in detail, but as the distinction between (1) chemotherapy-free protocols and (2) ATRA + ATO protocols with reduced chemotherapy is somewhat blurred, it is appropriate to briefly discuss these regimens here.

Pioneering work at the MD Anderson Hospital showed that a chemotherapy-free protocol involving ATRA + ATO was highly effective in patients with standard-risk disease [72, 73]. That experience has been validated conclusively in a GIMEMA-AMLSG-SAL prospective randomized study (APL0406) which demonstrated the superiority of ATRA + ATO over ATRA + chemotherapy for EFS, CIR, DFS, and OS in patients with standard-risk disease up to the age of 70 [74, 75]. A comparable NCRI study (AML17) [76] also showed superiority for ATRA + ATO over ATRA + chemotherapy as demonstrated by significantly fewer relapses.

Whereas the APL0406 study was restricted to patients with standard-risk disease, high-risk patients were included in both the MD Anderson program and in AML17. Consequently, in order to minimize the consequences of hyperleukocytosis in high-risk patients, both induction protocols included gemtuzumab ozogamicin (GO), a recombinant humanized anti-CD33 monoclonal antibody covalently linked to the cytotoxic antitumor antibiotic calicheamicin. Despite the addition of GO, compared to patients with standard-risk disease, high-risk patients had inferior DFS and OS in the MD Anderson study, and OS was also lower in AML17. Together with the excellent DFS of high-risk patients in APML4, it seems reasonable to conclude that there is still a role for limited chemotherapy combined with ATRA and ATO in patients with high-risk APL. Table 9.2 summarizes the treatment programs and outcomes of patients with high-risk APL, grouped according to ATO and chemotherapy content.

Table 9.2 Selected treatment programs and outcomes for patients with high-risk APL, grouped according to ATO and chemotherapy content

Reference — trial	Upper age limit (years)	Number of high-risk patients	Median follow-up (months)	Induction drugs[a]	Consolidation drugs	Maintenance drugs	Cumulative[b] idarubicin-equivalent dose (mg/m²)[c]	Cumulative cytarabine dose (g/m²)	Cumulative ATO dose (mg/kg)[d]	CR	ED	Time of outcome estimates (years)	CIR	DFS	OS
Trials combining ATRA with chemotherapy															
Lengfelder, 2009 [91] German AMLCG	≤60	37	72	ATRA, 6TG, DNR, ARAC, HIDAC, MIT	DNR, ARAC, 6TG	DNR, ARAC, 6TG, CPX	133	56.8	–	84%	16%	10	11%	80%	73%
Lo-Coco, 2010 [110] GIMEMA AIDA2000	≤61	129	59	ATRA, IDA	ATRA, IDA, HIDAC, MIT, ETOP, ARAC, 6TG	ATRA, 6MP, MTX	122	6.3	–	ns[e]	ns	6	9%	85%	83%
Sanz, 2010 [113] PETHEMA LPA2005	–	118	28	ATRA, IDA	ATRA, IDA, HIDAC, MIT, ARAC	ATRA, 6MP, MTX	122	5.8	–	83%	17%	4	14%	82%	79%
Ades, 2013 [92] French-Belgian-Swiss APL2000	≤60	74	103	ATRA, DNR, ARAC	DNR, ARAC, HIDAC	ATRA, 6MP, MTX	99	22.8	–	97%	3%	7	7%	ns	88%
Shinagawa, 2014 [115] JALSG APL204	≤70	70	52	ATRA, IDA, ARAC	MIT, ARAC, DNR, IDA	ATRA vs. TAMI	119.5	3.4	–	87%	11%	4	ns	58% (ATRA) vs. 87% (TAMI)	ns
Röllig, 2015 [116] SAL AIDA2000	–	41	55	ATRA, IDA	DNR, ARAC, HIDAC, MIT	ATRA, 6MP, MTX	109 (age ≤ 60) 100 (age > 60)	25.4 (age ≤ 60) 8.7 (age > 60)	–	88%	ns	6	ns	78%	71%
Trials combining ATO with ATRA and chemotherapy															
Powell, 2010 [58] North American Leukemia Intergroup C9710 (ATO arm)	–	113	29	ATRA, DNR, ARAC	ATRA, DNR, ATO	ATRA ±6MP, MTX	100	1.4	7.5	71%	20%	4	ns	87%[f]	ns

(continued)

Table 9.2 (continued)

Reference — trial	Upper age limit (years)	Number of high-risk patients	Median follow-up (months)	Induction drugs[a]	Consolidation drugs	Maintenance drugs	Cumulative[b] idarubicin-equivalent dose (mg/m^2)[c]	Cumulative cytarabine dose (g/m^2)	Cumulative ATO dose (mg/kg)[d]	CR	ED	Time of outcome estimates (years)	CIR	DFS	OS
Huang, 2012 [117] Nantong University Affiliated Hospital, Jiangsu	–	33	37	ATRA, ATO, DNR	DNR, ARAC, HIDAC	ATRA, ATO, MTX, 6MP	72	11.0	18.88	88%	12%	4	7%	ns	85%
Zhu, 2015 [55] Shanghai Institute of Hematology	–	53	72	ATRA, ATO, IDA or OHU	IDA, ARAC, HIDAC, HHT	ATRA, ATO, 6MP or MTX	48	7.4	26.88	87%	ns	10	27%	73%	78%
Trials combining ATRA and ATO with reduced chemotherapy															
Ravandi, 2009 [73] MD Anderson	–	26	23	ATRA, ATO, GO	ATRA, ATO	–	Not calculable (GO 9 mg/m^2)	0	16.2	81%	19%	4	ns	56%[f]	57%[f]
Iland, 2015 [71] ALLG APML4	–	23	50	ATRA, ATO, IDA	ATRA, ATO	ATRA, 6MP, MTX	48	0	12.15	87%[g]	9%[g]	5	5%	95%	87%
Burnett, 2015 [76] NCRI AML17 (ATRA + ATO arm)	–	30	31	ATRA, ATO, GO	ATRA, ATO	–	Not calculable (GO 6–12 mg/m^2)	0	17.0	ns	ns	4	ns	ns	87%

[a]*ARAC* conventional dose cytarabine (<1 g/m^2/day), *ATO* arsenic trioxide, *ATRA* all-*trans* retinoic acid, *CPX* cyclophosphamide, *IDA* idarubicin, *DNR* daunorubicin, *GO* gemtuzumab ozogamicin, *HHT* homoharringtonine, *HIDAC* intermediate- or high-dose cytarabine (≥1 g/m^2/day), *MIT* mitoxantrone, *6MP* 6-mercaptopurine, *MTX* methotrexate, *OHU* hydroxyurea, *TAMI* tamibarotene, *6TG* 6-thioguanine, *VP16* etoposide

[b]Cumulative dose for idarubicin (or equivalent), cytarabine, and ATO includes all exposure during induction, consolidation, and maintenance

[c]Idarubicin equivalence calculated as 10 mg idarubicin = 12 mg mitoxantrone = 50 mg daunorubicin [3, 114]

[d]Where ATO was given to CR during induction, the median time to CR has been used to estimate the number of days of ATO used during induction

[e]Not stated in the original publication

[f]Estimated from the survival curves in the original publication

[g]Not previously published

ATRA + ATO ± Reduced Chemotherapy: The New Standard of Care

The successes associated with the ATRA + ATO ± reduced chemotherapy studies have resulted in a number of changes to standard practice. In Australia, the Therapeutic Goods Administration has approved the use of ATO as initial therapy for all risk categories of APL based primarily on data from the APML4 and APL0406 studies. Frontline approval for standard-risk APL has also been secured in Europe but not yet in the USA. Despite that, the US National Comprehensive Cancer Network (NCCN Guidelines: Acute Myeloid Leukemia, version 3.2017; www.nccn.org, cited 3-Oct-2017) has endorsed the ATRA + ATO arms of APL0406 and AML17 for standard-risk disease, and APML4 for high-risk disease, and a panel of Canadian experts [77] has also recommended ATRA + ATO (APL0406) and APML4 for standard-risk and high-risk disease, respectively.

The Spectrum of Arsenic Toxicity

Consistent with its unique antileukemic activity in APL, ATO therapy is also characterized by a spectrum of distinguishing toxic effects [78]. APL DS can occur with ATO [79], though it is generally less severe than with ATRA, despite comparable degrees of hyperleukocytosis. Dose reduction from 0.15 to 0.08 mg/kg is recommended for mild-moderate DS, but ATO should be temporarily suspended if severe DS develops. Prophylactic prednisone has gained popularity in some protocols employing ATRA + ATO [66, 74], despite the lack of high-quality randomized trials proving its efficacy, and the use of intravenous (IV) dexamethasone 10 mg bid is recommended for established DS. Biochemical hepatotoxicity is common, particularly elevation of ALT and AST, though resolution usually occurs promptly after cessation of ATO, and dose reduction strategies for hepatotoxicity are well established [66, 74].

The potential for cardiac conduction abnormalities, particularly QT prolongation with an associated risk of polymorphic ventricular arrhythmias such as torsade de pointes [80], dominates intravenous administration of ATO. The concomitant use of other drugs that prolong QT [81], and electrolyte depletion (especially of K^+ and Mg^{2+}), accentuates the risk of QT prolongation. Frequent monitoring of electrolytes and intravenous or oral replacement is essential with the aim of keeping the serum K^+ above 4 mmol/L and the serum Mg^{2+} above 0.9 mmol/L. Since the QT interval is also rate dependent, several algorithms for calculation of corrected QT (QTc) are available. A detailed review of these algorithms has recommended the Framingham (Sagie), Hodges, or Fredericia algorithms rather than the commonly employed Bazett formula, since the latter was associated with substantially higher QTc values than the other methods [82]. ATO should be withheld if the QTc exceeds 500 ms until the relevant corrective measures have been instituted and the QTc normalizes.

Other ATO side effects include dermatological problems (rashes, hyperpigmentation), neurological disorders, particularly peripheral neuropathy [83], gastrointestinal disturbances, and metabolic abnormalities such as hyperglycemia. An increased risk of herpetic infections has also been reported [84], though this was not evident in the APML4 [66], APL0406 [74], or AML17 trials [76], despite the lack of protocol-specified antiviral prophylaxis. Not surprisingly, the toxicity of ATO is to some extent dependent on scheduling and on the concomitant use of other drugs [66].

Chronic environmental exposure to arsenic (e.g., by long-term ingestion of contaminated groundwater) has been associated with a range of nonmalignant disorders and with an increased risk of cancers [85, 86], especially involving the skin, lung, liver, kidney, and bladder. Reversible myelodysplastic features following arsenic poisoning have also been described [87]. Arsenic has been designated a human carcinogen by the US Environmental Protection Agency and by the International Agency for Research on Cancer. Whether short-term therapeutic arsenic exposure used in the treatment of APL, as opposed to chronic environmental exposure, will result in an increased risk of secondary malignancies is still uncertain [88], but to date no appreciable increase has been reported. The long-term safety of therapeutic ATO exposure has been assessed by the Shanghai group in a detailed survey of 112 ATO-treated APL patients and an age- and gender-matched control group [89]. A significant increase in grade 1 liver dysfunction and hepatic steatosis was observed in the APL patients, but there was no appreciable increase in second malignancies, diabetes, neurological, renal, or electrocardiographic disorders. Based on currently available data, the benefits of therapeutic ATO outweigh the potential risks.

Central Nervous System Relapse with ATO-Based Protocols

High-risk disease and central nervous system (CNS) hemorrhage during induction are associated with an increased risk of CNS relapse after ATRA and anthracycline-based chemotherapy [90]. However, there is no clear consensus on whether intrathecal chemoprophylaxis is of benefit. Intermediate- and high-dose cytarabine may provide some CNS protection, especially when total cytarabine administration exceeds 10 g/m^2 [91, 92]. Protocols that rely almost exclusively on ATRA and ATO also appear to be associated with a low risk of CNS relapse, despite the omission of CNS prophylaxis. Only one instance of CNS relapse was observed in each of the MD Anderson [73], APML4 [71], and AML17 [76] studies, and this may be related to the fact that, even when given orally, ATO is detectable in cerebrospinal fluid at therapeutically meaningful levels [93]. Concomitant administration of idarubicin, as in the APML4 protocol, may provide additional protection, since idarubicinol (its major active metabolite) has been detected at potentially antileukemic concentrations in the cerebrospinal fluid of children treated for acute lymphoblastic leukemia [94].

Maintenance in the ATO Era

Another area of controversy is the role of maintenance, which was associated with significantly better outcomes in both the European APL93 [95] and North American Intergroup APL [96] trials. In contrast, the GIMEMA AIDA0493 [97] study showed no advantage for maintenance, and it proved disadvantageous in the Japan Adult Leukemia Study Group (JALSG) APL97 trial [98]. A Cochrane meta-analysis [99] of 10 studies and over 2000 patients concluded that maintenance improved DFS but not OS, and maintenance with ATRA + chemotherapy was superior to ATRA alone.

While randomized studies comparing maintenance with no maintenance in the context of ATRA + ATO have not been conducted, the APL0406 [75] trial demonstrated that ATRA + ATO without maintenance was superior to ATRA + chemotherapy with maintenance. Accordingly, there seems no role for maintenance in standard-risk patients treated with ATRA + ATO. Whether that conclusion can be extrapolated to high-risk patients is unclear, but it is conceivable that merging APML4-style induction (ATRA + ATO + idarubicin) with the more prolonged ATRA + ATO consolidation utilized in APL0406 will eliminate the need for maintenance in high-risk patients.

Alternative Arsenic Formulations

The vast majority of the published arsenic data in APL relate to IV ATO, which is administered by daily 2-h infusions spanning several weeks/months, presenting considerable logistic issues for patients and hospital resources. A liquid oral ATO formulation developed in Hong Kong has shown efficacy in the relapsed setting [100–102] and has also been used extensively as maintenance after first remission [103]. Although oral ATO is more convenient and much less resource intensive [104], the CML experience with tyrosine kinase inhibitors indicates compliance may be a problem [105]. Limited pharmacokinetic data suggest that in comparison with IV administration, oral ATO is associated with lower peak blood levels, but exposure is comparable as estimated by area under the curve (AUC) [106]. Accordingly, it has been claimed that oral ATO may have an improved cardiac safety profile [101], but a clear safety benefit has not yet been proven.

Realgar is well established in traditional Chinese medicine, and its major constituent is tetra-arsenic tetra-sulfide (As_4S_4). It is administered orally and has been shown to be effective in previously untreated and relapsed APL and as long-term maintenance therapy [107]. The Chinese APL Cooperative Group has conducted a multicenter 2-year DFS non-inferiority study in which ATRA and IV ATO were compared with ATRA and oral realgar-*Indigo naturalis* formula (RIF) in induction and maintenance [108]. DFS with ATRA + RIF was non-inferior, and there were no significant differences in CR rates, OS, or toxicity. In a follow-up pilot study of 20 standard-risk patients, investigators from Beijing utilized a chemotherapy-free protocol combining ATRA and RIF in a schedule that mimicked the ATRA + ATO arm of APL0406 [109]. The primary endpoint, molecular CR, was achieved in 100% of patients, and with very limited follow-up (median 14 months), no relapses had occurred. That program has now been extended to two multicenter phase III studies comparing ATRA + RIF with ATRA + IV ATO in standard-risk APL (ChiCTR-TRC-13004054 and NCT02899169). RIF is not available outside China, and therefore the development of a convenient and high-quality oral ATO formulation is eagerly awaited. A novel capsule formulation, developed in Australia, is being evaluated by the ALLG in a phase I bioavailability study (APML5) which opened for accrual in June 2017 (ACTRN12616001022459).

Conclusion

The standard of care for APL has evolved dramatically in the last few years. While ATRA remains a fundamental part of treatment, chemotherapy has largely been replaced by ATO. In patients with standard-risk disease, a chemotherapy-free approach has been validated, but for patients with high-risk disease, current evidence suggests that an additional cytotoxic agent, typically idarubicin, is still required during induction but is no longer necessary in consolidation. If available, gemtuzumab ozogamicin is an appropriate alternative. The need for maintenance in high-risk disease is increasingly doubtful, though definitive studies have not yet been performed. Simplification of therapy through the substitution of oral for intravenous formulations of arsenic will further improve the therapeutic experience of patients with APL.

References

1. Sanz MA, Lo Coco F, Martín G, Avvisati G, Rayón C, Barbui T, et al. Definition of relapse risk and role of nonanthracycline drugs for consolidation in patients with acute promyelocytic leukemia: a joint study of the PETHEMA and GIMEMA cooperative groups. Blood. 2000;96(4):1247–53.
2. Iland HJ, Seymour JF, Wei A. Optimal approach for high-risk acute promyelocytic leukemia. Curr Opin Hematol. 2014;21(2):102–13.
3. Sanz MA, Martin G, Lo Coco F. Choice of chemotherapy in induction, consolidation and maintenance in acute promyelocytic leukaemia. Baillieres Best Pract Res Clin Haematol. 2003;16(3):433–51.
4. Le Deley M-C, Leblanc T, Shamsaldin A, Raquin M-A, Lacour B, Sommelet D, et al. Risk of secondary leukemia after a solid tumor in childhood according to the dose of Epipodophyllotoxins and Anthracyclines: a case-control study by the Société Française d'Oncologie Pédiatrique. J Clin Oncol. 2003;21(6):1074–81.
5. Praga C, Bergh J, Bliss J, Bonneterre J, Cesana B, Coombes RC, et al. Risk of acute myeloid leukemia and myelodysplastic syndrome in trials of adjuvant epirubicin for early breast cancer: correlation with doses of epirubicin and cyclophosphamide. J Clin Oncol. 2005;23(18):4179–91.
6. Ojeda-Uribe M, Schneider A, Luquet I, Berceanu A, Cornillet-Lefebvre P, Jeandidier E, et al. Therapy-related acute myeloid leukemia (t-AML) with poor-risk cytogenetics in two patients with persistent molecular complete remission of acute promyelocytic leukemia. Eur J Haematol. 2012;89(3):267–72.
7. Betancourt-Garcia RD, Castro J, Fernandez AC, Lopez-Enriquez A, Fradera J, Pacheco E. Acquired acute myelogenous leukemia after therapy for acute promyelocytic leukemia with t(15;17): a case report and review of the literature. P R Health Sci J. 2009;28(2):146–50.
8. Lee GY, Christina S, Tien SL, Ghafar ABA, Hwang W, Lim LC, et al. Acute promyelocytic leukemia with PML-RARA fusion on i(17q) and therapy-related acute myeloid leukemia. Cancer Genet Cytogenet. 2005;159(2):129–36.
9. Panizo C, Patino A, Lecumberri R, Calasanz MJ, Odero MD, Bendandi M, et al. Secondary myelodysplastic syndrome after treatment for promyelocytic

leukemia: clinical and genetic features of two cases. Cancer Genet Cytogenet. 2003;143(2):178–81.
10. Zompi S, Viguie F. Therapy-related acute myeloid leukemia and myelodysplasia after successful treatment of acute promyelocytic leukemia. Leuk Lymphoma. 2002;43(2):275–80.
11. Garcia-Manero G, Kantarjian H, Kornblau S, Estey E. Therapy-related myelodysplastic syndrome or acute myelogenous leukemia in patients with acute promyelocytic leukemia (APL). Leukemia. 2002;16(9):1888.
12. Andersen MK, Pedersen-Bjergaard J. Therapy-related MDS and AML in acute promyelocytic leukemia. Blood. 2002;100(5):1928–9.
13. Au WY, Lam CC, Ma ES, Man C, Wan T, Kwong YL. Therapy-related myelodysplastic syndrome after eradication of acute promyelocytic leukemia: cytogenetic and molecular features. Hum Pathol. 2001;32(1):126–9.
14. Todisco E, Testi AM, Avvisati G, Moleti ML, Cedrone M, Cimino G, et al. Therapy-related acute myelomonocytic leukemia following successful treatment for acute promyelocytic leukemia. Leukemia. 1995;9(9):1583–5.
15. Latagliata R, Petti MC, Fenu S, Mancini M, Spiriti MAA, Breccia M, et al. Therapy-related myelodysplastic syndrome-acute myelogenous leukemia in patients treated for acute promyelocytic leukemia: an emerging problem. Blood. 2002;99(3):822–4.
16. Lobe I, Rigal-Huguet F, Vekhoff A, Desablens B, Bordessoule D, Mounier C, et al. Myelodysplastic syndrome after acute promyelocytic leukemia: the European APL group experience. Leukemia. 2003;17(8):1600–4.
17. Batzios C, Hayes LA, He SZ, Quach H, McQuilten ZK, Wall M, et al. Secondary clonal cytogenetic abnormalities following successful treatment of acute promyelocytic leukemia. [Erratum appears in Am J Hematol. 2010 Jul;85(7):550]. Am J Hematol. 2009;84(11):715–9.
18. Imagawa J, Harada Y, Shimomura T, Tanaka H, Okikawa Y, Hyodo H, et al. Clinical and genetic features of therapy-related myeloid neoplasms after chemotherapy for acute promyelocytic leukemia. Blood. 2010;116(26):6018–22.
19. Harada Y, Harada H. Molecular mechanisms that produce secondary MDS/AML by RUNX1/AML1 point mutations. J Cell Biochem. 2011;112(2):425–32.
20. Snijder S, Mellink CH, van der Lelie H. Translocation (2;11)(q37;q23) in therapy-related myelodysplastic syndrome after treatment for acute promyelocytic leukemia. Cancer Genet Cytogenet. 2008;180(2):149–52.
21. Park TS, Choi JR, Yoon SH, Song J, Kim J, Kim SJ, et al. Acute promyelocytic leukemia relapsing as secondary acute myelogenous leukemia with translocation t(3;21)(q26;q22) and RUNX1-MDS1-EVI1 fusion transcript. Cancer Genet Cytogenet. 2008;187(2):61–73.
22. Jeddi R, Gouider E, Benneji H, Mnif S, Ben Abid H, Belhadjali Z, et al. Secondary chronic myelomonocytic leukemia with monosomy 7 after successful treatment of acute promyelocytic leukemia. Pathol Biol. 2008;56(3):162–3.
23. Pawarode A, Finlay E, Sait SNJ, Barcos M, Baer MR. Isochromosome 1q in a myelodysplastic syndrome after treatment for acute promyelocytic leukemia. Cancer Genet Cytogenet. 2006;167(2):155–60.
24. Athanasiadou A, Saloum R, Zorbas I, Tsompanakou A, Batsis I, Fassas A, et al. Therapy-related myelodysplastic syndrome with monosomy 5 and 7 following successful therapy for acute promyelocytic leukemia with anthracyclines. Leuk Lymphoma. 2002;43(12):2409–11.
25. Tan TC, Neilan TG, Francis S, Plana JC, Scherrer-Crosbie M. Anthracycline-induced cardiomyopathy in adults. Compr Physiol. 2015;5(3):1517–40.
26. Pellicori P, Calicchia A, Lococo F, Cimino G, Torromeo C. Subclinical anthracycline cardiotoxicity in patients with acute promyelocytic leukemia in long-term remission after the AIDA protocol. Congest Heart Fail. 2012;18(4):217–21.
27. Shimizu H, Nakadate H, Taga T, Utsumi J, Nishikawa K, Gushiken T, et al. Clinical characteristics and treatment results of acute promyelocytic leukemia in children (Children's Cancer and Leukemia Study Group). Rinsho Ketsueki. 1993;34(9):989–96.
28. ISSI Consulting Group. Arsenic occurrence in public drinking water supplies. Washington, DC: US Environmental Protection Agency. EPA publication no. 815-R-00-023.; 2000.
29. Kitchin KT. Recent advances in arsenic carcinogenesis: modes of action, animal model systems, and methylated arsenic metabolites. Toxicol Appl Pharmacol. 2001;172(3):249–61.
30. Chen S-J, Zhou G-B, Zhang X-W, Mao J-H, de Thé H, Chen Z. From an old remedy to a magic bullet: molecular mechanisms underlying the therapeutic effects of arsenic in fighting leukemia. Blood. 2011;117(24):6425–37.
31. Au WY. A biography of arsenic and medicine in Hong Kong and China. Hong Kong Med J. 2011;17(6):507–13.
32. Forkner C, Scott T. Arsenic as a therapeutic agent in chronic myelogenous leukemia: preliminary report. JAMA. 1931;97:3–5.
33. Zhang T, Sun H, Hu H. Treatment of acute promyelocytic leukemia with Ailing number one combination therapy: a study of 73 cases [in Chinese]. Heilongjiang J Tradit Chin Med. 1981;4:40–4.
34. Sun H, Ma L, Hu X, Zhang T. Ai-Lin I treated 32 cases of acute promyelocytic leukemia. Chin J Integrat Chin West Med. 1992;12:170–1.
35. Zhang P, Wang SY, Hu LH. Arsenic trioxide treated 72 cases of acute promyelocytic leukemia. Chin J Hematol. 1996;17:58–62.
36. Shen ZX, Chen GQ, Ni JH, Li XS, Xiong SM, Qiu QY, et al. Use of arsenic trioxide (As2O3) in the treatment of acute promyelocytic leukemia

(APL): II. Clinical efficacy and pharmacokinetics in relapsed patients. Blood. 1997;89(9):3354–60.

37. Niu C, Yan H, Yu T, Sun HP, Liu JX, Li XS, et al. Studies on treatment of acute promyelocytic leukemia with arsenic trioxide: remission induction, follow-up, and molecular monitoring in 11 newly diagnosed and 47 relapsed acute promyelocytic leukemia patients. Blood. 1999;94(10):3315–24.
38. Spencer A, Firkin F. Arsenic trioxide treatment of relapsed acute promyelocytic leukaemia: initial Australian experience. Aust N Z J Med. 1999;29(3):385–6.
39. Soignet SL, Maslak P, Wang ZG, Jhanwar S, Calleja E, Dardashti LJ, et al. Complete remission after treatment of acute promyelocytic leukemia with arsenic trioxide. N Engl J Med. 1998;339(19):1341–8.
40. Soignet SL, Frankel SR, Douer D, Tallman MS, Kantarjian H, Calleja E, et al. United States multicenter study of arsenic trioxide in relapsed acute promyelocytic leukemia. J Clin Oncol. 2001;19(18):3852–60.
41. Kwong YL, Au WY, Chim CS, Pang A, Suen C, Liang R. Arsenic trioxide- and idarubicin-induced remissions in relapsed acute promyelocytic leukaemia: clinicopathological and molecular features of a pilot study. Am J Hematol. 2001;66(4):274–9.
42. Leoni F, Gianfaldoni G, Annunziata M, Fanci R, Ciolli S, Nozzoli C, et al. Arsenic trioxide therapy for relapsed acute promyelocytic leukemia: a bridge to transplantation. Haematologica. 2002;87(5):485–9.
43. Au WY, Lie AKW, Chim CS, Liang R, Ma SK, Chan CH, et al. Arsenic trioxide in comparison with chemotherapy and bone marrow transplantation for the treatment of relapsed acute promyelocytic leukaemia. Ann Oncol. 2003;14(5):752–7.
44. Raffoux E, Rousselot P, Poupon J, Daniel M-T, Cassinat B, Delarue R, et al. Combined treatment with arsenic trioxide and all-trans-retinoic acid in patients with relapsed acute promyelocytic leukemia. J Clin Oncol. 2003;21(12):2326–34.
45. Lazo G, Kantarjian H, Estey E, Thomas D, O'Brien S, Cortes J. Use of arsenic trioxide (As2O3) in the treatment of patients with acute promyelocytic leukemia: the M. D. Anderson experience. Cancer. 2003;97(9):2218–24.
46. Carmosino I, Latagliata R, Avvisati G, Breccia M, Finolezzi E, Lo Coco F, et al. Arsenic trioxide in the treatment of advanced acute promyelocytic leukemia. Haematologica. 2004;89(5):615–7.
47. Shigeno K, Naito K, Sahara N, Kobayashi M, Nakamura S, Fujisawa S, et al. Arsenic trioxide therapy in relapsed or refractory Japanese patients with acute promyelocytic leukemia: updated outcomes of the phase II study and postremission therapies. Int J Hematol. 2005;82(3):224–9.
48. Thomas X, Pigneux A, Raffoux E, Huguet F, Caillot D, Fenaux P. Superiority of an arsenic trioxide-based regimen over a historic control combining all-trans retinoic acid plus intensive chemotherapy in the treatment of relapsed acute promyelocytic leukemia. Haematologica. 2006;91(7):996–7.
49. Aribi A, Kantarjian HM, Estey EH, Koller CA, Thomas DA, Kornblau SM, et al. Combination therapy with arsenic trioxide, all-trans retinoic acid, and gemtuzumab ozogamicin in recurrent acute promyelocytic leukemia. Cancer. 2007;109(7):1355–9.
50. Shen Y, Shen ZX, Yan H, Chen J, Zeng XY, Li JM, et al. Studies on the clinical efficacy and pharmacokinetics of low-dose arsenic trioxide in the treatment of relapsed acute promyelocytic leukemia: a comparison with conventional dosage. Leukemia. 2001;15(5):735–41.
51. Westervelt P, Brown RA, Adkins DR, Khoury H, Curtin P, Hurd D, et al. Sudden death among patients with acute promyelocytic leukemia treated with arsenic trioxide. Blood. 2001;98(2):266–71.
52. Shen Z-X, Shi Z-Z, Fang J, Gu B-W, Li J-M, Zhu Y-M, et al. All-trans retinoic acid/As2O3 combination yields a high quality remission and survival in newly diagnosed acute promyelocytic leukemia. Proc Natl Acad Sci U S A. 2004;101(15):5328–35.
53. Shao W, Fanelli M, Ferrara FF, Riccioni R, Rosenauer A, Davison K, et al. Arsenic trioxide as an inducer of apoptosis and loss of PML/RAR alpha protein in acute promyelocytic leukemia cells. J Natl Cancer Inst. 1998;90(2):124–33.
54. Hu J, Liu Y-F, Wu C-F, Xu F, Shen Z-X, Zhu Y-M, et al. Long-term efficacy and safety of all-trans retinoic acid/arsenic trioxide-based therapy in newly diagnosed acute promyelocytic leukemia. Proc Natl Acad Sci U S A. 2009;106(9):3342–7.
55. Zhu H, Hu J, Li X, Chen L, Zhao H, Zhou W, et al. All-trans retinoic acid and arsenic combination therapy benefits low-to-intermediate-risk patients with newly diagnosed acute promyelocytic leukaemia: a long-term follow-up based on multivariate analysis. Br J Haematol. 2015;171(2):277–80.
56. Wang G, Li W, Cui J, Gao S, Yao C, Jiang Z, et al. An efficient therapeutic approach to patients with acute promyelocytic leukemia using a combination of arsenic trioxide with low-dose all-trans retinoic acid. Hematol Oncol. 2004;22(2):63–71.
57. Dai C-W, Zhang G-S, Shen J-K, Zheng W-L, Pei M-F, Xu Y-X, et al. Use of all-trans retinoic acid in combination with arsenic trioxide for remission induction in patients with newly diagnosed acute promyelocytic leukemia and for consolidation/maintenance in CR patients. [Erratum appears in Acta Haematol. 2009;121(4):243]. Acta Haematol. 2009;121(1):1–8.
58. Powell BL, Moser B, Stock W, Gallagher RE, Willman CL, Stone RM, et al. Arsenic trioxide improves event-free and overall survival for adults with acute promyelocytic leukemia: North American Leukemia Intergroup Study C9710. Blood. 2010;116(19):3751–7.
59. Gore SD, Gojo I, Sekeres MA, Morris L, Devetten M, Jamieson K, et al. Single cycle of arsenic trioxide-based consolidation chemotherapy spares anthracycline exposure in the primary management

of acute promyelocytic leukemia. J Clin Oncol. 2010;28(6):1047–53.
60. Leech M, Morris L, Stewart M, Smith BD, Bashey A, Holland K, et al. Real-life experience of a brief arsenic trioxide-based consolidation chemotherapy in the management of acute promyelocytic leukemia: favorable outcomes with limited anthracycline exposure and shorter consolidation therapy. Clin Lymphoma Myeloma Leuk. 2015;15(5):292–7.
61. Mathews V, George B, Lakshmi KM, Viswabandya A, Bajel A, Balasubramanian P, et al. Single-agent arsenic trioxide in the treatment of newly diagnosed acute promyelocytic leukemia: durable remissions with minimal toxicity. Blood. 2006;107(7):2627–32.
62. Ghavamzadeh A, Alimoghaddam K, Ghaffari SH, Rostami S, Jahani M, Hosseini R, et al. Treatment of acute promyelocytic leukemia with arsenic trioxide without ATRA and/or chemotherapy. Ann Oncol. 2006;17(1):131–4.
63. Mathews V, George B, Chendamarai E, Lakshmi KM, Desire S, Balasubramanian P, et al. Single-agent arsenic trioxide in the treatment of newly diagnosed acute promyelocytic leukemia: long-term follow-up data. J Clin Oncol. 2010;28(24):3866–71.
64. Ghavamzadeh A, Alimoghaddam K, Rostami S, Ghaffari SH, Jahani M, Iravani M, et al. Phase II study of single-agent arsenic trioxide for the front-line therapy of acute promyelocytic leukemia. J Clin Oncol. 2011;29(20):2753–7.
65. Pei R, Cao J, Ma J, Zhang P, Liu X, Du X, et al. Long term curative effects of sequential therapy with all-trans retinoic acid, arsenious oxide and chemotherapy on patients with acute promyelocytic leukemia. Hematology. 2012;17(6):311–6.
66. Iland HJ, Bradstock K, Supple SG, Catalano A, Collins M, Hertzberg M, et al. All-trans-retinoic acid, idarubicin, and IV arsenic trioxide as initial therapy in acute promyelocytic leukemia (APML4). Blood. 2012;120(8):1570–80.
67. Iland H, Bradstock K, Seymour J, Hertzberg M, Grigg A, Taylor K, et al. Results of the APML3 trial incorporating all-trans-retinoic acid and idarubicin in both induction and consolidation as initial therapy for patients with acute promyelocytic leukemia. Haematologica. 2012;97(2):227–34.
68. Wiley JS, Firkin FC. Reduction of pulmonary toxicity by prednisolone prophylaxis during all-trans retinoic acid treatment of acute promyelocytic leukemia. Australian Leukaemia Study Group. Leukemia. 1995;9(5):774–8.
69. Sanz MA, Grimwade D, Tallman MS, Lowenberg B, Fenaux P, Estey EH, et al. Management of acute promyelocytic leukemia: recommendations from an expert panel on behalf of the European LeukemiaNet. Blood. 2009;113(9):1875–91.
70. Sanz MA, Martin G, Gonzalez M, Leon A, Rayon C, Rivas C, et al. Risk-adapted treatment of acute promyelocytic leukemia with all-trans-retinoic acid and anthracycline monochemotherapy: a multicenter study by the PETHEMA group. Blood. 2004;103(4):1237–43.
71. Iland HJ, Collins M, Bradstock K, Supple SG, Catalano A, Hertzberg M, et al. Use of arsenic trioxide in remission induction and consolidation therapy for acute promyelocytic leukaemia in the Australasian Leukaemia and Lymphoma Group (ALLG) APML4 study: a non-randomised phase 2 trial. Lancet Haematol. 2015;2(9):e357–e66.
72. Estey E, Garcia-Manero G, Ferrajoli A, Faderl S, Verstovsek S, Jones D, et al. Use of all-trans retinoic acid plus arsenic trioxide as an alternative to chemotherapy in untreated acute promyelocytic leukemia. Blood. 2006;107(9):3469–73.
73. Ravandi F, Estey E, Jones D, Faderl S, O'Brien S, Fiorentino J, et al. Effective treatment of acute promyelocytic leukemia with all-trans-retinoic acid, arsenic trioxide, and gemtuzumab ozogamicin. J Clin Oncol. 2009;27(4):504–10.
74. Lo-Coco F, Avvisati G, Vignetti M, Thiede C, Orlando SM, Iacobelli S, et al. Retinoic acid and arsenic trioxide for acute promyelocytic leukemia. N Engl J Med. 2013;369(2):111–21.
75. Platzbecker U, Avvisati G, Cicconi L, Thiede C, Paoloni F, Vignetti M, et al. Improved outcomes with retinoic acid and arsenic trioxide compared with retinoic acid and chemotherapy in non-high-risk acute promyelocytic leukemia: final results of the randomized Italian-German APL0406 trial. J Clin Oncol. 2017;35(6):605–12.
76. Burnett AK, Russell NH, Hills RK, Bowen D, Kell J, Knapper S, et al. Arsenic trioxide and all-trans retinoic acid treatment for acute promyelocytic leukaemia in all risk groups (AML17): results of a randomised, controlled, phase 3 trial. Lancet Oncol. 2015;16(13):1295–305.
77. Seftel MD, Barnett MJ, Couban S, Leber B, Storring J, Assaily W, et al. A Canadian consensus on the management of newly diagnosed and relapsed acute promyelocytic leukemia in adults. Curr Oncol. 2014;21(5):234–50.
78. Au W-Y, Kwong Y-L. Arsenic trioxide: safety issues and their management. Chung Kuo Yao Li Hsueh Pao. 2008;29(3):296–304.
79. Camacho LH, Soignet SL, Chanel S, Ho R, Heller G, Scheinberg DA, et al. Leukocytosis and the retinoic acid syndrome in patients with acute promyelocytic leukemia treated with arsenic trioxide. J Clin Oncol. 2000;18(13):2620–5.
80. Barbey JT, Pezzullo JC, Soignet SL. Effect of arsenic trioxide on QT interval in patients with advanced malignancies. J Clin Oncol. 2003;21(19):3609–15.
81. Gowda RM, Khan IA, Wilbur SL, Vasavada BC, Sacchi TJ. Torsade de pointes: the clinical considerations. Int J Cardiol. 2004;96(1):1–6.
82. Roboz GJ, Ritchie EK, Carlin RF, Samuel M, Gale L, Provenzano-Gober JL, et al. Prevalence, management,

and clinical consequences of QT interval prolongation during treatment with arsenic trioxide. J Clin Oncol. 2014;32(33):3723–8.
83. Huang S-Y, Chang C-S, Tang J-L, Tien H-F, Kuo T-L, Huang S-F, et al. Acute and chronic arsenic poisoning associated with treatment of acute promyelocytic leukaemia. Br J Haematol. 1998;103(4):1092–5.
84. Au W-Y, Kwong Y-L. Frequent varicella zoster reactivation associated with therapeutic use of arsenic trioxide: portents of an old scourge. J Am Acad Dermatol. 2005;53(5):890–2.
85. Tchounwou PB, Patlolla AK, Centeno JA. Invited reviews: carcinogenic and systemic health effects associated with arsenic exposure—a critical review. Toxicol Pathol. 2003;31(6):575–88.
86. Firkin F. Carcinogenic risk of retained arsenic after successful treatment of acute promyelocytic leukemia with arsenic trioxide: a cause for concern? Leuk Lymphoma. 2014;55(5):977–8.
87. Rezuke WN, Anderson C, Pastuszak WT, Conway SR, Firshein SI. Arsenic intoxication presenting as a myelodysplastic syndrome: a case report. Am J Hematol. 1991;36(4):291–3.
88. Au W-Y, Lang BH, Fong BMW, Mao KJ, Tam S. Thyroid arsenic content and papillary thyroid carcinoma arising 10 years after oral arsenic trioxide therapy for refractory acute promyelocytic leukemia. Leuk Lymphoma. 2014;55(5):1184–5.
89. Zhu H, Hu J, Chen L, Zhou W, Li X, Wang L, et al. The 12-year follow-up of survival, chronic adverse effects, and retention of arsenic in patients with acute promyelocytic leukemia. Blood. 2016;128(11):1525–8.
90. Montesinos P, Diaz-Mediavilla J, Deben G, Prates V, Tormo M, Rubio V, et al. Central nervous system involvement at first relapse in patients with acute promyelocytic leukemia treated with all-trans retinoic acid and anthracycline monochemotherapy without intrathecal prophylaxis. Haematologica. 2009;94(9):1242–9.
91. Lengfelder E, Haferlach C, Saussele S, Haferlach T, Schultheis B, Schnittger S, et al. High dose ara-C in the treatment of newly diagnosed acute promyelocytic leukemia: long-term results of the German AMLCG. Leukemia. 2009;23(12):2248–58.
92. Adès L, Chevret S, Raffoux E, Guerci-Bresler A, Pigneux A, Vey N, et al. Long-term follow-up of European APL 2000 trial, evaluating the role of cytarabine combined with ATRA and Daunorubicin in the treatment of nonelderly APL patients. Am J Hematol. 2013;88(7):556–9.
93. Au W-Y, Tam S, Fong BM, Kwong Y-L. Determinants of cerebrospinal fluid arsenic concentration in patients with acute promyelocytic leukemia on oral arsenic trioxide therapy. Blood. 2008;112(9):3587–90.
94. Reid JM, Pendergrass TW, Krailo MD, Hammond GD, Ames MM. Plasma pharmacokinetics and cerebrospinal-fluid concentrations of idarubicin and idarubicinol in pediatric leukemia patients—a Childrens Cancer Study-Group report. Cancer Res. 1990;50(20):6525–8.
95. Adès L, Guerci A, Raffoux E, Sanz M, Chevallier P, Lapusan S, et al. Very long-term outcome of acute promyelocytic leukemia after treatment with all-trans retinoic acid and chemotherapy: the European APL Group experience. Blood. 2010;115(9):1690–6.
96. Tallman MS, Andersen JW, Schiffer CA, Appelbaum FR, Feusner JH, Woods WG, et al. All-trans retinoic acid in acute promyelocytic leukemia: long-term outcome and prognostic factor analysis from the North American Intergroup protocol. Blood. 2002;100(13):4298–302.
97. Avvisati G, Lo-Coco F, Paoloni FP, Petti MC, Diverio D, Vignetti M, et al. AIDA 0493 protocol for newly diagnosed acute promyelocytic leukemia: very long-term results and role of maintenance. Blood. 2011;117(18):4716–25.
98. Asou N, Kishimoto Y, Kiyoi H, Okada M, Kawai Y, Tsuzuki M, et al. A randomized study with or without intensified maintenance chemotherapy in patients with acute promyelocytic leukemia who have become negative for PML-RARalpha transcript after consolidation therapy: the Japan Adult Leukemia Study Group (JALSG) APL97 study. Blood. 2007;110(1):59–66.
99. Muchtar E, Vidal L, Ram R, Gafter-Gvili A, Shpilberg O, Raanani P. The role of maintenance therapy in acute promyelocytic leukemia in the first complete remission. Cochrane Database Syst Rev. 2013;(3):CD009594.
100. Au WY, Kumana CR, Kou M, Mak R, Chan GC, Lam CW, et al. Oral arsenic trioxide in the treatment of relapsed acute promyelocytic leukemia. Blood. 2003;102(1):407–8.
101. Siu C-W, Au W-Y, Yung C, Kumana CR, Lau C-P, Kwong Y-L, et al. Effects of oral arsenic trioxide therapy on QT intervals in patients with acute promyelocytic leukemia: implications for long-term cardiac safety. Blood. 2006;108(1):103–6.
102. Au WY, Li C-K, Lee V, Yuen HL, Yau J, Chan GCF, et al. Oral arsenic trioxide for relapsed acute promyelocytic leukemia in pediatric patients. Pediatr Blood Cancer. 2012;58(4):630–2.
103. Au W-Y, Kumana CR, Lee HKK, Lin S-Y, Liu H, Yeung DYM, et al. Oral arsenic trioxide-based maintenance regimens for first complete remission of acute promyelocytic leukemia: a 10-year follow-up study. Blood. 2011;118(25):6535–43.
104. Firkin F. Oral administration of arsenic trioxide in the treatment of acute promyelocytic leukaemia and accelerated phase chronic myeloid leukaemia: an Australian single-centre study. Intern Med J. 2012;42(8):948–52.
105. Ibrahim AR, Eliasson L, Apperley JF, Milojkovic D, Bua M, Szydlo R, et al. Poor adherence is the main reason for loss of CCyR and imatinib failure for chronic myeloid leukemia patients on long-term therapy. Blood. 2011;117(14):3733–6.
106. Kumana CR, Au WY, Lee NSL, Kou M, Mak RWM, Lam CW, et al. Systemic availability of arsenic

from oral arsenic-trioxide used to treat patients with hematological malignancies. Eur J Clin Pharmacol. 2002;58(8):521–6.

107. Lu D-P, Qiu J-Y, Jiang B, Wang Q, Liu K-Y, Liu Y-R, et al. Tetra-arsenic tetra-sulfide for the treatment of acute promyelocytic leukemia: a pilot report. Blood. 2002;99(9):3136–43.

108. Zhu HH, Wu DP, Jin J, Li JY, Ma J, Wang JX, et al. Oral tetra-arsenic tetra-sulfide formula versus intravenous arsenic trioxide as first-line treatment of acute promyelocytic leukemia: a multicenter randomized controlled trial. J Clin Oncol. 2013;31(33):4215–21.

109. Zhu H-H, Huang X-J. Oral arsenic and retinoic acid for non-high-risk acute promyelocytic leukemia. N Engl J Med. 2014;371(23):2239–41.

110. Lo-Coco F, Avvisati G, Vignetti M, Breccia M, Gallo E, Rambaldi A, et al. Front-line treatment of acute promyelocytic leukemia with AIDA induction followed by risk-adapted consolidation for adults younger than 61 years: results of the AIDA-2000 trial of the GIMEMA Group. Blood. 2010;116(17):3171–9.

111. Burnett AK, Hills RK, Grimwade D, Jovanovic JV, Craig J, McMullin MF, et al. Inclusion of chemotherapy in addition to anthracycline in the treatment of acute promyelocytic leukaemia does not improve outcomes: results of the MRC AML15 trial. Leukemia. 2013;27(4):843–51.

112. Adès L, Sanz MA, Chevret S, Montesinos P, Chevallier P, Raffoux E, et al. Treatment of newly diagnosed acute promyelocytic leukemia (APL): a comparison of French-Belgian-Swiss and PETHEMA results. Blood. 2008;111(3):1078–84.

113. Sanz MA, Montesinos P, Rayon C, Holowiecka A, de la Serna J, Milone G, et al. Risk-adapted treatment of acute promyelocytic leukemia based on all-trans retinoic acid and anthracycline with addition of cytarabine in consolidation therapy for high-risk patients: further improvements in treatment outcome. Blood. 2010;115(25):5137–46.

114. Mandelli F, Vignetti M, Suciu S, Stasi R, Petti MC, Meloni G, et al. Daunorubicin versus mitoxantrone versus Idarubicin as induction and consolidation chemotherapy for adults with acute myeloid leukemia: the EORTC and GIMEMA Groups Study AML-10. J Clin Oncol. 2009;27(32):5397–403.

115. Shinagawa K, Yanada M, Sakura T, Ueda Y, Sawa M, Miyatake J, et al. Tamibarotene as maintenance therapy for acute promyelocytic leukemia: results from a randomized controlled trial. J Clin Oncol. 2014;32(33):3729–35.

116. Röllig C, Schäfer-Eckardt K, Hänel M, Kramer M, Schaich M, Thiede C, et al. Two cycles of risk-adapted consolidation therapy in patients with acute promyelocytic leukemia. Results from the SAL-AIDA2000 trial. Ann Hematol. 2015;94(4):557–63.

117. Huang H, Qin Y, Xu R, You X, Teng R, Yang L, et al. Combination therapy with arsenic trioxide, all-trans retinoic acid, and chemotherapy in acute promyelocytic leukemia patients with various relapse risks. Leuk Res. 2012;36(7):841–5.

Cure of Acute Promyelocytic Leukemia Without Chemotherapy

10

Mary-Elizabeth M. Percival and Elihu H. Estey

Introduction

Acute promyelocytic leukemia (APL) is an uncommon subtype of acute myeloid leukemia (AML) which accounts for around 5–10% of all AML cases in adults and children. APL is characterized by a recurrent translocation between chromosome 15 (the promyelocytic gene or *PML*) and chromosome 17 (the retinoic receptor alpha gene or *RARA*); the resulting fusion protein PML-RARα leads to specific morphologic, molecular, and biologic properties that distinguish APL from other subtypes of AML. In particular, because of complications such as the thrombohemorrhagic syndrome, APL has a high early death rate [1, 2]. High-risk APL is defined as having an initial WBC count $\geq 10 \times 10^9$ cells/L (which occurs in approximately one-quarter of patients) [3]; all other cases are considered standard risk. As with all acute leukemia, the first step in the treatment of APL is induction therapy. This chapter will focus on the options for a chemotherapy-free approach to APL induction. The combination of all-*trans* retinoic acid (ATRA) and arsenic trioxide (ATO) has been widely adopted since the seminal randomized trial first reported by Lo-Coco et al. in 2013 [4]. The drugs are both naturally occurring, leading to the description of treatment with "a vitamin and a mineral." However, the development of this chemotherapy-free combination took over four decades of intensive research and clinical trials before becoming the current standard of care for most APL patients.

M.-E.M. Percival, M.D. (✉) • E.H. Estey, M.D.
Department of Medicine, University of Washington, 825 Eastlake Ave E, MS G3200, Seattle, WA 98109-1023, USA

Clinical Research Division, Fred Hutchinson Cancer Research Center, Seattle, WA, USA
e-mail: mperciva@uw.edu

ATRA Monotherapy

ATRA, also known as tretinoin, is the agent most associated with APL (though ATO is more efficacious when used as a single agent). ATRA is a derivative of vitamin A; vitamin A and its analogues are generically known as retinoids. ATRA became the backbone of treatment for newly diagnosed APL based on a series of seminal trials in the 1980s, primarily from China. ATRA is often heralded as the first "targeted" therapy in human cancer, thereby preceding the use of imatinib in chronic myeloid leukemia (CML) in the following decade. This description is not completely borne out by the historical record, since retinoic acid derivatives were identified as differentiating agents for cell lines during drug screens (which led to clinical trials); only later was it

O. Abla et al. (eds.), *Acute Promyelocytic Leukemia*, https://doi.org/10.1007/978-3-319-64257-4_10

determined that the target of ATRA was the fusion protein PML-RARα. However, as reviewed by some of the principal Chinese scientists involved in initial trials, investigators began to seek a novel treatment for APL that did not involve traditional chemotherapy, perhaps based on Confucian principles, and the newly identified drug ATRA which led to differentiation of APL cells seemed to be an excellent candidate [5].

Early Experimentation with ATRA

Retinoic acid derivatives were first discovered in the early 1980s through drug screens examining promyelocyte differentiation. Preclinical work by Breitman et al. demonstrated that continuous exposure to retinoic acid led to optimal terminal cellular differentiation in an AML cell line (HL-60) [6, 7]. Only later were the mechanisms worked out by which retinoic acid was effective in APL cell lines. The PML-RARα fusion protein undergoes a conformational change in the presence of ATRA, which leads to significant changes at the transcriptome and proteome levels in addition to gain of apoptotic potential [8]. Additionally, ATRA leads to destruction of the PML-RARα fusion protein. Interestingly, early in vitro studies with retinoids were performed in other subtypes of AML, using both cell lines and primary patient samples, and retinoids appeared to effect differentiation and inhibit growth in non-APL AML cells as well [9], a finding that has not been borne out in subsequent clinical practice.

The provocative findings in APL cell lines were quickly taken into the clinic. In one of the earliest clinical publications, bone marrow promyelocytes were harvested from a patient with chemotherapy-refractory APL and treated with retinoic acid in vitro [10]. After the cultured cells were found to exhibit differentiation without active proliferation, the patient was treated with oral 13-*cis*-retinoic acid at a dose of 100 mg/m^2/day for 13 days. Preliminary analysis suggested that the patient had a response to the retinoic acid, with a higher percentage of maturing cells in the blood and bone marrow, but unfortunately the patient died on day 13 from disseminated candidiasis [10]. Subsequent case studies were reported for patients with refractory APL treated with 13-*cis*-retinoic acid; this single-agent treatment led to normalization of peripheral blood counts for 20 weeks and 1 year, respectively [11–13]. Notably, 13-*cis*-retinoic acid is a retinoic acid isomer identical to ATRA except for the orientation of its carboxy terminus. Subsequent reports demonstrated that outcomes with ATRA were superior to those with 13-*cis*-retinoic acid [14, 15].

Induction of APL with Single-Agent ATRA

Because of the accessibility of ATRA and the promising published case reports, the Shanghai group began clinical trials with this agent in APL. Many of the patients had relapsed/refractory (R/R) disease, but this chapter will focus on the patients with newly diagnosed APL receiving their first treatment. The studies of single-agent ATRA in newly diagnosed APL are summarized in Table 10.1. The first six patients enrolled by the Shanghai group who received ATRA were described in 1987, though importantly ATRA was co-administered with cytarabine [16]. A larger trial, with single-agent ATRA, was conducted by Huang et al. in a cohort of 24 APL patients, 16 with newly diagnosed APL and 6 with R/R disease [17]. The untreated patients ranged in age from 18 to 61 years and had peripheral white blood cell (WBC) counts ranging from 0.9 to 15.8×10^9 cells/L. The doses of ATRA in the untreated patients ranged from 45 to 50 mg/m^2/day for induction therapy, which is in line with the current recommended dosing of 45 mg/m^2/day in a divided dose. Remarkably, of the newly diagnosed patients, all but one achieved CR (defined as <5% blasts plus promyelocytes in a normo cellular marrow with normal peripheral blood counts); the final newly diagnosed patient achieved a CR when cytarabine was added to induction, and all eight of the R/R patients achieved CR. The description of the treatment course of the patients in the trial closely resembles what is seen in current clinical practice: "The total WBC count rose progressively starting with initia-

Table 10.1 Summary of patient outcomes for studies using single-agent retinoic acid derivatives for induction treatment of newly diagnosed APL

Reference	Patients (n)	Induction treatment	CR rate	Overall survival	Comments
Huang ME et al. 1988 [17]	16	ATRA	94% (15/16)	Not reported	1 patient achieved CR with addition of cytarabine; all patients received chemotherapy consolidation
Castaigne S et al. 1990 [19]	4	ATRA	50% (2/4)	Not reported	2 patients had early death (days +6 and +12); all patients received chemotherapy consolidation
Warrell RP et al. 1991 [20]	6	ATRA	83% (5/6)	Not reported	1 patient who did not achieve CR did not have t(15;17); all patients received chemotherapy consolidation
Chen ZX et al. 1991 [21]	47	ATRA	94% (44/47)	Not reported	3 patients had early death (days +4, +4, +5); all patients received chemotherapy consolidation
Frankel SR et al. 1994 [22]	34	ATRA	87% (26/30)	31 months (median)	5 patients had early death; most patients (22) received chemotherapy consolidation
Kanamaru A et al. 1995 [23]	28	ATRA	89% (25/28)	Not reported	Other patients on the study received ATRA plus chemotherapy
Fenaux P et al. 1993 [24]	54	ATRA	91% (49/54)	91% at 1 year	5 patients had early death; study patients were randomized to ATRA vs. chemotherapy, with both arms followed by chemotherapy consolidation
Tallman MS et al. 1997 [26]	124	ATRA	72% (124/172)	71% at 3 years	19 patients had early death; study patients were randomized to ATRA vs. chemotherapy, with both arms followed by chemotherapy consolidation
Estey E et al. 2001 [83]	34	lipoATRA	79% (27/34)	Not reported	6 patients had early death; consolidation was also with lipoATRA

Abbreviations: all-trans retinoic acid (ATRA), complete remission (CR), liposomal ATRA (lipoATRA)

tion of treatment and reaching a peak between 7 and 14 days. The WBC count then fell with the progressive maturation of granulocytes. Increase in platelets was most prominent after 3 weeks. Elevation of the hemoglobin concentration appeared reluctant and slow. Bone marrow aspirate revealed that hypercellularity existed throughout RA [retinoic acid] treatment." The responses were transient, however, and patients relapsed after a period of months, though it should be noted that patients received a variety of maintenance regimens that are not routinely used today (ATRA at 20–30 mg/m^2/day, ATRA plus low-dose cytarabine or harringtonine, low-dose cytarabine, or multidrug consolidation followed by maintenance chemotherapy) [17]. This trial would change the treatment algorithm for APL, ultimately turning APL into a disease curable in 90% of people treated in academic centers [1]. Further enrollment on the clinical trial demonstrated a CR rate of 84% at 42 days after initiation of ATRA (48 out of 57 total patients), with the caveat that the study population contained both newly diagnosed and R/R patients and many patients received chemotherapy as consolidation [18].

The remarkable findings from the Shanghai group using single-agent ATRA were quickly replicated in a worldwide series of studies in the early 1990s. The French group induced 22 patients with single-agent ATRA, but only 4 of these were previously untreated; only 2 of the 4 untreated patients achieved CR, with the other 2 dying at day 6 and day 12 after initiation of treatment with a pronounced, and unusual, hyperleukocytosis [19]. A similar study treated 11 patients with single-agent ATRA; five of the six previously untreated patients achieved CR [20]. Patients in both of these studies went on to receive consolidation therapy with chemotherapy and sometimes hematopoietic stem cell transplantation (HSCT).

Another Chinese study, from the Jiangsu Institute of Hematology, examined induction treatment with single-agent ATRA in 50 patients, 47 of whom were newly diagnosed [21]. The CR rate for this group was a remarkable 94%, with only three patients not achieving a CR because they died within the first week after treatment initiation (two of hemorrhagic complications). The CR1 duration ranged from 3 to 30 months, though it should be noted that patients generally received subsequent chemotherapy with a variety of agents (homoharringtonine, vincristine, cytarabine, and prednisone) [21]. A subsequent study from Memorial Sloan Kettering examined 56 consecutive patients treated with ATRA at 45 mg/m^2/day in New York; 26 out of the 30 newly diagnosed patients with a confirmed reverse transcriptase polymerase chain reaction (RT-PCR) *PML-RARA* gene rearrangement achieved CR (86%) [22]. Twenty-two of these patients received consolidation chemotherapy; the group as a whole had a median relapse-free survival of over 28 months (range 1–34) with an overall survival of over 31 months (range 0.4–36). The New York group performed a comparison to a historical control cohort of 80 patients treated with conventional chemotherapy, demonstrating the superiority of induction with ATRA ($p = 0.014$) [22]. The Japan Adult Leukemia Study Group also investigated ATRA induction, but only 28 of 109 patients received ATRA alone because daunorubicin and cytarabine were administered if patients had a WBC > 3 × 10^9/L at diagnosis; the CR rate for these 28 patients was 89%, and the survival data were favorable in a retrospective comparison to a previous study [23]. The conclusion from these studies as a whole was that ATRA was highly effective at inducing CR in patients with untreated APL, but that remissions were transient if patients were not consolidated with chemotherapy because ATRA resistance developed rapidly.

The next series of studies confirming the effectiveness of ATRA as induction therapy included randomized comparisons of ATRA followed by chemotherapy versus ATRA plus simultaneous chemotherapy in newly diagnosed APL patients. Two large intergroup studies compared these approaches. The goal was to decrease the risk of the so-called ATRA differentiation syndrome, as well as to prolong the duration of CR. The European APL 91 study included 101 patients from 46 centers, who were randomized to receive 7 + 3 chemotherapy (with cytarabine 200 mg/m^2/day on days 1–7 plus daunorubicin 60 mg/m^2/day on days 1–3) versus ATRA 45 mg/m^2/day until CR, followed by 7 + 3 chemotherapy [24].

Both arms were consolidated with two further courses of combination chemotherapy (one 7 + 3 and one with intermediate-dose cytarabine). The study was terminated early because the event-free survival was significantly higher in the ATRA group, and 49 patients (91%) achieved CR [24]. The North American Intergroup examined a slightly different question of the effect of ATRA maintenance chemotherapy after initial induction, to determine if the early benefits seen with ATRA were sustained at the time of long-term follow-up. Three hundred fifty patients were randomized to receive induction with ATRA 45 mg/m^2/day until CR or one to two cycles of 7 + 3 chemotherapy (with cytarabine 100 mg/m^2/day on days 1–7 plus daunorubicin 45 mg/m^2/day on days 1–3); consolidation was similar to the APL 91 study with two further courses of combination chemotherapy [25, 26]. Patients in CR following consolidation underwent a second randomization to receive maintenance ATRA for 1 year of observation. The CR rate was not significantly different between the two groups (70% in the ATRA group and 73% in the chemotherapy group); however, long-term follow-up demonstrated that the 5-year disease-free survival and overall survival were significantly longer for the ATRA maintenance group (69% for both in the ATRA group, but with relapse-free survival of only 29% and overall survival of 45% in the chemotherapy cohort) [25].

Toxicity of ATRA

The initial toxicities of ATRA described in the Shanghai study by Huang et al. closely resemble those identified in clinical practice today. The drug is extremely well tolerated, but common toxicities included "dryness of the lips and skin (100%), headache (25%), nausea or vomiting (20.8%), moderate bone or joint pain (12.5%), and mild exfoliation (8.3%)" [17]. Two other notable toxicities of ATRA include teratogenicity (part of the black box warning for tretinoin) and development of intracranial hypertension (pseudotumor cerebri, PTC). The latter was first identified in a small early study of ATRA in 2 of 11 patients [20]. Though it is a recognized toxicity of ATRA, PTC is likely much less common than initially observed; a large analysis of 240 patients treated with ATRA on an intergroup protocol showed that only 1.7% of patients had "probable" PTC [27]. However, the incidence of PTC appears to be higher in children with APL (16% in the APL93 trial, which combined ATRA and chemotherapy), particularly in those aged <10 years [28].

The most concerning toxicity of ATRA is that of the differentiation syndrome (DS), which was first described by Frankel et al. in 1992 [29] and is identified in approximately 25% of patients treated with ATRA. Symptoms include fever, respiratory distress, weight gain, edema, pleural or pericardial effusions, and hypotension, occurring between 2 and 21 days after initiation of treatment in the initial description of the syndrome. Then as now, steroids were the mainstay of treatment; prompt administration of dexamethasone at 10 mg every 12 h led to symptomatic improvement in three of four patients [29]. Multiorgan failure and even death can occur as a result of DS, leading to a black box warning on tretinoin formulations. A retrospective analysis of patients from the European APL group described the "ATRA syndrome" or DS in 15% of patients (64 of 413) during induction; though steroids and supportive care led to a low rate of death, patients with DS still had lower event-free and overall survival rates [30]. Interestingly, though pretreatment WBC count has been posited as an important factor in the development of differentiation syndrome based on a previous analysis of data from the New York Group [31], no predictive significant factors (including WBC count) could be identified in the larger European group [30]. As will be discussed later, ATO can also lead to a differentiation syndrome.

Current Use of ATRA in APL

Single-agent ATRA is highly effective at inducing CR in patients with newly diagnosed APL. Since these remissions are transient, however, it is generally combined with other agents; we will next discuss the most significant of these,

ATO. However, because of the low level of toxicity, high level of efficacy, and ease of administration with oral gelatin capsules, ATRA is frequently administered as a single agent to patients with a new diagnosis of AML while awaiting confirmatory testing for APL, usually by fluorescence in situ hybridization.

Arsenic Trioxide (ATO) Monotherapy

ATO, also known by its chemical compound As_2O_3, is more effective than ATRA in APL. It is a naturally occurring metallic element, analogous to phosphorus on the periodic table, and arsenic's inorganic forms are known to be poisonous to humans and animals. In large doses, arsenic and many of its commonly occurring compounds disrupt signaling pathways, glutathione conjugation, and the intracellular production of adenosine triphosphate (ATP) through a variety of mechanisms, leading to cellular necrosis and fairly rapid death [32]. In smaller doses, which can affect humans through contaminated groundwater or foods such as seafood, rice, and mushrooms, arsenic has been reported to adversely and permanently affect hematologic, cardiovascular, and neurologic systems, among others [33–35].

However, despite the fact that it is a toxic chemical, arsenic has a long history as an ancient remedy. Arsenic has been described in a comprehensive review of its medicinal uses as moving from "notoriety to respectability" [36]. Medicinal use of arsenic was described by Hippocrates, and arsenic-containing compounds have been a mainstay of traditional Chinese medicine for thousands of years [37]. Fowler solution (which contains 1% potassium arsenite) was developed in the 1700s and used for the treatment of malignant, rheumatologic, and infectious diseases, including the treatment of chronic myeloid leukemia (CML) for over a century [37]. ATO, currently the most clinically relevant arsenic-containing compound, is under investigation for the treatment of multiple non-APL malignancies. Data demonstrating activity in phase 2 trials for patients with multiple myeloma and other diseases have been reviewed previously [38], and there are multiple active or recently closed trials in other non-hematologic malignancies.

Mechanism of Action of ATO

Interestingly, the mechanism of action of ATO was discovered only after the clinical benefit was observed. Two arsenic-containing compounds (ATO and arsenic disulfide) were found to be components of traditional Chinese medicine that seemed to be beneficial in APL patients, particularly in those who were resistant to ATRA. Later studies were conducted to help determine the mechanism of action of ATO in APL. In vitro analysis of the NB_4 cell line (derived from an APL patient) showed that ATO led to selective apoptosis of malignant cells, likely through downregulation of BCL-2 expression and modulation of the PML-RARα fusion protein [39]. Importantly, this pathway is independent of the mechanism of ATRA and was not affected by ATRA pretreatment. Later work, also by the Shanghai group, examined an ATRA-resistant cell line (MR2 subclone) and primary patient samples and found what appeared to be a dose-dependent effect of ATO: induction of apoptosis at higher doses and differentiation at lower doses, with both likely mediated by degradation of the PML-RARα fusion protein [40]. The induction of apoptosis may be the most important effect of ATO, but there is no doubt that it can also act as an agent to promote differentiation in APL [41]. ATO also seemed to have a negative effect on other leukemia cell lines, similar to preclinical studies of ATRA that have not been borne out in clinical practice (at least not for use as a single agent) [42].

Treatment of APL with ATO

ATO had been used for the treatment of CML in the Western world, as previously mentioned, but it became a compound of interest when it was found to be a component of traditional Chinese medicines. A systematic study of the effect of ATO was begun in the 1970s by the Harbin group in Northeastern China, and APL was found to be particularly responsive to ATO in a series of publications starting in 1992 [43, 44].

ATO was not widely applied to the treatment of APL outside of the northernmost part of China until the 1990s. The studies of single-agent ATO in the induction treatment of newly diagnosed APL are summarized in Table 10.2. In 1997, the Shanghai group reported on the use of ATO in 15 patients with R/R APL [45], along with accompanying laboratory-based study that was mentioned previously [40]. Ten of these patients had been induced with ATRA and received single-agent ATO at the time of first relapse (the remaining five patients had received multi-agent therapy including ATO); 90% (9 out of 10) achieved CR with single-agent ATO [45]. This study confirmed the efficacy of ATO as a single agent in APL and paved the way for larger studies in the future.

Shortly afterward, ATO was studied in the Western world, again in patients with R/R APL [46]. Twelve patients were studied, who had relapsed between one and three times, and 11 achieved CR. The current standard dosing of ATO (0.15 mg/kg) was derived from this study as well; the first few patients received a fixed dose, but the investigators moved to weight-based dosing after the enrollment of two pediatric patients [46]. With correlative studies on patient samples, the investigators confirmed that ATO led to the so-called nonterminal differentiation followed by apoptosis of leukemic cells.

Investigators from the Harbin and Shanghai groups next began to include patients with newly diagnosed APL in their studies of ATO. This drug that appeared to be so effective in the R/R state might lead to profound improvements in the upfront treatment of APL as well. Eleven patients with newly diagnosed APL were included in the study of Niu et al. which was published in 1999, though only seven were treated with ATO alone (the remaining four received chemotherapy in addition) [47]. Six of seven achieved CR (86%), after a range of 30 to 36 days receiving ATO. Consolidation consisted of further courses of ATO and chemotherapy. Three of

Table 10.2 Summary of patient outcomes for studies using single-agent arsenic compounds for induction treatment of newly diagnosed APL

Reference	Patients (*n*)	Induction treatment	CR rate	Overall survival	Comments
Niu C et al. 1999 [47]	7	ATO	86% (6/7)	Not reported	1 patient had early death; most patients received chemotherapy consolidation
Mathews V et al. 2010 [52]	72	ATO	86% (62/72)	74% at 5 years	10 patients had early death (8 from intracranial bleeding); 8 patients received anthracycline; consolidation was also with ATO
Ghavamzadeh A et al. 2011 [54]	197	ATO	86% (169/197)	64% at 5 years	Early death more common in high-risk patients
Zhu HH et al. 2013 [98]	112	ATO	97% (114/117)	97% at 3 years	Patients received chemotherapy consolidation and maintenance
Zhu HH et al. 2013 [98]	108	RIF	99% (113/114)	99% at 3 years	Patients received chemotherapy consolidation and maintenance

Abbreviations: arsenic trioxide (ATO), complete remission (CR), Realgar-Indigo naturalis (RIF)

the 11 newly diagnosed patients had early death within the first 15 days of treatment, but the remaining 8 remained in CR for a period of 8–20 months with a median follow-up of 12 months [47].

Many studies were conducted to cement the role of ATO as an effective agent for R/R APL, even showing that it was as effective as consolidative HCT [48, 49], but the Indian and Iranian groups asked the question of whether single-agent ATO could be an effective treatment for newly diagnosed patients. The Indian group first demonstrated the efficacy of single-agent ATO in 2002, with the publication of a small series of 14 patients treated with ATO at a fixed dose of 10 mg/day [50]. Three patients died within the first 4 days, and one died at day 21; impressively, the remaining 10 attained CR (71%). This study confirmed that ATO was a highly effective agent in the treatment of APL and that the major risk associated with the disease at the time of diagnosis was early death. Notably, part of the impetus of these studies was the expense of ATRA in the setting of the relative affordability of ATO on clinical trial. The positive results were extended in a 2006 study [51] and further updated in the large 2010 analysis by Mathews et al. [52]. In all of these studies, ATO was administered as a single-agent induction therapy until approximately day 60 or CR. After a 4-week interval, another 4-week course was administered; finally, after another 4-week interval, ATO was administered 10 days per month for 6 months. Occasional patients were treated with anthracycline (at the clinician's discretion if there was profound leukocytosis, or concern for differentiation syndrome), and many received concurrent hydroxyurea. Seventy-two patients were treated, and 62 achieved CR (86%); the remaining 10 patients died during induction, the majority of bleeding complications. What is most remarkable is that the 5-year OS is 74% ± SE 5.2%, meaning that the large majority of patients were cured with this powerful single-agent regimen [52].

Similar impressive findings for single-agent ATO were shown in the same timeframe by the Iranian group. The Iranian group treated 111 patients with single-agent ATO, 94 of whom were previously untreated [53]. The dose of ATO was 0.15 mg/kg daily for a 2-h IV infusion until CR or day 60; consolidation consisted of ATO at the same dose 6 days/week for 28 doses. CR was achieved in 82 of the 94 newly diagnosed patients (86%). Notably, 23 patients had the APL differentiation syndrome, and 8 died of this complication. Approximately half of the patients in the study were followed for minimal residual disease (MRD) by RT-PCR, and 92% had no evidence of MRD. Interestingly, 24 patients relapsed; 5 died during re-induction with ATO, but the remaining 19 achieved a second CR with the same ATO induction regimen [53]. Long-term follow-up of 197 newly diagnosed patients treated with ATO alone demonstrated impressive survival results [54], with the accompanying editorial noting that ATO is moving "front and center" in the treatment of APL and that results with single-agent ATO surpassed those seen with single-agent ATRA [55]. The study population consisted of 197 patients enrolled between 1999 and 2010. These patients received the same induction as previously described but starting in 2006 received a total of four courses of 28-day consolidation with ATO: one that started 1 month after CR, another that started 1 month later, and then repeat courses at 1 and 2 years after CR. The CR rate was 86% (169 of 197 patients); the major reason for not achieving CR was early death, which occurred in 29 patients (15%), primarily as a result of bleeding complications. The disease-free survival was 66.7% ± 4% at 5 years, and the overall survival at 5 years was 64.4% ± 4% [54].

Controversy exists about the conduct of the clinical trials utilizing single-agent ATO in the upfront treatment setting, since the impetus for moving this agent into the frontline was because of cost concerns related to ATRA [56]. However, ATO has clearly been shown through these comprehensive studies to be a highly effective and well-tolerated drug for APL induction as a single agent.

Toxicity of ATO in APL

From the first clinical trials of ATO in APL, it is clear that the drug has recurrent side effects aside from its history as a toxic chemical. As the dosing was being established, some patients had evidence of acute and chronic arsenic toxicity while being treated for APL [57], and some studies had analysis of hair and nail clippings built in for analysis of dosing, toxicity, and timing of arsenic exposure [52]. Predictably, since it leads to in vitro differentiation in tissue culture, ATO leads to a differentiation syndrome quite similar to that seen with single-agent ATRA, which is also treated with high-dose steroids and which also had led to a black box warning. It was first described in patients with R/R APL treated with single-agent ATO, and, as for patients with ATRA differentiation syndrome, symptoms were found in 31% of patients and appeared more likely to develop in those with leukocytosis [58].

The cardiac toxicity of ATO is also notable, with most current protocols requiring regular electrocardiographic monitoring and aggressive electrolyte (potassium and magnesium) repletion of patients while receiving ATO to help prevent toxicity. A black box warning also exists for this cardiac toxicity, noting the QT-interval prolongation and complete atrioventricular block that can develop with ATO exposure [59]. Many physicians will limit the use of concomitant QT-interval prolonging drugs. At least two reports have suggested that the ATO-associated cardiac toxicity has a genetic basis, with African-American patients having a predisposition to sudden cardiac death [60, 61]. Cardiac toxicity can usually be mitigated with a decrease in the ATO dose.

Hepatotoxicity was reported in some of the early studies of single-agent ATO, including two cases of fulminant liver failure [47]. However, this study was published before the dose of ATO was standardized, and the frequency of hepatotoxicity appears lower in subsequent clinical practice than previously noted.

Combination of ATRA and ATO in APL

The next logical step in the progression of treatment of APL was to combine ATRA and ATO, each highly efficacious on their own, into one regimen. The ultimate goal of such a regimen would be to minimize or completely remove chemotherapy and complete the transformation of APL from a highly lethal subtype of AML into the most highly curable one.

Preclinical Studies

ATRA and ATO were found to act in synergistic ways through a variety of elegant experiments. One early report suggested that ATO caused apoptosis without differentiation [41], but subsequent experiments (and clinical experience) have borne out the claim that ATO is a potent agent of differentiation for promyelocytes. Later in vitro work showed that the ATRA/ATO combination appeared to lead to differentiation and apoptosis in the ATO-resistant NB4 cell line, though it was not clear if sequential or concurrent therapy would be most beneficial [62]. In vivo mouse models transplanted with APL leukemic blasts further suggested that ATRA and ATO in combination led to improved responses and survival when compared to either agent alone [63, 64].

ATO and ATRA in Standard-Risk APL

The promising combination of ATRA and ATO, which has now become the standard for all patients with newly diagnosed standard-risk APL, was investigated in a fascinating case report of a Jehovah's Witness with newly diagnosed APL [65]. The patient presented with pancytopenia and refused all blood product support; since anthracycline chemotherapy was contraindicated, the investigators administered single-agent ATRA (at a reduced dose of 25 mg/m^2/day), followed by repeated courses of concurrent ATRA and ATO consolidation therapy. Remarkably, the patient achieved a molecular remission without requiring blood product support.

This case report, along with the preclinical data showing that ATRA and ATO targeted different intracellular pathways, laid the groundwork for the development of clinical trials with combination induction therapy (summarized in Table 10.3). The Shanghai group published a randomized trial of 61 patients, who received ATRA alone at 25 mg/m^2/

Table 10.3 Summary of patient outcomes for studies using retinoic acid and arsenic derivatives together for induction treatment of newly diagnosed APL

Reference	Patients (*n*)	Induction treatment	CR rate	Overall survival	Comments
Shen ZX et al. 2004 [66]	21	ATRA/ATO	95% (20/21)	Not reported	1 patient had early death; patients received chemotherapy consolidation and maintenance; disease-free survival was 100%
Estey EH et al. 2006 [67]	44	ATRA/ATO	89% (39/44)	Not reported	GO was given for high WBC count during induction; only 3 patients relapsed
Burnett AK et al. 2015 [72]	116	ATRA/ATO	94% (109/116)	93% at 4 years	Included standard- and high-risk APL; study patients were randomized to ATRA/ATO vs. ATRA/chemotherapy; GO was given for high WBC count during induction
Platzbecker U et al. 2016 [69]	127	ATRA/ATO	100% (127/127)	99% at 50 months	Included only standard-risk APL; study patients were randomized to ATRA/ATO vs. ATRA/chemotherapy
Zhu HH et al. 2014 [98]	20	ATRA/RIF	100% (20/20)	Not reported	10 patients completed all therapy on an outpatient basis; this combination is the basis of an ongoing larger clinical trial (NCT02899169)

Abbreviations: all-trans retinoic acid (ATRA), arsenic trioxide (ATO), Realgar-Indigo naturalis (RIF), complete remission (CR)

day, ATO alone at 0.16 mg/kg/day, or ATRA/ATO concurrently at the same doses as single agent for induction therapy [66]. Notably, the trial was not free of chemotherapy. Patients with high WBC count (>10 × 10^9 cells/L) received cytarabine and idarubicin in a 7 + 3 pattern during induction; also, all patients received three consolidation cycles with chemotherapy (7 + 3, intermediate-dose cytarabine, and homoharringtonine plus cytarabine). Nearly all patients achieved CR after induction, including 20 of 21 patients in the ATRA/ATO arm; the four who did not all died of cerebral hemorrhage. Remission induction was significantly faster in the combination arm (median 25.5 days) than in the other two (median 40.5 days in the ATRA arm and 31 days in the ATO arm); the combination arm also led to the greatest decrease in the levels of *PML-RARA* transcript when assessed by RT-PCR [66].

Spurred onward by these provocative results, Estey et al. performed the first clinical trial in newly diagnosed APL that did not include required chemotherapy [67]. The 44 evaluable patients received ATRA at 45 mg/m^2/day starting on day 1; ATO was added at 0.15 mg/kg on day 10. Once in CR, patients received consolidation therapy with alternating courses of ATRA and ATO (see Fig. 10.1). Patients received chemotherapy with the CD33-targeted antibody-drug conjugate gemtuzumab ozogamicin (GO) only in certain predefined circumstances: (1) high-risk APL with initial WBC > 10 × 10^9 cells/L, (2) PCR positivity for *PML-RARA* transcript 3 months after morphologic CR, (3) molecular relapse, or (4) ATRA or ATO toxicity forcing discontinuation. Eighteen patients received chemotherapy, primarily due to having a high WBC count at diagnosis and thus falling into the high-risk APL group; three patients also received idarubicin due to individual physicians' discomfort with the GO prescribed by the study. The CR rate was an impressive 89% (39 of 44), with four early deaths in the first 3 days on study [67]. This

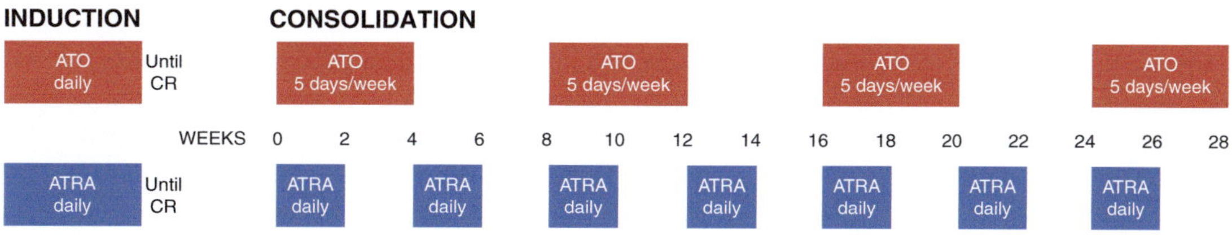

Fig. 10.1 Schema of ATRA and ATO induction in newly diagnosed APL, as published by Lo-coco et al. [4]. The dose of ATO is 0.15 mg/kg/day, and the dose of ATRA is 45 mg/m²/day administered in a divided dose. After complete remission (CR) is established, patients enter consolidation for 28 weeks. The regimen leads to cure rates in excess of 95% for standard-risk APL

groundbreaking study set up future trials with the combination of ATRA and ATO without traditional chemotherapy, while demonstrating that high-risk APL patients could have similar and excellent outcomes.

The large randomized trial by Lo-Coco et al. confirmed that the chemotherapy-free approach to induction was non-inferior (and likely superior) to the standard incorporation of chemotherapy [4]. This cooperative multicenter phase 3 study was conducted through Gruppo Italiano Malattie Ematologiche dell'Adulto, the German-Austrian Acute Myeloid Leukemia Study Group, and the Study Alliance Leukemia. The study randomized 162 standard-risk newly diagnosed APL patients to receive induction and consolidation ATRA and ATO alone, as per the study of Estey et al. [67] or to receive ATRA and idarubicin at 12 mg/m² on days 2, 4, 6, and 8 of induction (the AIDA regimen, plus further anthracycline therapy during consolidation) [68]. Of the 156 evaluable patients, all 77 (100%) in the ATRA/ATO group achieved CR, and 75/79 (95%) in the ATRA/chemotherapy group achieved CR ($p = 0.12$). EFS was significantly different between the two groups (97% vs. 85%, $p < 0.001$ for non-inferiority), as was the 2-year OS probability of 99% (95% CI 96, 100) in the ATRA/ATO group versus 91% (95% CI 94, 100) in the ATRA/chemotherapy group ($p = 0.02$). These remarkable findings of high CR rates and impressive OS in the ATRA/ATO group have been borne out by the final follow-up data [69].

What is perhaps most noteworthy about this series of studies is that the investigators were not content with the known high cure rate with ATRA plus chemotherapy in APL (over 80%) and instead strove for (and achieved) an even higher goal. In the final results, the OS in the ATRA/ATO arm at 50 months is 99.2% (compared to 92.6% in the ATRA/chemotherapy arm, $p = 0.0073$) [69]. The superiority of ATRA/ATO compared to ATRA/chemotherapy has been confirmed by a meta-analysis, in terms of improved CR rate, EFS, and OS [70]. Additionally, by not receiving traditional cytotoxic chemotherapy, patients may have fewer short-term complications (viz., decreased myelosuppression) and long-term side effects (such as less anthracycline-related cardiac toxicity and a decreased rate of therapy-related AML). It is worth noting that patients still require the inconvenience of daily ATO infusions, in the setting of the known manageable toxicities of ATRA and ATO.

ATO and ATRA in High-Risk APL

Though the aforementioned study of Estey et al. included all patients with APL [67], as did the follow-up analysis from MD Anderson Cancer Center [71], the Lo-coco et al. randomized study did not, instead limiting the study to standard-risk patients with a WBC < 10×10^9 cells/L at diagnosis [4]. The Medical Research Council (MRC) in the United Kingdom included all-risk APL patients in their AML17 trial [72]. Patients were randomized to receive ATRA/chemotherapy ($n = 119$, using idarubicin in the AIDA regimen) or ATRA/ATO ($n = 116$, with the option for high-risk patients to receive an initial dose of GO 6 mg/m² for rapid cytoreduction). In the ATRA/ATO group,

28 of 30 high-risk patients ultimately received GO (the remaining two received idarubicin because GO was not available). Seven low-risk patients were administered a dose of GO due to increasing WBC count. Therefore, 30% of patients in the ATRA/ATO group received GO (35 of 116). Though the CR rates were not different between the two groups, the 4-year EFS was significantly different and superior in the ATRA/ATO arm; differences in OS and quality of life outcome measures did not reach statistical significance [72].

The role and efficacy of GO in the treatment of APL will be discussed next in this chapter, but in short, high-risk APL may require initial cytoreduction during induction, but patients can then likely receive maximal benefit with a chemotherapy-free consolidation.

Combination Therapy with Gemtuzumab Ozogamicin (GO) in APL

The combination of ATRA and ATO, as described previously, leads to impressive response rates and survival with limited toxicity in newly diagnosed APL patients. The antibody-drug conjugate GO, a monoclonal antibody against CD33 which is targeted to the potent calicheamicin chemotherapeutic agent, has been explored in APL as another alternative to traditional cytotoxic chemotherapy. Because of the nearly ubiquitous expression of CD33 on the surface of APL cells, GO was suspected to be particularly effective in the treatment of APL. GO also holds a role in the treatment of relapsed APL patients, and its use in APL (both upfront and R/R) has been previously reviewed [73]. GO received accelerated approval for the treatment of older patients with AML. However, this medication with significant efficacy in APL was voluntarily withdrawn from the market in the United States in 2010 after required post-marketing surveillance suggested minimal benefit in unselected patients with AML, despite a positive meta-analysis and public pleas for its reinstatement [74, 75]. In 2017, the United States Food and Drug Administration approved GO for the treatment of AML, but the label makes no particular reference to APL.

In APL, GO was first studied in the consolidation phase of treatment for newly diagnosed patients who had achieved CR with ATRA and/or chemotherapy; addition of GO led to a high response rate with a low level of detection of RT-PCR transcript [76]. GO was quickly moved into the upfront treatment of APL [77]. This study combined ATRA (45 mg/m^2/day during induction, then switched to an alternating 14 days on/14 days off schedule) with GO (9 mg/m^2) administered during induction on day 1 or 5, then in CR every 4–5 weeks for 8 further doses. Nineteen patients were enrolled, and 16 achieved CR (84%, the remaining three died early before marrow evaluation) [77].

A follow-up study from MD Anderson Cancer Center confirmed that the administration of GO with ATRA and ATO for newly diagnosed APL patients was safe and effective, with 74 of 85 patients achieving CR (92%) [71]. Twenty-five patients received GO on the first day of treatment, and four received a dose later in induction because their WBC count increased to >30 × 10^9 cells/L. This study suggested that the chemotherapy-free treatment option for APL (ATRA/ATO plus or minus GO) could be expanded to include a larger patient population, including those who are traditionally considered unfit for intensive (aka, anthracycline-containing) chemotherapy.

Special Populations

The use of ATO in children and the elderly with APL is discussed in Chaps. 14 and 15, respectively.

Emerging Therapies

A number of interesting non-chemotherapy drugs may modify the treatment of APL upfront or may have utility in the setting of relapse. These include retinoic acid variants (liposomal ATRA and tamibarotene) and oral arsenic formulations.

Liposomal ATRA

Early studies identified single-agent ATRA as a powerful agent for attaining CR in newly diagnosed APL, as has been discussed previously. However, since pharmacokinetic analyses indicated that the drug levels of ATRA decreased after a few days of administration [78], a novel liposomal formulation of ATRA was developed (lipoATRA). Preclinical data suggested lipoATRA-circumvented hepatic clearance of oral ATRA, leading to sustained high levels after intravenous (IV) administration [79, 80]. A phase 1 study of lipoATRA was conducted in patients with R/R APL at MD Anderson Cancer Center, which showed that the drug was well tolerated in 19 patients [81]. Investigators quickly moved the drug as a single agent to induction therapy for newly diagnosed APL [82]. Eighteen patients were enrolled and received single-agent lipoATRA at 90 mg/m^2; twelve achieved CR (67%), with four dying of hemorrhagic complications within the first weeks of treatment. Three patients required the addition of idarubicin to their treatment regimen (all after 6 months) because of persistent PCR positivity for the *PML-RARA* fusion product. This and a follow-up study which described a total of 34 newly diagnosed patients treated with single-agent lipoATRA in induction and consolidation noted a high percentage of long-term PCR-negative CR rates [83, 84]. Eleven of 26 evaluable patients remained PCR negative at a median follow-up of 18 months (and up to 34 months) [83]; in contrast, administration of single-agent oral ATRA invariably leads to relapse, usually within 1 year of attainment of CR for newly diagnosed APL. A final update of the MD Anderson experience showed that 10 of 26 responders to lipoATRA who never received idarubicin remained in CR at a median of 6.4 years (range 3.1–7.7 years) [85]. Despite these impressive results, lipoATRA was never approved for the treatment of APL.

Tamibarotene

Tamibarotene, also known as Am80, is a highly potent novel synthetic retinoid. This oral drug is currently approved in Japan for the treatment of APL and was initially developed for use in patients who relapsed after previous treatment with ATRA [86, 87]. The drug has shown striking responses in relapsed patients, even in those with unusual manifestations such as extramedullary disease [88, 89]. A recent trial studied 14 patients who had relapsed after induction with ATRA/ATO, and the overall response rate was 64% [90]. Tamibarotene has been studied for APL maintenance [91]. Patients received single-agent ATRA induction, followed by chemotherapy courses, the composition of which depends on initial peripheral WBC count and blast count. A total of 344 patients were enrolled upfront, and 269 ultimately completed the three planned courses of consolidation and were randomly assigned to maintenance therapy with ATRA (45 mg/m^2/day) or tamibarotene (6 mg/m^2/day) for 14 days every 3 months for a total of 2 years. No difference was found for relapse-free survival (RFS) between the two maintenance groups, though an exploratory analysis of the 52 high-risk APL patients showed a 4 year RFS of 58% in the ATRA arm and 87% in the tamibarotene arm (HR 0.26; 95% CI, 0.07–0.95) [91]. None of the patients in the study received ATO, limiting applicability of the results in the modern era when ATO has been moved to frontline therapy. Additionally, the current chemotherapy-free paradigm of ATRA and ATO for induction and consolidation does not include maintenance therapy. Whether tamibarotene will be incorporated into future trials in the setting of newly diagnosed APL remains to be determined. In 2017, tamibarotene received orphan drug approval in the United States for certain subtypes of AML.

Oral Arsenic Formulations

The agent perhaps most likely to be widely adopted for induction therapy of APL is oral arsenic, which is particularly attractive because it may improve patient compliance due to ease of administration; the use of oral arsenic trioxide in APL has been recently reviewed [92]. An oral formulation of arsenic was first published in 2002; Chinese investigators manipulated commercial grade ATO to create an oral solution and then administered the resulting compound to nine patients with R/R AML [93]. Oral and IV arsenic trioxide have not been compared head to head in a randomized fashion, though the oral formulation appears to achieve similar drug levels [93, 94]. Long-term follow-up of 76 patients with APL who received chemotherapy-based induction followed by oral ATO maintenance has been published, with a 3-year OS of 91% [95].

Another inorganic oral formulation of arsenic has been studied in APL, tetra-arsenic tetra-sulfide (As_4S_4), which can be isolated from a mined ore known as realgar. The pharmacokinetics of tetra-arsenic tetra-sulfide were first studied in APL patients by a Chinese group who described 129 APL patients at all stages of the disease (19 with new diagnosis, 7 with first relapse, and 103 in hematologic CR) [96]. The most widely available formulation of tetra-arsenic tetra-sulfide is the Realgar-Indigo naturalis formula (RIF), which was recently studied in a randomized phase 3 trial versus an IV ATO formulation in 242 patients with APL receiving induction and maintenance [97]. The RIF solution confirmed non-inferiority to IV ATO with disease-free survival of 98.1% vs. 95.5% at 2 years; CR rate and OS were not significantly different [97]. Patients in this study received combination therapy with ATRA during induction and then after CR received consolidation chemotherapy with homoharringtonine, cytarabine, and daunorubicin.

A large follow-up study is ongoing in China to evaluate oral arsenic (administered as the RIF solution) and ATRA without chemotherapy for newly diagnosed APL (NCT02899169). A pilot study of 20 patients with standard-risk APL showed 100% CR rate (20 out of 20 patients) at a median of 29.5 days [98]. The regimen was administered on an almost entirely outpatient basis, which can decrease healthcare-related costs [98–100]. Oral formulations of arsenic, whether oral ATO or tetra-arsenic tetra-sulfide, seem likely to convert the treatment of standard-risk APL to a completely oral regimen. Whether such a regimen can be safely administered on an outpatient basis remains to be seen; patients may benefit from a period of hospitalization, since the risk of complications from coagulation cascade dysfunction and differentiation syndrome is highest in the first 2–3 weeks after initiation of treatment [101].

Conclusions

Through 40 years of clinical trials, APL has progressed from being the most lethal subtype of AML to the most curable. ATRA and ATO are the two most active agents in the induction treatment of APL; ATO was identified in China as a component of traditional medicine in the 1970s with activity in APL and ATRA in the 1980s. Both ATRA and arsenic compounds lead to differentiation of promyelocytes through distinct, complementary mechanisms. The drugs were moved initially into clinical trials as single agents or in combination with chemotherapy, but treatment of standard-risk newly diagnosed APL has moved into a chemotherapy-free era. Patients with high-risk APL due to a high WBC count as presentation should still receive leukodepletion, whether with GO or anthracycline, in addition to ATRA and arsenic therapy. The cure rates are so high for patients treated with ATRA and ATO, especially for patients with low-risk disease that there seems to be little utility for routine PCR monitoring of the *PML-RARA* transcript after the completion of therapy.

Single-agent ATO is highly efficacious in the treatment of APL and leads to long-term cure in somewhere between two-thirds and three-quarters of all patients [52, 54]. Single-agent ATRA, in contrast, has a high rate of CR during induction, but patients invariably relapse after approximately 1 year; though lipoATRA can lead to long-term disease-free survival and even cure as a single agent, the rates of both are lower than for ATO. Taking together with the very high early death rate in APL, these findings suggest that patients might benefit from the initiation of both ATRA and ATO for initial treatment when APL is suspected clinically, before final confirmation of the diagnosis.

The role of the newer agents, including lipoATRA, tamibarotene, and oral arsenic preparations, has yet to be fully established. However, the current standard of ATRA and ATO in the chemotherapy-free induction of APL is a collaborative, international success leading to cure in over 95% of patients.

References

1. Park JH, Qiao B, Panageas KS, Schymura MJ, Jurcic JG, Rosenblat TL, et al. Early death rate in acute promyelocytic leukemia remains high despite all-trans retinoic acid. Blood. 2011;118(5):1248–54. https://doi.org/10.1182/blood-2011-04-346437.
2. Lehmann S, Ravn A, Carlsson L, Antunovic P, Deneberg S, Mollgard L, et al. Continuing high early death rate in acute promyelocytic leukemia: a population-based report from the Swedish Adult Acute Leukemia Registry. Leukemia. 2011;25(7):1128–34. https://doi.org/10.1038/leu.2011.78.
3. Sanz MA, Lo Coco F, Martin G, Avvisati G, Rayon C, Barbui T, et al. Definition of relapse risk and role of nonanthracycline drugs for consolidation in patients with acute promyelocytic leukemia: a joint study of the PETHEMA and GIMEMA cooperative groups. Blood. 2000;96(4):1247–53.
4. Lo-Coco F, Avvisati G, Vignetti M, Thiede C, Orlando SM, Iacobelli S, et al. Retinoic acid and arsenic trioxide for acute promyelocytic leukemia. N Engl J Med. 2013;369(2):111–21. https://doi.org/10.1056/NEJMoa1300874.
5. Wang ZY, Chen Z. Acute promyelocytic leukemia: from highly fatal to highly curable. Blood. 2008;111(5):2505–15. https://doi.org/10.1182/blood-2007-07-102798.
6. Breitman TR, Selonick SE, Collins SJ. Induction of differentiation of the human promyelocytic leukemia cell line (HL-60) by retinoic acid. Proc Natl Acad Sci U S A. 1980;77(5):2936–40.
7. Breitman TR, Collins SJ, Keene BR. Terminal differentiation of human promyelocytic leukemic cells in primary culture in response to retinoic acid. Blood. 1981;57(6):1000–4.
8. Zheng PZ, Wang KK, Zhang QY, Huang QH, Du YZ, Zhang QH, et al. Systems analysis of transcriptome and proteome in retinoic acid/arsenic trioxide-induced cell differentiation/apoptosis of promyelocytic leukemia. Proc Natl Acad Sci U S A. 2005;102(21):7653–8. https://doi.org/10.1073/pnas.0502825102.
9. Douer D, Koeffler HP. Retinoic acid. Inhibition of the clonal growth of human myeloid leukemia cells. J Clin Invest. 1982;69(2):277–83.
10. Flynn PJ, Miller WJ, Weisdorf DJ, Arthur DC, Brunning R, Branda RF. Retinoic acid treatment of acute promyelocytic leukemia: in vitro and in vivo observations. Blood. 1983;62(6):1211–7.
11. Nilsson B. Probable in vivo induction of differentiation by retinoic acid of promyelocytes in acute promyelocytic leukaemia. Br J Haematol. 1984;57(3):365–71.
12. Fontana JA, Rogers JS 2nd, Durham JP. The role of 13 cis-retinoic acid in the remission induction of a patient with acute promyelocytic leukemia. Cancer. 1986;57(2):209–17.
13. Daenen S, Vellenga E, van Dobbenburgh OA, Halie MR. Retinoic acid as antileukemic therapy in a patient with acute promyelocytic leukemia and Aspergillus pneumonia. Blood. 1986;67(2):559–61.
14. Runde V, Aul C, Sudhoff T, Heyll A, Schneider W. Retinoic acid in the treatment of acute promyelocytic leukemia: inefficacy of the 13-cis isomer and induction of complete remission by the all-trans isomer complicated by thromboembolic events. Ann Hematol. 1992;64(6):270–2.
15. Chomienne C, Ballerini P, Balitrand N, Amar M, Bernard JF, Boivin P, et al. Retinoic acid therapy for promyelocytic leukaemia. Lancet. 1989;2(8665):746–7.
16. Huang ME, Ye YC, Chen SR, Zhao JC, Gu LJ, Cai JR, et al. All-trans retinoic acid with or without low dose cytosine arabinoside in acute promyelocytic leukemia. Report of 6 cases. Chin Med J (Engl). 1987;100(12):949–53.
17. Huang ME, Ye YC, Chen SR, Chai JR, Lu JX, Zhoa L, et al. Use of all-trans retinoic acid in the treatment of acute promyelocytic leukemia. Blood. 1988;72(2):567–72.
18. Wang ZY, Sun GL, Lu JX, Gu LJ, Huang ME, Chen SR. Treatment of acute promyelocytic leukemia with all-trans retinoic acid in China. Nouv Rev Fr Hematol. 1990;32(1):34–6.
19. Castaigne S, Chomienne C, Daniel MT, Ballerini P, Berger R, Fenaux P, et al. All-trans retinoic acid as a differentiation therapy for acute promyelocytic leukemia. I. Clinical results. Blood. 1990;76(9):1704–9.
20. Warrell RP Jr, Frankel SR, Miller WH Jr, Scheinberg DA, Itri LM, Hittelman WN, et al. Differentiation therapy of acute promyelocytic leukemia with tretinoin (all-trans-retinoic acid). N Engl J Med. 1991;324(20):1385–93. https://doi.org/10.1056/NEJM199105163242002.
21. Chen ZX, Xue YQ, Zhang R, Tao RF, Xia XM, Li C, et al. A clinical and experimental study on all-trans retinoic acid-treated acute promyelocytic leukemia patients. Blood. 1991;78(6):1413–9.
22. Frankel SR, Eardley A, Heller G, Berman E, Miller WH Jr, Dmitrovsky E, et al. All-trans retinoic acid for acute promyelocytic leukemia. Results of the New York Study. Ann Intern Med. 1994;120(4):278–86.
23. Kanamaru A, Takemoto Y, Tanimoto M, Murakami H, Asou N, Kobayashi T, et al. All-trans retinoic acid for the treatment of newly diagnosed acute promyelocytic leukemia. Japan Adult Leukemia Study Group. Blood. 1995;85(5):1202–6.
24. Fenaux P, Le Deley MC, Castaigne S, Archimbaud E, Chomienne C, Link H, et al. Effect of all transretinoic acid in newly diagnosed acute promyelocytic leukemia. Results of a multicenter randomized trial. European APL 91 Group. Blood. 1993;82(11):3241–9.

25. Tallman MS, Andersen JW, Schiffer CA, Appelbaum FR, Feusner JH, Woods WG, et al. All-trans retinoic acid in acute promyelocytic leukemia: long-term outcome and prognostic factor analysis from the North American Intergroup protocol. Blood. 2002;100(13):4298–302. https://doi.org/10.1182/blood-2002-02-0632.
26. Tallman MS, Andersen JW, Schiffer CA, Appelbaum FR, Feusner JH, Ogden A, et al. All-trans-retinoic acid in acute promyelocytic leukemia. N Engl J Med. 1997;337(15):1021–8. https://doi.org/10.1056/NEJM199710093371501.
27. Coombs CC, DeAngelis LM, Feusner JH, Rowe JM, Tallman MS. Pseudotumor cerebri in acute promyelocytic leukemia patients on Intergroup Protocol 0129: clinical description and recommendations for new diagnostic criteria. Clin Lymphoma Myeloma Leuk. 2016;16(3):146–51. https://doi.org/10.1016/j.clml.2015.11.018.
28. de Botton S, Coiteux V, Chevret S, Rayon C, Vilmer E, Sanz M, et al. Outcome of childhood acute promyelocytic leukemia with all-trans-retinoic acid and chemotherapy. J Clin Oncol. 2004;22(8):1404–12. https://doi.org/10.1200/JCO.2004.09.008.
29. Frankel SR, Eardley A, Lauwers G, Weiss M, Warrell RP Jr. The "retinoic acid syndrome" in acute promyelocytic leukemia. Ann Intern Med. 1992;117(4):292–6.
30. De Botton S, Dombret H, Sanz M, Miguel JS, Caillot D, Zittoun R, et al. Incidence, clinical features, and outcome of all trans-retinoic acid syndrome in 413 cases of newly diagnosed acute promyelocytic leukemia. The European APL Group. Blood. 1998;92(8):2712–8.
31. Vahdat L, Maslak P, Miller WH Jr, Eardley A, Heller G, Scheinberg DA, et al. Early mortality and the retinoic acid syndrome in acute promyelocytic leukemia: impact of leukocytosis, low-dose chemotherapy, PMN/RAR-alpha isoform, and CD13 expression in patients treated with all-trans retinoic acid. Blood. 1994;84(11):3843–9.
32. Watanabe T, Hirano S. Metabolism of arsenic and its toxicological relevance. Arch Toxicol. 2013;87(6):969–79. https://doi.org/10.1007/s00204-012-0904-5.
33. Tchounwou PB, Centeno JA, Patlolla AK. Arsenic toxicity, mutagenesis, and carcinogenesis—a health risk assessment and management approach. Mol Cell Biochem. 2004;255(1–2):47–55.
34. Hughes MF. Arsenic toxicity and potential mechanisms of action. Toxicol Lett. 2002;133(1):1–16.
35. Caito S, Aschner M. Neurotoxicity of metals. Handb Clin Neurol. 2015;131:169–89. https://doi.org/10.1016/B978-0-444-62627-1.00011-1.
36. Doyle D. Notoriety to respectability: a short history of arsenic prior to its present day use in haematology. Br J Haematol. 2009;145(3):309–17. https://doi.org/10.1111/j.1365-2141.2009.07623.x.
37. Chen SJ, Zhou GB, Zhang XW, Mao JH, de The H, Chen Z. From an old remedy to a magic bullet: molecular mechanisms underlying the therapeutic effects of arsenic in fighting leukemia. Blood. 2011;117(24):6425–37. https://doi.org/10.1182/blood-2010-11-283598.
38. Kritharis A, Bradley TP, Budman DR. The evolving use of arsenic in pharmacotherapy of malignant disease. Ann Hematol. 2013;92(6):719–30. https://doi.org/10.1007/s00277-013-1707-3.
39. Chen GQ, Zhu J, Shi XG, Ni JH, Zhong HJ, Si GY, et al. In vitro studies on cellular and molecular mechanisms of arsenic trioxide (As2O3) in the treatment of acute promyelocytic leukemia: As2O3 induces NB4 cell apoptosis with downregulation of Bcl-2 expression and modulation of PML-RAR alpha/PML proteins. Blood. 1996;88(3):1052–61.
40. Chen GQ, Shi XG, Tang W, Xiong SM, Zhu J, Cai X, et al. Use of arsenic trioxide (As2O3) in the treatment of acute promyelocytic leukemia (APL): I. As2O3 exerts dose-dependent dual effects on APL cells. Blood. 1997;89(9):3345–53.
41. Shao W, Fanelli M, Ferrara FF, Riccioni R, Rosenauer A, Davison K, et al. Arsenic trioxide as an inducer of apoptosis and loss of PML/RAR alpha protein in acute promyelocytic leukemia cells. J Natl Cancer Inst. 1998;90(2):124–33.
42. Wang ZG, Rivi R, Delva L, Konig A, Scheinberg DA, Gambacorti-Passerini C, et al. Arsenic trioxide and melarsoprol induce programmed cell death in myeloid leukemia cell lines and function in a PML and PML-RARalpha independent manner. Blood. 1998;92(5):1497–504.
43. Sun HD, Ma L, Hu XC, Zhang TD. Ai-Lin I treated 32 cases of acute promyelocytic leukemia. Chin J Integrat Chin West Med. 1992;12:170–1.
44. Zhang P, Wang SY, Hu LH. Arsenic trioxide treated 72 cases of acute promyelocytic leukemia. Chin J Hematol. 1996;17:58–62.
45. Shen ZX, Chen GQ, Ni JH, Li XS, Xiong SM, Qiu QY, et al. Use of arsenic trioxide (As2O3) in the treatment of acute promyelocytic leukemia (APL): II. Clinical efficacy and pharmacokinetics in relapsed patients. Blood. 1997;89(9):3354–60.
46. Soignet SL, Maslak P, Wang ZG, Jhanwar S, Calleja E, Dardashti LJ, et al. Complete remission after treatment of acute promyelocytic leukemia with arsenic trioxide. N Engl J Med. 1998;339(19):1341–8. https://doi.org/10.1056/NEJM199811053391901.
47. Niu C, Yan H, Yu T, Sun HP, Liu JX, Li XS, et al. Studies on treatment of acute promyelocytic leukemia with arsenic trioxide: remission induction, follow-up, and molecular monitoring in 11 newly diagnosed and 47 relapsed acute promyelocytic leukemia patients. Blood. 1999;94(10):3315–24.
48. Soignet SL, Frankel SR, Douer D, Tallman MS, Kantarjian H, Calleja E, et al. United States multicenter study of arsenic trioxide in relapsed acute promyelocytic leukemia. J Clin Oncol. 2001;19(18):3852–60.
49. Au WY, Lie AK, Chim CS, Liang R, Ma SK, Chan CH, et al. Arsenic trioxide in comparison with

chemotherapy and bone marrow transplantation for the treatment of relapsed acute promyelocytic leukaemia. Ann Oncol. 2003;14(5):752–7.

50. Mathews V, Balasubramanian P, Shaji RV, George B, Chandy M, Srivastava A. Arsenic trioxide in the treatment of newly diagnosed acute promyelocytic leukemia: a single center experience. Am J Hematol. 2002;70(4):292–9. https://doi.org/10.1002/ajh.10138.
51. Mathews V, George B, Lakshmi KM, Viswabandya A, Bajel A, Balasubramanian P, et al. Single-agent arsenic trioxide in the treatment of newly diagnosed acute promyelocytic leukemia: durable remissions with minimal toxicity. Blood. 2006;107(7):2627–32. https://doi.org/10.1182/blood-2005-08-3532.
52. Mathews V, George B, Chendamarai E, Lakshmi KM, Desire S, Balasubramanian P, et al. Single-agent arsenic trioxide in the treatment of newly diagnosed acute promyelocytic leukemia: long-term follow-up data. J Clin Oncol. 2010;28(24):3866–71. https://doi.org/10.1200/JCO.2010.28.5031.
53. Ghavamzadeh A, Alimoghaddam K, Ghaffari SH, Rostami S, Jahani M, Hosseini R, et al. Treatment of acute promyelocytic leukemia with arsenic trioxide without ATRA and/or chemotherapy. Ann Oncol. 2006;17(1):131–4. https://doi.org/10.1093/annonc/mdj019.
54. Ghavamzadeh A, Alimoghaddam K, Rostami S, Ghaffari SH, Jahani M, Iravani M, et al. Phase II study of single-agent arsenic trioxide for the front-line therapy of acute promyelocytic leukemia. J Clin Oncol. 2011;29(20):2753–7. https://doi.org/10.1200/JCO.2010.32.2107.
55. Estey EH, Hutchinson F. Newly diagnosed acute promyelocytic leukemia: arsenic moves front and center. J Clin Oncol. 2011;29(20):2743–6. https://doi.org/10.1200/JCO.2011.35.1031.
56. Mahmoudi N. Research on acute promyelocytic leukemia conducted in Iran. J Clin Oncol. 2012;30(2):217–8; author reply 8–20; discussion 20–2. doi:https://doi.org/10.1200/JCO.2011.38.8785.
57. Huang SY, Chang CS, Tang JL, Tien HF, Kuo TL, Huang SF, et al. Acute and chronic arsenic poisoning associated with treatment of acute promyelocytic leukaemia. Br J Haematol. 1998;103(4):1092–5.
58. Camacho LH, Soignet SL, Chanel S, Ho R, Heller G, Scheinberg DA, et al. Leukocytosis and the retinoic acid syndrome in patients with acute promyelocytic leukemia treated with arsenic trioxide. J Clin Oncol. 2000;18(13):2620–5.
59. Ohnishi K, Yoshida H, Shigeno K, Nakamura S, Fujisawa S, Naito K, et al. Prolongation of the QT interval and ventricular tachycardia in patients treated with arsenic trioxide for acute promyelocytic leukemia. Ann Intern Med. 2000;133(11):881–5.
60. Westervelt P, Brown RA, Adkins DR, Khoury H, Curtin P, Hurd D, et al. Sudden death among patients with acute promyelocytic leukemia treated with arsenic trioxide. Blood. 2001;98(2):266–71.
61. Patel SP, Garcia-Manero G, Ferrajoli A, Faderl S, Verstovek S, Kantarjian H, et al. Cardiotoxicity in African-American patients treated with arsenic trioxide for acute promyelocytic leukemia. Leuk Res. 2006;30(3):362–3. https://doi.org/10.1016/j.leukres.2005.08.002.
62. Gianni M, Koken MH, Chelbi-Alix MK, Benoit G, Lanotte M, Chen Z, et al. Combined arsenic and retinoic acid treatment enhances differentiation and apoptosis in arsenic-resistant NB4 cells. Blood. 1998;91(11):4300–10.
63. Lallemand-Breitenbach V, Guillemin MC, Janin A, Daniel MT, Degos L, Kogan SC, et al. Retinoic acid and arsenic synergize to eradicate leukemic cells in a mouse model of acute promyelocytic leukemia. J Exp Med. 1999;189(7):1043–52.
64. Jing Y, Wang L, Xia L, Chen GQ, Chen Z, Miller WH, et al. Combined effect of all-trans retinoic acid and arsenic trioxide in acute promyelocytic leukemia cells in vitro and in vivo. Blood. 2001;97(1):264–9.
65. Kennedy GA, Marlton P, Cobcroft R, Gill D. Molecular remission without blood product support using all-trans retinoic acid (ATRA) induction and combined arsenic trioxide/ATRA consolidation in a Jehovah's Witness with de novo acute promyelocytic leukaemia. Br J Haematol. 2000;111(4):1103–5.
66. Shen ZX, Shi ZZ, Fang J, Gu BW, Li JM, Zhu YM, et al. All-trans retinoic acid/As2O3 combination yields a high quality remission and survival in newly diagnosed acute promyelocytic leukemia. Proc Natl Acad Sci U S A. 2004;101(15):5328–35. https://doi.org/10.1073/pnas.0400053101.
67. Estey E, Garcia-Manero G, Ferrajoli A, Faderl S, Verstovsek S, Jones D, et al. Use of all-trans retinoic acid plus arsenic trioxide as an alternative to chemotherapy in untreated acute promyelocytic leukemia. Blood. 2006;107(9):3469–73. https://doi.org/10.1182/blood-2005-10-4006.
68. Lo-Coco F, Avvisati G, Vignetti M, Breccia M, Gallo E, Rambaldi A, et al. Front-line treatment of acute promyelocytic leukemia with AIDA induction followed by risk-adapted consolidation for adults younger than 61 years: results of the AIDA-2000 trial of the GIMEMA Group. Blood. 2010;116(17):3171–9. https://doi.org/10.1182/blood-2010-03-276196.
69. Platzbecker U, Avvisati G, Cicconi L, Thiede C, Paoloni F, Vignetti M, et al. Improved outcomes with retinoic acid and arsenic trioxide compared with retinoic acid and chemotherapy in non-high-risk acute promyelocytic leukemia: final results of the randomized Italian-German APL0406 Trial. J Clin Oncol. 2017;35(6):605–12. https://doi.org/10.1200/JCO.2016.67.1982.
70. Ma Y, Liu L, Jin J, Lou Y. All-trans retinoic acid plus arsenic trioxide versus all-trans retinoic acid plus chemotherapy for newly diagnosed acute promyelocytic leukemia: a meta-analysis. PLoS One. 2016;11(7):e0158760. https://doi.org/10.1371/journal.pone.0158760.

71. Ravandi F, Estey E, Jones D, Faderl S, O'Brien S, Fiorentino J, et al. Effective treatment of acute promyelocytic leukemia with all-trans-retinoic acid, arsenic trioxide, and gemtuzumab ozogamicin. J Clin Oncol. 2009;27(4):504–10. https://doi.org/10.1200/JCO.2008.18.6130.
72. Burnett AK, Russell NH, Hills RK, Bowen D, Kell J, Knapper S, et al. Arsenic trioxide and all-trans retinoic acid treatment for acute promyelocytic leukaemia in all risk groups (AML17): results of a randomised, controlled, phase 3 trial. Lancet Oncol. 2015;16(13):1295–305. https://doi.org/10.1016/S1470-2045(15)00193-X.
73. Breccia M, Lo-Coco F. Gemtuzumab ozogamicin for the treatment of acute promyelocytic leukemia: mechanisms of action and resistance, safety and efficacy. Expert Opin Biol Ther. 2011;11(2):225–34. https://doi.org/10.1517/14712598.2011.543895.
74. Clarke WT, Marks PW. Gemtuzumab ozogamicin: is there room for salvage? Blood. 2010;116(14):2618–9. https://doi.org/10.1182/blood-2010-08-300871.
75. Hills RK, Castaigne S, Appelbaum FR, Delaunay J, Petersdorf S, Othus M, et al. Addition of gemtuzumab ozogamicin to induction chemotherapy in adult patients with acute myeloid leukaemia: a meta-analysis of individual patient data from randomised controlled trials. Lancet Oncol. 2014;15(9):986–96. https://doi.org/10.1016/S1470-2045(14)70281-5.
76. Jurcic JG, DeBlasio T, Dumont L, Yao TJ, Scheinberg DA. Molecular remission induction with retinoic acid and anti-CD33 monoclonal antibody HuM195 in acute promyelocytic leukemia. Clin Cancer Res. 2000;6(2):372–80.
77. Estey EH, Giles FJ, Beran M, O'Brien S, Pierce SA, Faderl SH, et al. Experience with gemtuzumab ozogamycin ("mylotarg") and all-trans retinoic acid in untreated acute promyelocytic leukemia. Blood. 2002;99(11):4222–4. https://doi.org/10.1182/blood-2001-12-0174.
78. Muindi J, Frankel SR, Miller WH Jr, Jakubowski A, Scheinberg DA, Young CW, et al. Continuous treatment with all-trans retinoic acid causes a progressive reduction in plasma drug concentrations: implications for relapse and retinoid "resistance" in patients with acute promyelocytic leukemia. Blood. 1992;79(2):299–303.
79. Gokhale PC, Kshirsagar NA, Khan MU, Pandya SK, Merchant RH, Mehta KP, et al. Treatment of candiduria with liposomal amphotericin B (L-AmpB-LRC) in children. J Antimicrob Chemother. 1994;33(4):889–91.
80. Parthasarathy R, Mehta K. Altered metabolism of all-trans-retinoic acid in liposome-encapsulated form. Cancer Lett. 1998;134(2):121–8.
81. Estey E, Thall PF, Mehta K, Rosenblum M, Brewer T Jr, Simmons V, et al. Alterations in tretinoin pharmacokinetics following administration of liposomal all-trans retinoic acid. Blood. 1996;87(9):3650–4.
82. Estey EH, Giles FJ, Kantarjian H, O'Brien S, Cortes J, Freireich EJ, et al. Molecular remissions induced by liposomal-encapsulated all-trans retinoic acid in newly diagnosed acute promyelocytic leukemia. Blood. 1999;94(7):2230–5.
83. Estey E, Koller C, Cortes J, Reed P, Freireich E, Giles F, et al. Treatment of newly-diagnosed acute promyelocytic leukemia with liposomal all-trans retinoic acid. Leuk Lymphoma. 2001;42(3):309–16. https://doi.org/10.3109/10428190109064587.
84. Douer D, Estey E, Santillana S, Bennett JM, Lopez-Bernstein G, Boehm K, et al. Treatment of newly diagnosed and relapsed acute promyelocytic leukemia with intravenous liposomal all-trans retinoic acid. Blood. 2001;97(1):73–80.
85. Tsimberidou AM, Tirado-Gomez M, Andreeff M, O'Brien S, Kantarjian H, Keating M, et al. Single-agent liposomal all-trans retinoic acid can cure some patients with untreated acute promyelocytic leukemia: an update of The University of Texas M. D. Anderson Cancer Center Series. Leuk Lymphoma. 2006;47(6):1062–8. https://doi.org/10.1080/10428190500463932.
86. Tobita T, Takeshita A, Kitamura K, Ohnishi K, Yanagi M, Hiraoka A, et al. Treatment with a new synthetic retinoid, Am80, of acute promyelocytic leukemia relapsed from complete remission induced by all-trans retinoic acid. Blood. 1997;90(3):967–73.
87. Takeuchi M, Yano T, Omoto E, Takahashi K, Kibata M, Shudo K, et al. Re-induction of complete remission with a new synthetic retinoid, Am-80, for relapse of acute promyelocytic leukaemia previously treated with all-trans retinoic acid. Br J Haematol. 1997;97(1):137–40.
88. Di Veroli A, Ramadan SM, Divona M, Cudillo L, Gianni L, Wieland S, et al. Molecular remission in advanced acute promyelocytic leukaemia after treatment with the oral synthetic retinoid Tamibarotene. Br J Haematol. 2010;151(1):99–101. https://doi.org/10.1111/j.1365-2141.2010.08308.x.
89. Naina HV, Levitt D, Vusirikala M, Anderson LD Jr, Scaglioni PP, Kirk A, et al. Successful treatment of relapsed and refractory extramedullary acute promyelocytic leukemia with tamibarotene. J Clin Oncol. 2011;29(18):e534–6. https://doi.org/10.1200/JCO.2011.34.8953.
90. Sanford D, Lo-Coco F, Sanz MA, Di Bona E, Coutre S, Altman JK, et al. Tamibarotene in patients with acute promyelocytic leukaemia relapsing after treatment with all-trans retinoic acid and arsenic trioxide. Br J Haematol. 2015;171(4):471–7. https://doi.org/10.1111/bjh.13607.
91. Shinagawa K, Yanada M, Sakura T, Ueda Y, Sawa M, Miyatake J, et al. Tamibarotene as maintenance therapy for acute promyelocytic leukemia: results from a randomized controlled trial. J Clin Oncol. 2014;32(33):3729–35. https://doi.org/10.1200/JCO.2013.53.3570.
92. Torka P, Al Ustwani O, Wetzler M, Wang ES, Griffiths EA. Swallowing a bitter pill-oral arsenic trioxide for acute promyelocytic leukemia. Blood Rev. 2016;30(3):201–11. https://doi.org/10.1016/j.blre.2015.11.004.

93. Kumana CR, Au WY, Lee NS, Kou M, Mak RW, Lam CW, et al. Systemic availability of arsenic from oral arsenic-trioxide used to treat patients with hematological malignancies. Eur J Clin Pharmacol. 2002;58(8):521–6. https://doi.org/10.1007/s00228-002-0514-x.
94. Firkin F. Oral administration of arsenic trioxide in the treatment of acute promyelocytic leukaemia and accelerated phase chronic myeloid leukaemia: an Australian single-centre study. Intern Med J. 2012;42(8):948–52. https://doi.org/10.1111/j.1445-5994.2012.02852.x.
95. Au WY, Kumana CR, Lee HK, Lin SY, Liu H, Yeung DY, et al. Oral arsenic trioxide-based maintenance regimens for first complete remission of acute promyelocytic leukemia: a 10-year follow-up study. Blood. 2011;118(25):6535–43. https://doi.org/10.1182/blood-2011-05-354530.
96. Lu DP, Qiu JY, Jiang B, Wang Q, Liu KY, Liu YR, et al. Tetra-arsenic tetra-sulfide for the treatment of acute promyelocytic leukemia: a pilot report. Blood. 2002;99(9):3136–43.
97. Zhu HH, Wu DP, Jin J, Li JY, Ma J, Wang JX, et al. Oral tetra-arsenic tetra-sulfide formula versus intravenous arsenic trioxide as first-line treatment of acute promyelocytic leukemia: a multicenter randomized controlled trial. J Clin Oncol. 2013;31(33):4215–21. https://doi.org/10.1200/JCO.2013.48.8312.
98. Zhu HH, Huang XJ. Oral arsenic and retinoic acid for non-high-risk acute promyelocytic leukemia. N Engl J Med. 2014;371(23):2239–41. https://doi.org/10.1056/NEJMc1412035.
99. Falchi L, Verstovsek S, Ravandi-Kashani F, Kantarjian HM. The evolution of arsenic in the treatment of acute promyelocytic leukemia and other myeloid neoplasms: moving toward an effective oral, outpatient therapy. Cancer. 2016;122(8):1160–8. https://doi.org/10.1002/cncr.29852.
100. Jiang H, Liang GW, Huang XJ, Jiang Q, Han S, Shi LW, et al. Reduced medical costs and hospital days when using oral arsenic plus ATRA as the first-line treatment of acute promyelocytic leukemia. Leuk Res. 2015;39(12):1319–24. https://doi.org/10.1016/j.leukres.2015.09.007.
101. Lo-Coco F, Cicconi L. Outpatient oral treatment for acute promyelocytic leukemia. N Engl J Med. 2015;372(9):884–5. https://doi.org/10.1056/NEJMc1500125#SA1.

11 Minimal Residual Disease in Acute Promyelocytic Leukemia

Laura Cicconi and Eva Barragàn

Introduction

The genetic hallmark of acute promyelocytic leukemia (APL) is the balanced reciprocal translocation t(15;17)(q22;q11–12) leading to a fusion of the promyelocytic leukemia (*PML*) and the retinoic acid receptor alpha (*RARA*) gene. The fusion gene results in a chimeric PML-RARA oncoprotein which plays a causative role in APL pathogenesis [1]. The t(15;17) is present in almost all cases of morphologically defined APL, while a small minority of cases harbor variant rearrangements generally involving *RARA* and partner genes other than *PML* [2].

Detecting the unique PML-RARA fusion transcript is of utmost importance for the genetic diagnosis of APL, and its presence in leukemic cells predicts favorable response to targeted treatments including *all-trans*-retinoic acid (ATRA) and arsenic trioxide (ATO). The gene fusion is readily detectable with sensitive techniques such as reverse transcriptase-polymerase chain reaction (RT-PCR) or quantitative PCR (RQ-PCR), and its levels can be longitudinally monitored during patient follow-up to assess minimal residual disease (MRD). A number of well-designed prospective studies have now clearly established the clinical value of MRD in APL and provided a model for new outcome definitions and therapeutic measures in leukemia such as *molecular remission*, *molecular relapse*, and *preemptive treatment* of disease recurrence [3–5] (Table 11.1).

Molecular Remission as a Therapeutic End Point in APL

The identification of the APL-specific genetic lesion at diagnosis in leukemic cells is feasible at the chromosome, DNA, RNA, and protein levels with the use of conventional karyotyping, fluorescence in situ hybridization (FISH), RT-PCR, and anti-PML monoclonal antibodies, respectively [3, 4, 6–8]. Of the various molecular techniques available, RT-PCR remains mandatory because it offers the advantage of defining the PML-RARA isoform type and therefore enables precise and sensitive detection of residual PML-RARA transcript levels. The *PML-RARA* fusion gene is generated by the breakpoint within *RARA* intron 2 and the disruption of *PML* gene in three different breakpoint regions. *PML* breakpoint regions are located in intron 6 (bcr1), intron 3 (bcr3), and exon 6 (bcr2) and give rise to long isoform, short isoform, and variable PML-RARA isoform when rearranged with RARA exon 2 [7].

Early studies using RT-PCR suggested that this approach could improve outcome prediction

L. Cicconi, M.D. (✉)
Department of Biomedicine and Prevention, University Tor Vergata, Rome, Italy
e-mail: cicconi.laura@yahoo.it

E. Barragàn, Ph.D.
Department of Medical Biopathology, Hospital Universitario La Fe, Valencia, Spain

O. Abla et al. (eds.), *Acute Promyelocytic Leukemia*, https://doi.org/10.1007/978-3-319-64257-4_11

Table 11.1 Main prospective studies investigating MRD in APL

Study	N. pts	Therapy	Sampling source	Technique and control gene	Correlation between PCR status after induction and relapse risk	Correlation between PCR status after consolidation and relapse risk	Preemptive therapy of molecular relapse	Main findings
Diverio et al. [6]	163	ATRA + CHT	BM	RT-PCR (ABL)	None	Yes	No	• Conversion to PCR positivity during remission is highly predictive of subsequent hematologic relapse • High prognostic value of stringent molecular monitoring during the early post-consolidation
Burnett et al. [18]	239	ATRA + CHT	BM	RT-PCR (ABL)	None	Yes	No	• Molecular assessment after the third cons course was correlated with the relapse risk (57% if RT-PCR was positive vs. 27% if the RT-PCR was negative; $P = .006$)
Lo Coco et al. [22]	253	ATRA + CHT	BM	RT-PCR (ABL)	None	Yes	Yes	• 2-year OS survival from relapse was superior for patients treated in molecular relapse as compared to those treated at the time of hematologic recurrence (92% vs. 44%; $P < .05$)
Esteve et al. [23]	549	ATRA + CHT	BM	RT-PCR (ABL)	None	Yes	Yes	• Outcome after treatment of molecular relapse compared favorably to hematologic relapse, with longer survival (5-year OS: 64 vs. 24%, $P = 0.01$) and lower relapse risk (5-year relapse risk: 30 vs. 64%; $P = 0.044$)
Grimwade et al. [31]	406	ATRA + CHT	BM PB	RQ-PCR (ABL)	None	Yes	Yes	• Use of MRD monitoring to predict relapse and direct preemptive ATO therapy • RQ-PCR on BM precedes PB in detecting molecular relapse
Chendamarai et al. [39]	151	ATO	PB	RT-PCR (GADPDH)	Yes	–		• Relapse prediction by RT-PCR positivity after induction in 60% of monitored cases
Santamarìa et al. [30]	145	ATRA + CHT	BM PB	RQ-PCR (ABL)	None	Low % of positive cases	Yes	• During f-up monitoring, >10 PML-RARA NCN predict relapse
Cicconi et al. [40]	182	ATRA + CHT ATRA + ATO	BM	RQ-PCR (ABL)	None	Yes	Yes	• Higher % of positive RQ-PCR pts after induction in the ATO + ATRA vs. ATRA + CHT • Slower clearance of PML-RARA at the post-induction time point in ATO + ATRA, but better clearance after consolidation

in APL by providing relevant information on prognosis. The first data on longitudinal RT-PCR monitoring of APL were reported in the early 1990s and were mainly derived from retrospective studies [9–11]. The analysis of MRD conducted in large patient series using RT-PCR indicated that APL treatment with ATRA as a single agent was almost invariably associated with persistence of PML-RARA transcripts and that this agent alone was unable to eradicate the leukemic clone. By contrast, combining ATRA with chemotherapy as induction therapy was associated in approximately half of the cases with negativity of the PCR test for PML-RARA; furthermore, patients in long-term remission after ATRA plus chemotherapy approaches tested negative for the hybrid transcript [12–15]. Prospective molecular studies conducted in the late 1990s by Lo Coco et al. within the Gruppo Italiano Malattie Ematologiche dell'Adulto (GIMEMA) on APL patients homogeneously treated with standard AIDA therapy (ATRA plus anthracycline-based chemotherapy) demonstrated that the persistence of RT-PCR positivity for PML-RARA after the completion of treatment, in particular at the end of consolidation therapy, was almost invariably followed by relapse. In contrast, also in prospective studies, patients in long-term molecular remission were found to lack detectable PML-RARA [16]. Several studies conducted in the context of ATRA and chemotherapy-based regimens by European cooperative groups have confirmed that PML-RARA positivity at the end of consolidation therapy was detectable from 2 to 8% of APL patients and was highly predictive of impending relapse requiring additional intensification of therapy including allogeneic hematopoietic stem cell transplantation (HSCT) [16–19]. Based on these results, the revised recommendations of the International Working Group on acute myeloid leukemia included the achievement of "molecular remission" at the end of consolidation therapy as the therapeutic end point in APL. Molecular remission for APL was conventionally defined as the absence of the PML-RARA fusion transcript using RT-PCR methods with a sensitivity threshold of $10^{-3}/10^{-4}$ [5]. On the other hand, MRD studies conducted in patients receiving chemotherapy in addition to ATRA reported a very high proportion (>90–95%) of RT-PCR negative cases at the end of consolidation [6, 16, 18], implying that MRD evaluation at this sampling time failed to identify most patients who will eventually relapse (≈25–30%).

Regarding the post-induction time point, the majority of studies reported high rates of PML-RARA positivity, ranging from 40 to 64%. In particular, in the GIMEMA study employing the AIDA (<u>A</u>ll-*trans*-retinoic and <u>IDA</u>rubicin) scheme, a positive MRD analysis at the end of induction was not predictive of subsequent relapse [12–15]. This lack of correlation probably results from the effect of differentiation therapy. Indeed, the high rate of persistence of PML-RARA transcript at the end of induction may result from late maturation of leukemic cells undergoing subsequent apoptosis, rather than from the persistence of blasts that are resistant to therapy. Of note, APL resistance after induction chemotherapy is virtually absent in those patients treated with modern therapies including ATRA and anthracyclines and has not been reported in several series now including thousands of patients [4].

Subsequent studies have also explored the clinical value of analyzing the reciprocal fusion RARA-PML as target for MRD monitoring. Grimwade and colleagues reported that nested PCR for the RARA-PML fusion could increase by 20% the detection of the transcript in patients in morphologic CR either at the end of induction or end of consolidation therapy [18]. However, contrary to PML-RARA RT-PCR, the RARA-PML expression status after consolidation therapy was not predictive of subsequent relapse in the reported series [20, 21]. Furthermore, the RARA-PML fusion is transcribed in only 70% of APL patients; thus its use for longitudinal MRD studies has remained limited after the above mentioned initial studies.

Longitudinal Monitoring of Minimal Residual Disease and Molecular Relapse

The application of PCR strategies during patient follow-up introduced the novel concept of "molecular relapse," preceding the overt hematological reappearance of APL blasts and therefore clinical manifestations of the disease. Data from the GIMEMA group had already shown that the elimination of the RT-PCR signal after therapy was associated with long-term remission, whereas a confirmed positive assay after completion of therapy was highly predictive of relapse [16]. This strategy was applied to molecular monitoring during follow-up and after the end of therapy by the same GIMEMA investigators, with bone marrow RT-PCR for PML-RARA performed every 3 months after the completion of therapy. Diverio et al. prospectively analyzed a cohort of 163 APL patients receiving the AIDA protocol and detected conversion to PCR positivity during follow-up in 21 patients [6]. Twenty of these 21 patients developed hematologic relapse at a median time of 3 months (range, 1–14) from the first positive PCR test. In keeping with the GIMEMA results, several other studies demonstrated that conversion from negative to positive PML-RARA PCR test during remission was highly predictive of a subsequent hematological relapse [14, 15]. These data, together with the evidence that most relapses occur during the first 2 or 3 years after consolidation, allowed the implementation of molecular monitoring as an integral part of the treatment with PCR performed every 3 months at least for the first 3 years after the end of consolidation.

The ability to predict hematologic relapse at the molecular level was particularly important for APL patients, because overt disease is frequently accompanied in this condition by coagulopathy and potentially fatal thrombo-hemorrhagic complications. The advent of molecular strategies to prevent relapse prompted the design of preemptive strategies aimed at treating molecular relapse before hematologic manifestations of APL. Two major studies in the pre-ATO era have evaluated the survival benefit for patients treated either in molecular or in hematologic relapse with the combination of ATRA and various chemotherapy regimens [22, 23]. The first study performed by the GIMEMA group on 14 patients in molecular relapse showed a 2-year survival estimate from the time of first molecular relapse of 92% (95% CI: 61–98%), compared to the 44% (95% CI: 35–52%) 2-year survival rate of the historical series of 37 APL patients treated at the time of hematologic relapse [22]. A subsequent study conducted by the PETHEMA group substantially confirmed the GIMEMA data, with survival outcome of patients treated while in molecular relapse comparing favorably with those treated in hematologic relapse, with longer survival (5-year survival: 64% vs. 24%, $P = 0.01$) and lower risk of second relapse (5-year relapse risk: 30% vs. 64%; $P = 0.044$) [23].

Role of MRD Monitoring in the Setting of Hematopoietic Stem Cell Transplantation

Another context in which MRD assessment has emerged as an important tool for clinical decision-making is hematopoietic stem cell transplantation (HSCT). In this setting, the assessment of PCR status immediately prior to transplant represents a powerful predictor of the relapse-free probability after stem cell harvesting [24]. An Italian pivotal study prospectively studied by RT-PCR for PML-RARA transcript, a cohort of 15 APL patients undergoing autologous HSCT in second morphologic CR, achieved in the majority of cases with ATRA plus chemotherapy [24]. Seven out of 15 patients tested positive for PML-RARA before transplant and all remained PCR-positive post-HSCT, ultimately relapsing at a median time of 5 months after transplant. As to the remaining eight patients who tested RT-PCR negative before autologous stem cell harvesting, all but one who relapsed at 10 months maintained long-term remissions. This study suggested that patients undergoing autologous HSCT after obtaining a second molecular remission are likely to have prolonged clinical and molecular remissions. Conversely, a PCR positivity after salvage therapy would require a more aggressive approach such as allogeneic HSCT. Similar results were obtained by investigators of the British MRC group, who reported results on a small cohort of APL patients enrolled on the ATRA trial undergoing autologous HSCT in CR2 with stem cell collection performed in CR1 [25]. In this series, four patients who tested PCR negative prior to HSCT and received PCR-negative marrow remained disease-free at a median follow-up of 28 months. Similar data were obtained by Japanese investigators in a small series of APL patients undergoing autologous HSCT [26].

Only limited data are available on the MRD assessment pre-transplant in patients undergoing allogeneic HSCT, given the rarity of patients requiring this approach. A US multicenter study including 294 patients with APL in CR2 receiving either allogeneic (n = 232) or autologous (n = 62) HSCT was reported by the Center for International Blood and Marrow Transplantation Research (CIBMTR) [27]. In the 155 patients for whom PML-RARA pre-transplant status was available, a positive test either before allogeneic (17/114) or autologous (6/41) transplant did not seem to impact on probability of relapse or survival. However, a more recent pan-European registry study collecting outcome data on 155 relapsed APL patients reported that a transplantation approach including allogeneic or autologous in CR2 (n = 93) produced a superior 3-year overall survival (OS) compared with approaches not including transplantation (80 vs. 59%; P = 0.03) [28]. In this context, multivariable analysis demonstrated that beside the duration of first remission and the employment of transplant procedures, the achievement of molecular CR retained its impact both on OS and on leukemia-free survival.

As for the post-HSCT evaluation, studies reported that the presence of residual disease at 3 months after HSCT is predictive of relapse, suggesting a prognostic role for minimal residual disease after transplant. In line with this assumption, PCR negativity has been consistently documented in the marrow derived from patients in long-term remission following autologous and allogeneic HSCT. The successful eradication of residual disease in these patients suggests that molecular monitoring should be routinely performed post-transplant, particularly in view of the relatively large number of treatment options available for treating molecular relapse in this setting.

Results with Real-Time Quantitative PCR (RQ-PCR)

The advent of more sensitive PCR techniques in the molecular biology field has allowed their application in the context of minimal residual disease studies. Early molecular studies employing RT-PCR technique highlighted limitations in the use of conventional reverse RT-PCR assay for clinical decision-making [3, 4, 25]. In fact, poor-quality samples can escape detection using this technique, giving rise to false-negative results. In addition, RT-PCR lacks the capacity to distinguish between decreasing and increasing levels of leukemia-specific transcripts, which may help in guiding decision-making. Finally, the long post-PCR handling needed in nested RT-PCR procedure might be subject to contamination. An international effort to standardize RQ-PCR for most frequent leukemia fusion transcripts, including PML-RARA, was finalized by Gabert and colleagues in 2003 with the development of standardized protocols for RQ-PCR analysis, providing robust and well-established methods for molecular determination of MRD levels in leukemia [29]. In the context of ATRA and chemotherapy-based protocols as front-line therapy of APL, the use of standardized RQ-PCR assays led to a slightly increase in MRD detection rates compared to nested RT-PCR. Several small retrospective series and only few prospective studies evaluating the impact of RQ-PCR for PML-RARA have been reported. A study by Santamarìa and colleagues from the Spanish PETHEMA group analyzed by RQ-PCR bone marrow samples of APL patients enrolled in PETHEMA trials in different phases of treatment, and the results were compared with those obtained by conventional qualitative RT-PCR [30]. This study did not show correlations between positive RQ-PCR after induction therapy and risk of relapse. In contrast, there was a strong correlation between RQ-PCR positivity and subsequent overt relapse after the end of consolidation therapy or during maintenance therapy and off treatment for all patients with >10 *PML-RARA* normalized copy number (NCN). A more recent study by Grimwade and colleagues from the MRC cooperative group investigated the use of rigorous sequential MRD monitoring in APL by means of RQ-PCR in a large series of 406 patients treated with ATRA and chemotherapy [31]. Sequential MRD monitoring according to the upfront recommended schedule provided information on kinetics of PML-RARA clearance in response to therapy, role of peripheral blood in longitudinal MRD monitoring, risk of relapse, and role of preemptive therapy with arsenic trioxide in preventing overt relapse. In agreement with the previous study by Santamarìa and colleagues, the majority of patients tested positive for RQ-PCR after induction therapy despite being in morphologic CR, which indicates that the high-level fusion transcripts detected were predominantly related to APL blast differentiation. No association was found between the magnitude of PML-RARA log reduction after induction and relapse risk. At the end of consolidation, 13/259 (5%) patients tested positive by RQ-PCR; however, in only 4 of these patients RQ-PCR positivity was confirmed by rising PML-RARA transcripts in the subsequent sample indicating persistent disease. Longitudinal monitoring of MRD allowed the identification of most patients who subsequently underwent relapse and proved to be the most powerful tool to predict relapse-free survival (RFS) in multivariable analysis, even superior to presenting WBC, currently used to stratify patients at risk. In fact, in 11 out of 20 patients who experienced frank relapse, conversion to RQ-PCR positivity was detected in remission samples taken 24–650 days (median, 74 days) prior to hematologic relapse. In the remaining patients, the ability to predict molecular relapse was limited mostly by low compliance to scheduled monitoring. Kinetics of molecular relapse was different in the analyzed patients, with a median rise of 1.1 log of PML-RARA transcripts per month, and the doubling time was generally faster than that reported for other leukemia fusion genes [31, 32]. Interesting information was provided also by the comparison of the paired bone marrow and peripheral blood samples during patient follow-up. Despite the high concordance of the two sources for RQ-PCR results, conversion to PCR positivity for PML-RARA was detected earlier when performed on bone marrow as compared to peripheral blood in the majority of patients by 29 days (range: 14–72 days). Finally, the delivery of a preemptive approach with ATO for the therapy of molecular relapse was applied successfully in this study, confirming that such strategy is relevant to reduce rates of clinical relapse in patients with APL [4, 31].

MRD Evaluation in the Era of Arsenic Trioxide

ATO is currently considered the most effective single agent in the therapy of APL. The current clinical use of this compound alone or in combination with ATRA as front-line therapy in APL has prompted more investigation on its efficacy at the molecular level [33–37]. Molecular studies have been performed both in the therapeutic setting of ATO as single agent and, more recently, in the context of ATO combined with ATRA. The first comparative study was conducted by Chinese investigators who used the RQ-PCR technique to evaluate prospectively the ability of ATO alone, ATRA alone, or ATRA and ATO in combination to reduce PML-RARA transcript levels [38]. PML-RARA transcripts decreased quickly after exposure to ATRA, ATO, or ATRA-ATO, but the decrement was more pronounced in the combination arm. This enhanced molecular response in the ATRA-ATO combination arm was confirmed also after consolidation chemotherapy. The greater reduction of disease burden obtained with ATRA and ATO combination as compared to either ATRA or ATO monotherapy translated also into a better DFS outcome. In 2013, an Indian study prospectively evaluated MRD by means of RT-PCR in APL patients treated with single-agent ATO [39]. The results of this study by Chendamarai and colleagues were slightly different from those previously reported in patients treated with ATRA plus chemotherapy. At the end of induction, 63.8% of patients tested RT-PCR positive; differently most studies produced in the ATRA and chemotherapy context; a positive RT-PCR reading at the end of induction therapy was significantly associated in multivariate analysis with an increased risk of relapse. A more recent experience from the GIMEMA group reported the direct comparison of PML-RARA transcript clearance measured by RQ-PCR in patients treated with ATRA-ATO or ATRA and chemotherapy within the randomized trial APL0406 [34]. Cicconi et al. analyzed the kinetics of PML-RARA transcripts by RQ-PCR in bone marrow samples from 184 patients enrolled on this trial in Italy. After induction therapy, most patients tested positive for PML-RARA, but the log reduction of PML-RARA transcripts was significantly greater in patients receiving ATRA-CHT compared to those treated with ATRA-ATO (3.4 vs. 2.9 logs; $P = 0.0182$) [40]. Conversely, a greater log reduction of PML-RARA transcripts was observed at the end of consolidation in the ATRA-ATO group compared to the ATRA-CHT group (6.3 vs. 5.3 logs; $P = 0.0024$). In agreement with data published in the context of ATRA plus chemotherapy [31], PML-RARA levels at the time point of post-induction were not predictive of subsequent relapse. This study provided a formal proof of the efficacy of ATRA-ATO at the biologic level, showing that such combined therapy is able to exert a clearance of PML-RARA transcript similar if not superior to that exerted by ATRA-CHT.

Future Perspectives

Acute promyelocytic leukemia is currently a curable disease using targeted approaches. Occurrence of relapse, especially in the low and intermediate risk patients treated with modern ATO and ATRA based regimens, is very rare and does not exceed 2% in recent trials. These figures may put into question the cost-effectiveness of longitudinal molecular monitoring in such risk category. Thus, one reasonable policy could be to avoid routine monitoring in these patients (provided that adequate therapy with modern ATRA-ATO is in place). To date, only a small number of high-risk patients have been included in trials using ATO and ATRA with minimal chemotherapy, and their probability of relapse appears to be similar to that of lower-risk categories receiving ATO-ATRA. However, given the small numbers and limited data, the standard of care for high-risk APL remains at present ATRA plus chemotherapy. It is suggested that stringent monitoring be continued in this patient category within controlled clinical studies using well-standardized RQ-PCR approach.

References

1. Wang ZY, Chen Z. Acute promyelocytic leukemia: from highly fatal to highly curable. Blood. 2008;111:2505–15.
2. Mistry AR, Pedersen EW, Solomon E, Grimwade D. The molecular pathogenesis of acute promyelocytic leukaemia: implications for the clinical management of the disease. Blood Rev. 2003;17(2):71–97.
3. Lo-Coco F, Ammatuna E. The biology of acute promyelocytic leukemia and its impact on diagnosis and treatment. Hematol Am Soc Hematol Educ Program. 2006;156–61, 514.
4. Sanz MA, Grimwade D, Tallman MS, Lowenberg B, Fenaux P, Estey EH, et al. Management of acute promyelocytic leukemia: recommendations from an expert panel on behalf of the European LeukemiaNet. Blood. 2009;113:1875–91.
5. Cheson BD, Bennett JM, Kopecky KJ, Buchner T, Willman CL, Estey EH, et al. Revised recommendations of the International Working Group for Diagnosis, Standardization of Response Criteria, Treatment Outcomes, and Reporting Standards for Therapeutic Trials in Acute Myeloid Leukemia. J Clin Oncol. 2003;21(24):4642–9.
6. Diverio D, Rossi V, Avvisati G, De Santis S, Pistilli A, Pane F, et al. Early detection of relapse by prospective reverse transcriptase-polymerase chain reaction analysis of the PML/RARalpha fusion gene in patients with acute promyelocytic leukemia enrolled in the GIMEMA-AIEOP multicenter "AIDA" trial. GIMEMA-AIEOP Multicent. Blood. 1998;92(3):784–9.
7. van Dongen JJ, Macintyre EA, Gabert JA, Delabesse E, Rossi V, Saglio G, et al. Standardized RT-PCR analysis of fusion gene transcripts from chromosome aberrations in acute leukemia for detection of minimal

residual disease. Report of the BIOMED-1 Concerted Action: investigation of minimal residual disease in acute leukemia. Leukemia. 1999;13(12):1901–28.
8. Falini B, Flenghi L, Fagioli M, Lo Coco F, Cordone I, Diverio D, et al. Immunocytochemical diagnosis of acute promyelocytic leukemia (M3) with the monoclonal antibody PG-M3 (anti-PML). Blood. 1997;90(10):4046–53.
9. Lo Coco F, Diverio D, Pandolfi PP, Biondi A, Rossi V, Avvisati G, et al. Molecular evaluation of residual disease as a predictor of relapse in acute promyelocytic leukaemia. Lancet. 1992;340(8833):1437–8.
10. Miller WHJ, Kakizuka A, Frankel SR, Warrell RPJ, DeBlasio A, Levine K, et al. Reverse transcription polymerase chain reaction for the rearranged retinoic acid receptor alpha clarifies diagnosis and detects minimal residual disease in acute promyelocytic leukemia. Proc Natl Acad Sci U S A. 1992;89(7):2694–8.
11. Lo Coco F, Diverio D, Falini B, Biondi A, Nervi C, Pelicci PG. Genetic diagnosis and molecular monitoring in the management of acute promyelocytic leukemia. Blood. 1999;94(1):12–22.
12. Martinelli G, Remiddi C, Visani G, Farabegoli P, Testoni N, Zaccaria A, et al. Molecular analysis of PML-RAR alpha fusion mRNA detected by reverse transcription-polymerase chain reaction assay in long-term disease-free acute promyelocytic leukaemia patients. Br J Haematol. 1995;90(4):966–8.
13. Diverio D, Pandolfi PP, Biondi A, Avvisati G, Petti MC, Mandelli F, et al. Absence of reverse transcription-polymerase chain reaction detectable residual disease in patients with acute promyelocytic leukemia in long-term remission. Blood. 1993;82:3556–9.
14. Laczika K, Mitterbauer G, Korninger L, Knobl P, Schwarzinger I, Kapiotis S, et al. Rapid achievement of PML-RAR alpha polymerase chain reaction (PCR)-negativity by combined treatment with all-trans-retinoic acid and chemotherapy in acute promyelocytic leukemia: a pilot study. Leukemia. 1994;8(1):1–5.
15. Grimwade D, Howe K, Langabeer S, Burnett A, Goldstone A, Solomon E. Minimal residual disease detection in acute promyelocytic leukemia by reverse-transcriptase PCR: evaluation of PML-RAR alpha and RAR alpha-PML assessment in patients who ultimately relapse. Leukemia. 1996;10(1):61–6.
16. Mandelli F, Diverio D, Avvisati G, Luciano A, Barbui T, Bernasconi C, et al. Molecular remission in PML/RAR alpha-positive acute promyelocytic leukemia by combined all-trans retinoic acid and idarubicin (AIDA) therapy. Gruppo Italiano-Malattie Ematologiche Maligne dell'Adulto and Associazione Italiana di Ematologia ed Oncologia Pe. United States. Blood. 1997;90(3):1014–21.
17. Sanz MA, Martin G, Rayon C, Esteve J, Gonzalez M, Diaz-Mediavilla J, et al. A modified AIDA protocol with anthracycline-based consolidation results in high antileukemic efficacy and reduced toxicity in newly diagnosed PML/RARalpha-positive acute promyelocytic leukemia. PETHEMA group. Blood. 1999;94(9):3015–21. United States.
18. Burnett AK, Grimwade D, Solomon E, Wheatley K, Goldstone AH. Presenting white blood cell count and kinetics of molecular remission predict prognosis in acute promyelocytic leukemia treated with all-trans retinoic acid: result of the Randomized MRC Trial. Blood. 1999;93(12):4131–43.
19. Lengfelder E, Reichert A, Schoch C, Haase D, Haferlach T, Loffler H, et al. Double induction strategy including high dose cytarabine in combination with all-trans retinoic acid: effects in patients with newly diagnosed acute promyelocytic leukemia. German AML Cooperative Group. Leukemia. 2000;14(8):1362–70. England.
20. Tobal K, Saunders MJ, Grey MR, Yin JA. Persistence of RAR alpha-PML fusion mRNA detected by reverse transcriptase polymerase chain reaction in patients in long-term remission of acute promyelocytic leukaemia. Br J Haematol. 1995;90(3):615–8. England.
21. Borrow J, Goddard AD, Gibbons B, Katz F, Swirsky D, Fioretos T, et al. Diagnosis of acute promyelocytic leukaemia by RT-PCR: detection of PML-RARA and RARA-PML fusion transcripts. Br J Haematol. 1992;82(3):529–40.
22. Lo Coco F, Diverio D, Avvisati G, Petti MC, Meloni G, Pogliani EM, et al. Therapy of molecular relapse in acute promyelocytic leukemia. Blood. 1999;94(7):2225–9.
23. Esteve J, Escoda L, Martin G, Rubio V, Diaz-Mediavilla J, Gonzalez M, et al. Outcome of patients with acute promyelocytic leukemia failing to front-line treatment with all-trans retinoic acid and anthracycline-based chemotherapy (PETHEMA protocols LPA96 and LPA99): benefit of an early intervention. Leukemia. 2007;21(3):446–52.
24. Meloni G, Diverio D, Vignetti M, Avvisati G, Capria S, Petti MC, et al. Autologous bone marrow transplantation for acute promyelocytic leukemia in second remission: prognostic relevance of pretransplant minimal residual disease assessment by reverse-transcription polymerase chain reaction of the PML/RAR alpha fusion gene. Blood. 1997;90(3):1321–5.
25. Grimwade D, Lo Coco F. Acute promyelocytic leukemia: a model for the role of molecular diagnosis and residual disease monitoring in directing treatment approach in acute myeloid leukemia. Leukemia. 2002;16(10):1959–73.
26. Takatsuki H, Umemura T, Sadamura S, Yamashita S, Goto T, Abe Y, et al. Detection of minimal residual disease by reverse transcriptase polymerase chain reaction for the PML/RAR alpha fusion mRNA: a study in patients with acute promyelocytic leukemia following peripheral stem cell transplantation. Leukemia. 1995;9(5):889–92.
27. Holter Chakrabarty JL, Rubinger M, Le-Rademacher J, Wang H-L, Grigg A, Selby GB, et al. Autologous is superior to allogeneic hematopoietic cell transplantation for acute promyelocytic leukemia in second

complete remission. Biol Blood Marrow Transplant. 2014;20(7):1021–5.
28. Lengfelder E, Lo-Coco F, Ades L, Montesinos P, Grimwade D, Kishore B, et al. Arsenic trioxide-based therapy of relapsed acute promyelocytic leukemia: registry results from the European LeukemiaNet. Leukemia. 2015;29(5):1084–91.
29. Gabert J, Beillard E, van der Velden VHJ, Bi W, Grimwade D, Pallisgaard N, et al. Standardization and quality control studies of "real-time" quantitative reverse transcriptase polymerase chain reaction of fusion gene transcripts for residual disease detection in leukemia—a Europe Against Cancer program. Leukemia. 2003;17(12):2318–57.
30. Santamaria C, Chillon MC, Fernandez C, Martin-Jimenez P, Balanzategui A, Garcia Sanz R, et al. Using quantification of the PML-RARalpha transcript to stratify the risk of relapse in patients with acute promyelocytic leukemia. Haematologica. 2007;92(3):315–22. Italy.
31. Grimwade D, Jovanovic JV, Hills RK, Nugent EA, Patel Y, Flora R, et al. Prospective minimal residual disease monitoring to predict relapse of acute promyelocytic leukemia and to direct pre-emptive arsenic trioxide therapy. J Clin Oncol. 2009;27(22):3650–8.
32. Ommen HB, Schnittger S, Jovanovic JV, Ommen IB, Hasle H, Ostergaard M, et al. Strikingly different molecular relapse kinetics in NPM1c, PML-RARA, RUNX1-RUNX1T1, and CBFB-MYH11 acute myeloid leukemias. Blood. 2010;115(2):198–205.
33. Seftel MD, Barnett MJ, Couban S, Leber B, Storring J, Assaily W, et al. A Canadian consensus on the management of newly diagnosed and relapsed acute promyelocytic leukemia in adults. Curr Oncol. 2014;21(5):234–50.
34. Lo-Coco F, Avvisati G, Vignetti M, Thiede C, Orlando SM, Iacobelli S, et al. Retinoic acid and arsenic trioxide for acute promyelocytic leukemia. N Engl J Med. 2013;369(2):111–21.
35. Burnett AK, Russell NH, Hills RK, Bowen D, Kell J, Knapper S, et al. Arsenic trioxide and all-trans retinoic acid treatment for acute promyelocytic leukaemia in all risk groups (AML17): results of a randomised, controlled, phase 3 trial. Lancet Oncol. 2015;16(13):1295–305.
36. Iland HJ, Collins M, Bradstock K, Supple SG, Catalano A, Hertzberg M, et al. Use of arsenic trioxide in remission induction and consolidation therapy for acute promyelocytic leukaemia in the Australasian Leukaemia and Lymphoma Group (ALLG) APML4 study: a non-randomised phase 2 trial. Lancet Haematol. 2015;2(9):e357–66.
37. Mathews V, George B, Chendamarai E, Lakshmi KM, Desire S, Balasubramanian P, et al. Single-agent arsenic trioxide in the treatment of newly diagnosed acute promyelocytic leukemia: long-term follow-up data. J Clin Oncol. 2010;28(24):3866–71.
38. Shen Z-X, Shi Z-Z, Fang J, Gu B-W, Li J-M, Zhu Y-M, et al. All-trans retinoic acid/As2O3 combination yields a high quality remission and survival in newly diagnosed acute promyelocytic leukemia. Proc Natl Acad Sci U S A. 2004;101(15):5328–35.
39. Chendamarai E, Balasubramanian P, George B, Viswabandya A, Abraham A, Ahmed R, et al. Role of minimal residual disease monitoring in acute promyelocytic leukemia treated with arsenic trioxide in frontline therapy. Blood. 2012;119(15):3413–9.
40. Cicconi L, Divona M, Ciardi C, Ottone T, Ferrantini A, Lavorgna S, et al. PML-RARalpha kinetics and impact of FLT3-ITD mutations in newly diagnosed acute promyelocytic leukaemia treated with ATRA and ATO or ATRA and chemotherapy. Leukemia. 2016;30(10):1987–92.

12 Treatment of Refractory and Relapsed Acute Promyelocytic Leukemia

Eva Lengfelder

Abbreviations

AML	Acute myeloid leukemia
APL	Acute promyelocytic leukemia
Ara-C	Cytosine arabinoside
ATO	Arsenic trioxide
ATRA	All-trans retinoic acid
CIR	Cumulative incidence of relapse
CNS	Central nervous system
CR	Complete remission
EBMT	European Society for Blood and Marrow Transplantation
GVHD	Graft versus host disease
HSCT	Hematopoietic stem cell transplantation
NCCN	National Comprehensive Cancer Network
OS	Overall survival
PML	Promyelocytic leukemia
RARA	Retinoic acid receptor alpha
RT-PCR	Reverse transcriptase polymerase chain reaction
TRM	Transplant related mortality
WBC	White blood cell

E. Lengfelder, M.D.
Department of Hematology and Oncology, University Hospital Mannheim, Theodor-Kutzer-Ufer 1-3, 68167 Mannheim, Germany
e-mail: eva.lengfelder@umm.de

Introduction

The prognosis of patients with acute promyelocytic leukemia (APL) has significantly improved over the past decades. At least 80% of adult patients included in clinical trials can be cured. The first important step in the successful development of APL therapy was the availability of anthracyclines, the first drugs with a curative potential in APL [1]. The outcome was further improved by the introduction of the differentiating agent *all-trans*-retinoic acid (ATRA) and more recently by arsenic trioxide (ATO) [2]. Major challenges are the unresolved problem of early death and the optimal management of relapsed patients.

Although the recent use of ATO in frontline therapy was associated with an extremely low relapse rate [3, 4], the optimal management of relapse after ATO is not well defined. Current literature is mainly restricted to patients in first relapse after ATRA plus chemotherapy, and ATO-based salvage therapy enables cure in a considerable proportion of these patients. Further, current data suggest that long-term stabilization and cure may be possible even after subsequent relapses. This chapter focuses on current problems, treatment options, and outcome of patients with relapsed APL.

O. Abla et al. (eds.), *Acute Promyelocytic Leukemia*, https://doi.org/10.1007/978-3-319-64257-4_12

Molecular Monitoring for Early Detection of Relapse

The induction and persistence of a molecular remission (negative RT-PCR for *PML/RARA*) are the prerequisites for long-term remission and cure in APL. Molecular relapse is conventionally defined as recurrence of a positive reverse transcriptase (RT) PCR or real-time quantitative PCR confirmed in two tests of bone marrow samples taken 2–4 weeks apart. As shown by follow-up studies, patients with molecular relapse usually developed an overt hematological relapse after a median time of 3 months [5]. Therefore, PCR monitoring offers the possibility to detect the relapse earlier on the molecular level and to avoid the problems and risks of an overt hematological relapse.

The benefit of molecular monitoring and of early intervention at the time of molecular relapse was shown in two retrospective studies comparing patients with APL in molecular and hematological relapse [6, 7]. Treatment at the time of molecular relapse was associated with a lower rate of complications during therapy such as early death and APL differentiation syndrome with a positive impact on survival. In a prospective British study for newly diagnosed APL patients, preemptive therapy with ATO for patients with molecular relapse was integrated in the study design. The cumulative incidence of overt hematological relapse (CIR) at 3 years was only 5% (on the UK-MRC AML 15) as compared to 12% in a previous British APL (AML 12) study [8]. The results argue in favor of regular molecular monitoring in first remission at least in high-risk patients treated with conventional ATRA and chemotherapy.

Given the high rate of stable remission after ATO frontline therapy, the value of molecular follow-up in this setting is questioned; thus molecular monitoring and its duration have to be determined individually.

Results with Conventional Treatment Strategies in Relapsed APL

The primary objective of relapse therapy in APL is the re-induction of molecular remission. With conventional approaches based on ATRA and intensive chemotherapy, remission rates of around 90% can be achieved, similar to frontline therapy [9–11]. But in the setting of salvage therapy, ATRA plus chemotherapy is no longer curative, and cure is only possible with subsequent allogeneic or autologous hematopoietic stem cell transplantation (HSCT) [12]. Especially for allogeneic HSCT, this approach may be problematic due to the reduced feasibility and failure rate of transplantation due to the high toxicity of intensified chemotherapy associated with neutropenia and infections. This was represented by the results of a French study including 50 patients with relapsed APL treated with ATRA, mitoxantrone, etoposide, and higher doses of Ara-C. Of 11 patients who underwent allogeneic transplantation, the 3-year survival rate was only 11% and the median survival 8.2 months. Causes of death in remission were infections or GVHD. Among 34 patients who were scheduled to receive an autologous HSCT, only 22 patients could be transplanted [11]. This demonstrates the need for less toxic salvage therapies for relapsed APL.

Current Approaches with ATO-Based Salvage Therapy

ATO-Based Induction and Consolidation Therapy

In the 1990s, authors from China reported the first clinical results on the successful outcome of patients with relapsed APL treated with ATO. Prominent results were the ability of the drug to induce long-lasting second molecular remissions and the low toxicity profile [13]. Subsequently, the high efficacy of ATO in relapsed APL was confirmed by phase II studies (reviewed in [14]). The drug was approved in the United States and in Europe for relapsed APL based on the results of the US Intergroup pivotal study, the largest trial including 40 patients in first relapse of APL. In this study, patients reached a complete remission (CR) rate of 85% and an estimated overall survival of 66% at 18 months [15]. A literature review summarized the results of more than 300 patients with relapsed APL treated with ATO between 1997 and 2011.

Approximately 40% of patients were already in second or more advanced relapse. The patients uniformly received ATO induction therapy (mostly 0.15 mg/kg/day). Post-induction treatment comprised up to five ATO courses and was often combined with chemotherapy. In, total, 59 patients proceeded to autologous or allogeneic HSCT. The average hematological CR rate was 86%, while early death and resistance rates were both at 7%. The rate of molecular CR reached 86% in the largest study with consequent molecular monitoring. The overall survival probability at 2 years ranged between 50 and 81% [14].

The clinical efficacy of the combination of the two differentiating drugs ATO plus ATRA was investigated in newly diagnosed and relapsed APL. The advantage of this combination was demonstrated by a faster and more extensive reduction of the *PML/RARA* burden and by a lower relapse rate [16]. A benefit of the combination was further suggested by the results of a meta-analysis of seven studies. These data showed that the combination of ATRA and ATO induced higher rates of CR and overall survival compared to ATO or ATRA alone without increasing early mortality or toxicity [17].

A registry study from the European LeukemiaNet included 155 patients with APL treated with ATO-based salvage therapy in first relapse after state-of-the-art frontline therapy with ATRA and chemotherapy (104 patients with hematological, 40 with molecular, 11 with extramedullary, mainly central nervous system (CNS) relapse) [18]. Salvage therapy was uniformly performed with one induction cycle ATO ± ATRA, followed by at least one identical consolidation course. Post-consolidation therapy consisted of autologous (n = 60) or allogeneic (n = 33) HSCT or of further ATO or chemotherapy (n = 55). After a median follow-up of 3.2 years, 3-year overall survival (OS) and cumulative incidence of relapse (CIR) of the whole population were 70% and 44%, respectively (Fig. 12.1a, b). This suggests a survival improvement of approximately 20% compared to previous results with ATRA and chemotherapy [10]. Patients treated for molecular relapse had decreased early death rate and better tolerance of the therapy (significantly lower rates of APL differentiation syndrome and of infections) in comparison to patients treated for hematological relapse. However, the survival advantage of patients with molecular relapse disappeared with longer follow-up (Fig. 12.2a, b). The multivariable analysis of prognostic factors for overall and leukemia-free survival demonstrated a positive impact of CR1 duration ≥1.5 years and achievement of a second molecular remission and of transplantation in second CR (allogeneic or autologous) [18].

Options for Post-consolidation Therapy

There is evidence from the literature that post-consolidation therapy with autologous or allogeneic HSCT or with prolonged ATO plus ATRA improves the outcome as compared to no further therapy [14]. In lack of randomized studies, the presently available guidelines (Europe, USA, Canada) are based on consensus recommendations.

In 2009, a panel of European APL experts published recommendations for the management of relapses on the basis of the available literature. The European recommendations indicate two cycles of ATO ± ATRA for induction and consolidation therapy followed by autologous HSCT, if a molecular remission was achieved after consolidation. For patients who fail to obtain a second molecular remission or who relapse after short CR1 duration of less than 1–1.5 years, allogeneic HSCT should be favored. For patients who do not qualify for transplantation, prolonged ATO plus ATRA therapy or chemotherapy intensification is recommended (Fig. 12.3) [19]. For the latter group of patients, the Canadian guidelines provided detailed information and recommended a sequence of six cycles of ATO plus ATRA [20]. The NCCN guidelines 2016 for APL relapse recommend an ATO-containing regimen for patients not previously exposed to ATO and for patients with later relapse (>6 months) after previous ATO therapy. In patients with early relapse (<6 months) after an ATO/anthracycline containing regimen, standard ATRA plus idarubicin with the addition of ATO is recommended [21].

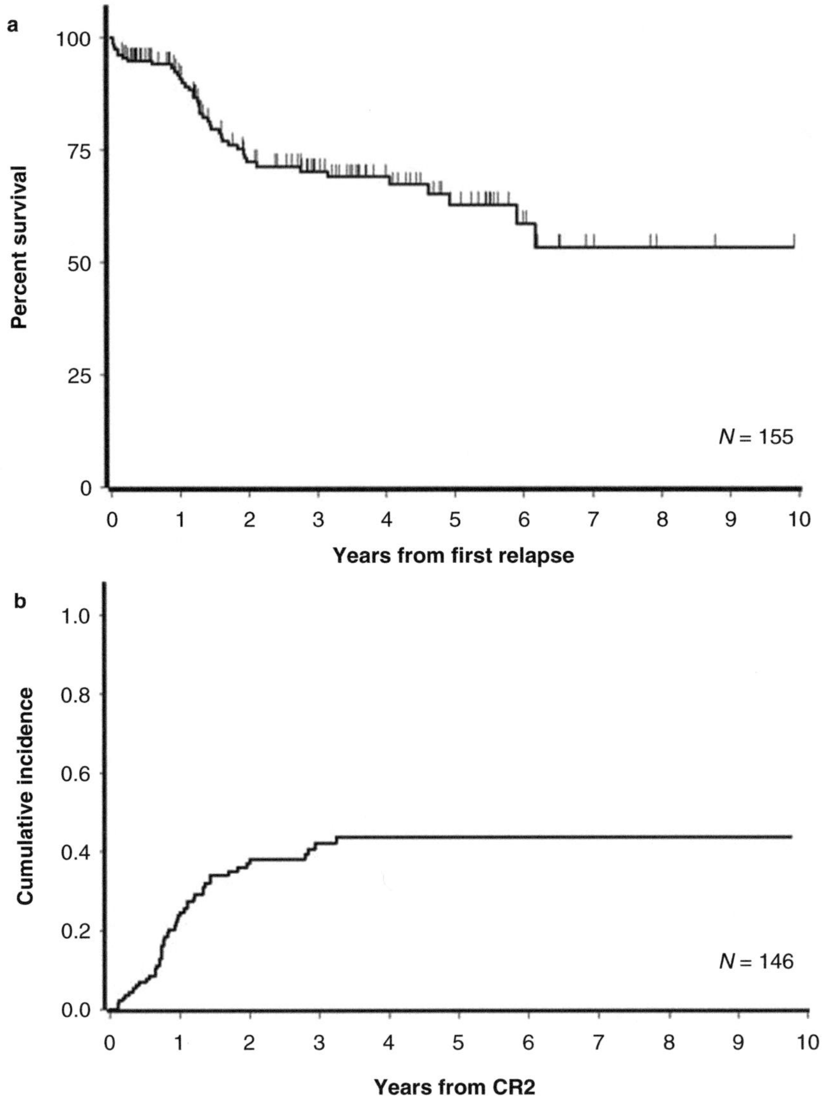

Fig. 12.1 Overall survival (**a**) and cumulative incidence of relapse (**b**) of all patients treated with ATO in first relapse of APL. Tics indicate the last follow-up of the living patients [18]

There are no randomized studies comparing autologous and allogeneic transplantation. Most data are available from retrospective comparisons. In general, autologous transplantation was associated with higher relapse probability but lower toxicity compared to allogeneic transplantation. The results of 122 relapsing patients included in the French/European APL91 and 93 trials showed a 7-year relapse-free survival rate of 79.4%, event-free survival of 60.6%, overall survival of 59.8%, and transplant-related mortality (TRM) of 6% in the autologous group. The respective results of the allogeneic group were 92.3%, 52.2%, and 51.8% and a TRM of 39% [22]. Similar data were reported from the EBMT registry and other smaller series [23]. A prospective Japanese study of 35 patients in first relapse treated with ATO and subsequent autologous transplantation showed a 5-year event-free and overall survival of 65% and 77%, respectively [24]. In a retrospective study of 31 Italian patients, who underwent allogeneic transplantation in CR2 or beyond, 4-year OS was 45%. Favorable prognostic factors for OS and CIR were molecular remission at transplantation and a lower number of relapses [25].

Other retrospective studies compared the outcome of transplantation, almost always

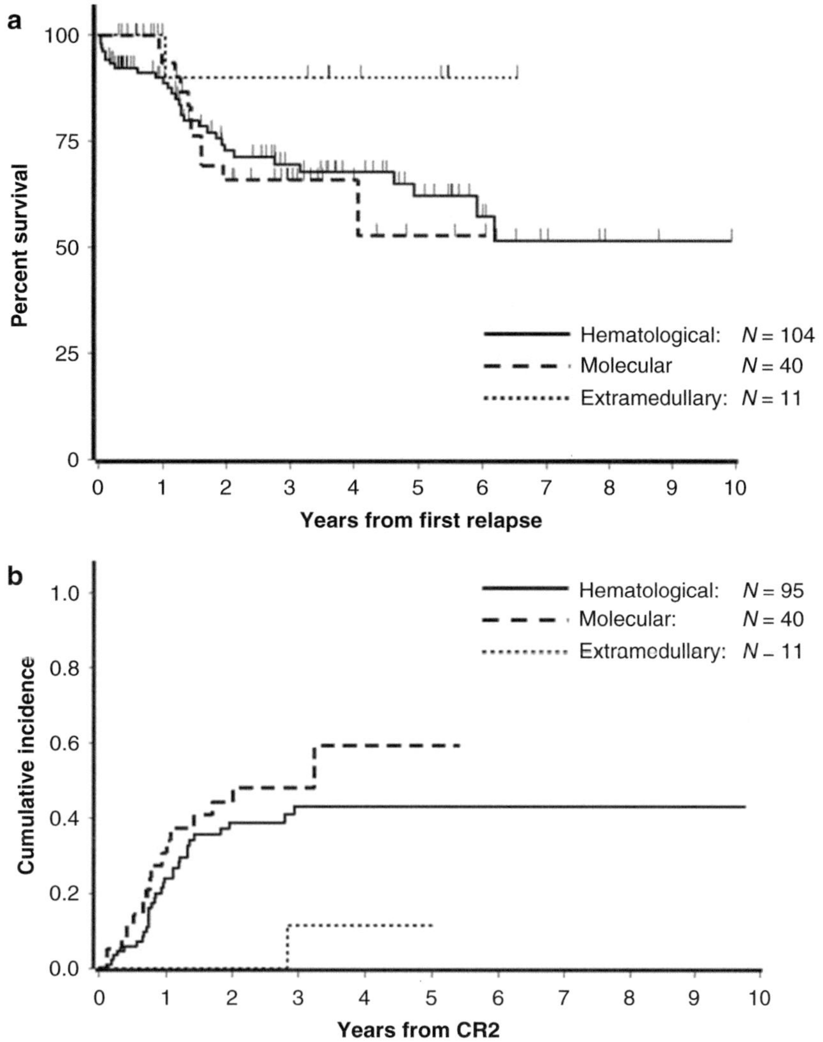

Fig. 12.2 Overall survival (**a**) and cumulative incidence of relapse (**b**) separated according to hematological, molecular, or extramedullary relapse (overall survival $p = 0.31$; cumulative incidence of relapse $p = 0.047$). Tics indicate the last follow-up of the living patients [18]

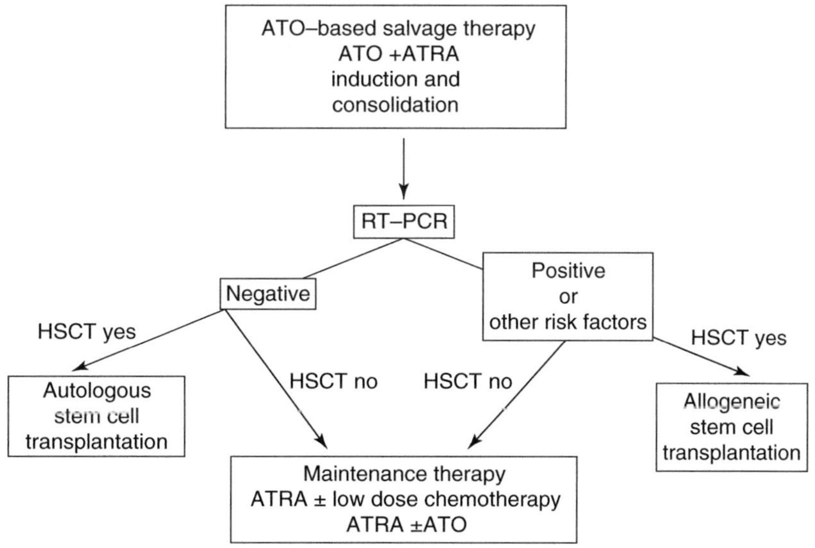

Fig. 12.3 Treatment algorithm for APL relapse. *HSCT* hematopoietic stem cell transplantation

autologous, with prolonged administration of ATO. Even if continuation of ATO therapy seems to prolong the remission duration, the majority of data suggests a longer survival after treatment intensification with autologous transplantation [26, 27].

Special Situations of Relapse

Extramedullary Relapse

Extramedullary APL relapses are rare, and most of them involve the CNS. Therapy mostly consisted of intrathecal chemotherapy (methotrexate ± Ara-C ± steroids) with or without cranial irradiation. Sporadic relapses in other locations (e.g., cutaneous, paraspinal mass, etc.) were published as case reports [28–31].

The Spanish PETHEMA group reported a 5-year cumulative incidence of 1.7% CNS relapses and a median survival of 13 months observed in 11 of 739 patients treated with ATRA and anthracyclines in the LPA96 and 99 trials. An initial high WBC count and intracranial hemorrhage at first diagnosis were independent prognostic factors for CNS relapse [32]. A combined analysis of 806 patients included in the studies of the French/European APL group and of the PETHEMA group showed a cumulative incidence of extramedullary relapse at 3 years of 1.1% ($n = 10$; nine in CNS, one cutaneous) compared to isolated bone marrow relapse of 15.5%, respectively. Median survival from time of extramedullary relapse was 6.7 months [33].

In the European relapsed APL registry, 11 patients in first relapse at extramedullary sites (CNS $n = 9$, other $n = 2$) were registered. Treatment consisted of ATO ± ATRA induction and consolidation with the addition of intrathecal chemotherapy. Post-consolidation therapy was variable including autologous transplantation in six cases and allogeneic transplantation in one case. The 3-year OS of these patients was 90% and the CIR 11% [18]. These results suggest an improvement of survival caused by ATO, as the drug was reported to penetrate the CNS over a broad range of plasma levels [34]. As reported by Chinese authors, arsenic concentration in the cerebrospinal fluid could be increased to the level of the peripheral blood, when intravenous mannitol was given prior to ATO administration [35].

Current Management of Advanced Relapses and Newer Treatment Options

Re-induction of remission, if possible, is still the main goal in advanced APL relapses. Despite reduced chances for another remission, patients may achieve a CR with various salvage approaches repeatedly. Patients pretreated with ATO may respond to ATO again. In those who became resistant after previous ATO therapy, mutations in the PML gene may be the underlying reason [36]. Allogeneic transplantation is currently the only curative chance for patients with advanced relapse.

Conservative treatment options include gemtuzumab ozogamicin (GO), which induced remissions in patients with several grades of molecular or hematological relapse [37, 38]. The synthetic retinoid tamibarotene (not approved in Europe) has a higher differentiation induction potential than conventional ATRA and induced remission in 58% of relapsed/refractory APL patients in an early study [39]. Recently tamibarotene monotherapy was reported to induce hematological remission in 65% and molecular remission in 21% of patients with advanced APL. The authors conclude that the efficacy of the drug warrants further studies in combination with ATO [40].

Conclusion

Despite improvement in the prognosis of relapsed APL with the introduction of ATO, the rate of subsequent relapses is still high. This requires further efforts to better define patients at risk of relapse and to improve the strategies for salvage therapy. Currently, ATO plus ATRA is the treatment of choice for patients in first relapse of APL after conventional therapy with ATRA and chemotherapy. Even in relapse after frontline therapy with

ATO, a second approach with ATO seems justified; however, the data in this setting are scarce. Treatment intensification with autologous HSCT remains an appropriate option for younger patients in molecular remission. In elderly patients with contraindications for HSCT, prolonged therapy with ATO may be an option. Patients with persistent positive RT-PCR or with higher degrees of relapse are candidates for allogeneic HSCT.

References

1. Bernard J, Weil M, Boiron M, Jacquillat C, Flandrin G, Gemon MF. Acute promyelocytic leukemia: results of treatment by daunorubicin. Blood. 1973;41:489–96.
2. Wang ZY, Chen Z. Acute promyelocytic leukemia: from highly fatal to highly curable. Blood. 2008;111:2505–15. https://doi.org/10.1182/blood-2007-07-102798
3. Lo-Coco F, Avvisati G, Vignetti M, Thiede C, Orlando SM, Iacobelli S, et al. Retinoic acid and arsenic trioxide for acute promyelocytic leukemia. N Engl J Med. 2013;369:111–21. https://doi.org/10.1056/NEJMoa1300874.
4. Burnett AK, Russell NH, Hills RK, Bowen D, Kell J, Knapper S, et al. Arsenic trioxide and all-trans retinoic acid treatment for acute promyelocytic leukaemia in all risk groups (AML17): results of a randomised, controlled, phase 3 trial. Lancet Oncol. 2015;16:1295–305. https://doi.org/10.1016/S1470-2045(15)00193-X.
5. Diverio D, Rossi V, Avvisati G, De Santis S, Pistilli A, Pane F, et al. Early detection of relapse by prospective reverse transcriptase-polymerase chain reaction analysis of the PML/RARalpha fusion gene in patients with acute promyelocytic leukemia enrolled in the GIMEMA-AIEOP multicenter "AIDA" trial. GIMEMA-AIEOP Multicenter "AIDA" Trial. Blood. 1998;92:784–9.
6. Lo Coco F, Diverio D, Avvisati G, Petti MC, Meloni G, Pogliani EM, et al. Therapy of molecular relapse in acute promyelocytic leukemia. Blood. 1999;94:2225–9.
7. Esteve J, Escoda L, Martín G, Rubio V, Díaz-Mediavilla J, González M, et al. Outcome of patients with acute promyelocytic leukemia failing to front-line treatment with all-trans retinoic acid and anthracycline-based chemotherapy (PETHEMA protocols LPA96 and LPA99): benefit of an early intervention. Leukemia. 2007;21:446–52.
8. Grimwade D, Jovanovic JV, Hills RK, Nugent EA, Patel Y, Flora R, et al. Prospective minimal residual disease monitoring to predict relapse of acute promyelocytic leukemia and to direct pre-emptive arsenic trioxide therapy. J Clin Oncol. 2009;27:3650–8. https://doi.org/10.1200/JCO.2008.20.1533.
9. Castagnola C, Lunghi M, Corso A, Tajana M, Zappasodi P, Dabusti M, et al. Management of acute promyelocytic leukemia relapse in the ATRA era. Haematologica. 1998;83:714–7.
10. Fenaux P, Chevret S, Guerci A, Fegueux N, Dombret H, Thomas X, et al. Long-term follow-up confirms the benefit of all-trans retinoic acid in acute promyelocytic leukemia. European APL group. Leukemia. 2000;14:1371–7.
11. Thomas X, Dombret H, Cordonnier C, Pigneux A, Gardin C, Guerci A, et al. Treatment of relapsing acute promyelocytic leukemia by all-trans retinoic acid therapy followed by timed sequential chemotherapy and stem cell transplantation. Leukemia. 2000;14:1006–13.
12. Degos L, Dombret H, Chomienne C, Daniel MT, Micléa JM, Chastang C, et al. All-trans-retinoic acid as a differentiating agent in the treatment of acute promyelocytic leukemia. Blood. 1995;85:2643–53.
13. Niu C, Yan H, Yu T, Sun HP, Liu JX, Li XS, et al. Studies on treatment of acute promyelocytic leukemia with arsenic trioxide: remission induction, follow-up, and molecular monitoring in 11 newly diagnosed and 47 relapsed acute promyelocytic leukemia patients. Blood. 1999;94:3315–24.
14. Lengfelder E, Hofmann WK, Nowak D. Impact of arsenic trioxide in the treatment of acute promyelocytic leukemia. Leukemia. 2012;26:433–42. https://doi.org/10.1038/leu.2011.245.
15. Soignet SL, Frankel SR, Douer D, Tallman MS, Kantarjian H, Calleja E, et al. United States multicenter study of arsenic trioxide in relapsed acute promyelocytic leukemia. J Clin Oncol. 2001;19:3852–60.
16. Shen ZX, Shi ZZ, Fang J, Gu BW, Li JM, Zhu YM, et al. All-trans retinoic acid/As2O3 combination yields a high quality remission and survival in newly diagnosed acute promyelocytic leukemia. Proc Natl Acad Sci U S A. 2004;101:5328–35.
17. Wang H, Chen XY, Wang BS, Rong ZX, Qi H, Chen HZ. The efficacy and safety of arsenic trioxide with or without all-trans retinoic acid for the treatment of acute promyelocytic leukemia: a meta-analysis. Leuk Res. 2011;35:1170–7. https://doi.org/10.1016/j.leukres.2011.06.002.
18. Lengfelder E, Lo-Coco F, Ades L, Montesinos P, Grimwade D, Kishore B, et al. Arsenic trioxide-based therapy of relapsed acute promyelocytic leukemia: registry results from the European LeukemiaNet. Leukemia. 2015;29:1084–91. https://doi.org/10.1038/leu.2015.12.
19. Sanz MA, Grimwade D, Tallman MS, Lowenberg B, Fenaux P, Estey EH, et al. Management of acute promyelocytic leukemia: recommendations from an expert panel on behalf of the European LeukemiaNet. Blood. 2009;113:1875–91. https://doi.org/10.1182/blood-2008-04-150250.

20. Seftel MD, Barnett MJ, Couban S, Leber B, Storring J, Assaily W, et al. A Canadian consensus on the management of newly diagnosed and relapsed acute promyelocytic leukemia in adults. Curr Oncol. 2014;21:234–50. https://doi.org/10.3747/co.21.2183.
21. NCCN. NCCN guidelines: acute myeloid leukemia, version 2.2016. Fort Washington: National Comprehensive Cancer Network; 2016. https://www.nccn.org/professionals/physician_gls/pdf/aml.pdf. Accessed 4 Aug 2016.
22. de Botton S, Fawaz A, Chevret S, Dombret H, Thomas X, Sanz M, et al. Autologous and allogeneic stem-cell transplantation as salvage treatment of acute promyelocytic leukemia initially treated with all-trans-retinoic acid: a retrospective analysis of the European acute promyelocytic leukemia group. J Clin Oncol. 2005;23:120–6.
23. Sanz MA, Labopin M, Gorin NC, de la Rubia J, Arcese W, Meloni G, et al. Hematopoietic stem cell transplantation for adults with acute promyelocytic leukemia in the ATRA era: a survey of the European Cooperative Group for Blood and Marrow Transplantation. Bone Marrow Transplant. 2007;39:461–9.
24. Yanada M, Tsuzuki M, Fujita H, Fujimaki K, Fujisawa S, Sunami K, et al. Phase 2 study of arsenic trioxide followed by autologous hematopoietic cell transplantation for relapsed acute promyelocytic leukemia. Blood. 2013;121:3095–102. https://doi.org/10.1182/blood-2012-11-466862.
25. Ramadan SM, Di Veroli A, Camboni A, Breccia M, Iori AP, Aversa F, et al. Allogeneic stem cell transplantation for advanced acute promyelocytic leukemia in the ATRA and ATO era. Haematologica. 2012;97:1731–5.
26. Thirugnanam R, George B, Chendamarai E, Lakshmi KM, Balasubramanian P, Viswabandya A, et al. Comparison of clinical outcomes of patients with relapsed acute promyelocytic leukemia induced with arsenic trioxide and consolidated with either an autologous stem cell transplant or an arsenic trioxide-based regimen. Biol Blood Marrow Transplant. 2009;15:1479–84. https://doi.org/10.1016/j.bbmt.2009.07.010.
27. Ganzel C, Mathews V, Alimoghaddam K, Ghavamzadeh A, Kuk D, Devlin S, et al. Autologous transplant remains the preferred therapy for relapsed APL in CR2. Bone Marrow Transplant. 2016;51:1180–3. https://doi.org/10.1038/bmt.2016.96.
28. Milone G, Inghilterra G, Li Gioi F, Peluso D, Giustolisi R. Testicular and cutaneous relapse after hematopoietic transplantation in a patient affected with APL. Bone Marrow Transplant. 1999;23:751.
29. Pacilli L, Lo Coco F, Ramadan SM, Giannì L, Pingi A, Remotti D, et al. Promyelocytic sarcoma of the spine: a case report and review of the literature. Adv Hematol. 2010;2010:137608. https://doi.org/10.1155/2010/137608.
30. Ochs RC, Gormley RH, Luger S, Bagg A. Isolated bowel relapse in acute promyelocytic leukemia: an unusual site of extramedullary recurrence. J Clin Oncol. 2010;28:e550–3. https://doi.org/10.1200/JCO.2010.29.7424.
31. Tirado CA, Chen W, Valdez F, Karandikar N, Arbini A, Acevedo I, et al. Unusual presentation of myeloid sarcoma in a case of acute promyelocytic leukemia with a cryptic PML-RARA rearrangement involving multiple sites including the atrium. Cancer Genet Cytogenet. 2010;200:47–53. https://doi.org/10.1016/j.cancergencyto.2010.03.016.
32. Montesinos P, Díaz-Mediavilla J, Debén G, Prates V, Tormo M, Rubio V, et al. Central nervous system involvement at first relapse in patients with acute promyelocytic leukemia treated with all-trans retinoic acid and anthracycline monochemotherapy without intrathecal prophylaxis. Haematologica. 2009;94:1242–9. https://doi.org/10.3324/haematol.2009.007872.
33. de Botton S, Sanz MA, Chevret S, Dombret H, Martin G, Thomas X, et al. Extramedullary relapse in acute promyelocytic leukemia treated with all-trans retinoic acid and chemotherapy. Leukemia. 2006;20:35–41.
34. Au WY, Tam S, Fong BM, Kwong YL. Elemental arsenic entered the cerebrospinal fluid during oral arsenic trioxide treatment of meningeal relapse of acute promyelocytic leukemia. Blood. 2006;107:3012–3.
35. Wang H, Cao F, Li J, Li L, Li Y, Shi C, et al. Arsenic trioxide and mannitol for the treatment of acute promyelocytic leukemia relapse in central nervous system. Blood. 2014;124:1998–2000. https://doi.org/10.1182/blood-2014-04-568121.
36. Zhu HH, Qin YZ, Huang XJ. Resistance to arsenic therapy in acute promyelocytic leukemia. N Engl J Med. 2014;370:1864–6. https://doi.org/10.1056/NEJMc1316382.
37. Lo-Coco F, Cimino G, Breccia M, Noguera NI, Diverio D, Finolezzi E, et al. Gemtuzumab ozogamicin (Mylotarg) as a single agent for molecularly relapsed acute promyelocytic leukemia. Blood. 2004;104:1995–9.
38. Breccia M, Cimino G, Diverio D, Gentilini F, Mandelli F, Lo Coco F. Sustained molecular remission after low dose gemtuzumab-ozogamicin in elderly patients with advanced acute promyelocytic leukemia. Haematologica. 2007;92:1273–4.
39. Tobita T, Takeshita A, Kitamura K, Ohnishi K, Yanagi M, Hiraoka A, et al. Treatment with a new synthetic retinoid, Am80, of acute promyelocytic leukemia relapsed from complete remission induced by all-trans retinoic acid. Blood. 1997;90:967–73.
40. Sanford D, Lo-Coco F, Sanz MA, Di Bona E, Coutre S, Altman JK, et al. Tamibarotene in patients with acute promyelocytic leukaemia relapsing after treatment with all-trans retinoic acid and arsenic trioxide. Br J Haematol. 2015;171:471–7. https://doi.org/10.1111/bjh.13607.

13 Hematopoietic Stem Cell Transplantation in Acute Promyelocytic Leukemia

Jaime Sanz and Miguel A. Sanz

Introduction

The outcome of patients with acute promyelocytic leukemia (APL) has improved dramatically during the recent decades with the introduction of all-trans retinoic acid (ATRA) and arsenic trioxide (ATO). The interest of hematopoietic stem cell transplantation (HSCT) in modern APL is marginal since most patients will be cured with front-line treatment without HSCT [1–3]. However, around 10–15% of APL patients will eventually relapse [4]. After salvage therapy, some kind of transplant strategy is recommended for relapsed APL patients [5].

Information on the role of HSCT in patients with APL is very limited and is based on small retrospective series [5–7] from single institutions or cooperative groups [6–8] and registry-based studies [9–12]. These studies can be classified according to the therapy available at that time, such as the pre-ATRA [9], ATRA [10], and ATO eras [6, 11]. Although some information can be withdrawn from older studies, these included patients in first remission that had not received differentiating agents and had no information on molecular status at time of transplantation. In addition to the most recent studies analyzing salvage strategies using ATO, there is no information on those patients failing ATO when used as front-line therapy. Well-designed studies are unlikely since the expected population that could potentially benefit from a transplant modality is small and diverse.

Role of HSCT in Front-Line Therapy

The indication of HSCT in patients with APL has evolved historically from a widespread use of this procedure in front-line therapy during the pre-ATRA era to a virtual rejection of this indication when patients are treated with modern treatments containing ATRA. Except for the beginning of the ATRA era, in which many groups still continued to indicate an HSCT in CR1 [9, 10], this has gradually been abandoned and explicitly rejected by the 2009 European LeukemiaNet recommendations [5]. The vast majority of patients with APL treated with modern front-line therapy with ATRA and either che-

J. Sanz, M.D.
Department of Hematology, Hospital Universitari i Politècnic La Fe, Valencia, Spain

Centro de Investigación Biomédica en Red de Cáncer, Instituto Carlos III, Madrid, Spain

M.A. Sanz, M.D. (✉)
Department of Medicine, Hospital Universitari i Politecnic La Fe, University of Valencia, Valencia, Spain

Centro de Investigacion Biomedica en Red de Cancer, Instituto Carlos III, Madrid, Spain
e-mail: msanz@uv.es

O. Abla et al. (eds.), *Acute Promyelocytic Leukemia*, https://doi.org/10.1007/978-3-319-64257-4_13

motherapy or ATO, without using HSCT, will achieve molecular remission at the end of consolidation (97–99%) [2], and more than 85% of APL patients will eventually be cured. Even in patients with high-risk disease [13], commonly defined as those with an initial white blood cell count (WBC) greater than 10×10^9 per liter, the probability of cure with risk-adapted strategies is around 90% [3]. There is therefore no role for HSCT for patients in first complete remission (CR), even in high-risk patients. The only exception is the very small fraction of patients with persistent minimal residual disease (MRD) at the end of consolidation, given that they have a very poor prognosis unless they are promptly managed aggressively prior to the occurrence of a hematologic relapse [14]. However, it should be noted that molecular persistence at this point was already rare in early studies (3–4%) [15] but has almost disappeared (<1%) in patients receiving state-of-the-art treatments with either ATRA plus ATO or ATRA plus chemotherapy-based approaches [3, 16]. Decisions based on molecular status are sometimes crucial and should therefore be made with caution and to rely on highly experienced laboratories. If confirmed in at least two different samples, allogeneic HSCT should be considered as the first option. For those candidates to allogeneic HSCT, it should be performed ideally after achieving molecular negativity before transplantation with additional chemotherapy, ATO or gemtuzumab ozogamycin. For patients unsuitable for allogeneic HSCT, due to poor overall performance and clinical condition, autologous HSCT can be considered as consolidation therapy provided that the patient achieves molecular remission in the bone marrow and has a PCR negative harvest [5].

Role of HSCT in Salvage Therapy for Relapsed APL

ELN recommendations for the management of relapsed APL are summarized in Table 13.1. Before the introduction of ATO as salvage therapy in relapsed APL, treatment usually consisted of the

Table 13.1 Management of relapse

Recommendation	Level of evidence	Grade of recommendation
1. For patients with confirmed molecular relapse (defined as two successive PCR positive assays, with stable or rising *PML-RARA* transcript levels detected in independent samples analyzed in two laboratories) preemptive therapy has to be started promptly to prevent frank relapse	IIa	B
2. Although ATRA in combination with chemotherapy can be used as salvage therapy, ATO-based regimens are presently regarded the first option for treatment of relapsed APL	IV	C
3. Patients achieving second CR should receive intensification with SCT or chemotherapy, if possible	IV	C
4. Allogeneic HSCT is recommended for patients failing to achieve a second molecular remission	IV	C
5. Autologous HSCT is a valid option for patients without detectable MRD in the marrow and with an adequate PCR negative harvest	IIa	B
6. For patients in whom HSCT is not feasible, the available options include repeated cycles of ATO with or without ATRA with or without chemotherapy	IV	C
7. For patients with CNS relapse, induction treatment consists of weekly triple intrathecal therapy (ITT) with methotrexate, hydrocortisone, and cytarabine until complete clearance of blasts in the cerebrospinal fluid, followed by 6–10 more spaced out ITT treatments as consolidation. Systemic treatment should also be given	IV	C

readministration of ATRA and chemotherapy for induction, generally containing high-dose cytarabine and an anthracycline, followed by further post-remission chemotherapy and/or HSCT [1, 8, 17, 18]. Nevertheless, although this combination can still be used as salvage therapy, ATO-based regimens are presently regarded as the first option for treatment of relapsed APL. The best consolidation strategy after ATO-induced second remission is unknown. Options include continued treatment with repeated cycles of ATO, the use of standard chemotherapy in combination with ATRA and/or ATO, and HSCT. The selection of the most appropriate post-remission treatment option for patients achieving second CR, as well as the modality of HSCT, depends on a range of prognostic and logistic variables (e.g., molecular status, duration of first remission, age, donor availability, etc.). The most relevant studies evaluating HSCT in relapsed APL during the ATRA era are shown in Table 13.2.

Several retrospective studies have suggested that treatment intensification with HSCT may improve outcomes of patients achieving second remission with ATO or chemotherapy [6, 7, 11, 19]. Overall survival (OS) ranged from 65 to 83% for transplanted patients (autologous or allogeneic) with increased antileukemic efficacy compared to 34–42% in non-transplanted patients. In all reports, due to the study design, the comparability of the different cohorts was limited, since there were important differences in patient characteristics. The non-transplanted group generally included an older and heterogeneously treated population of patients who probably did not qualify for transplantation in the majority of cases. Although a proportion of patients can maintain

Table 13.2 Selected studies evaluating HSCT in relapsed APL during the ATRA era

Reference	Study period	No. of patients	Salvage therapy	Type of HSCT	MR pre-HSCT, %	TRM, %	CIR, %	DFS, %	OS, %
De Botton et al. [7]	1992–2001	50	Chemotherapy	Autologous	93[a]	6	–	–	60 (7 years)
		23	Chemotherapy	Allogeneic	–	39	–	–	52 (7 years)
Sanz et al. [10]	1993–2003	195	Chemotherapy	Autologous	–	16	37 (5 years)	51 (5 years)	–
		137	Chemotherapy	Allogeneic	–	24	17 (5 years)	59 (5 years)	–
Yanada et al. [20]	2005–2009	35	ATO	Autologous	97	0	–[b]	–	77 (5 years)
Holter Chakrabarty et al. [12]	1995–2006	62	Chemotherapy	Autologous	–	7	30 (5 years)	63 (5 years)	75 (5 years)
		232	Chemotherapy	Allogeneic	–	31	18 (5 years)	50 (5 years)	54 (5 years)
Lengfelder et al. [6]	2003–2011	60	ATO based	Autologous	98	–	37 (3 years)	–	77 (3 years)
		33	ATO based	Allogeneic	48	–	39 (3 years)	–	79 (3 years)
Ganzel et al. [11]	<2000–2011	140	ATO	Autologous	–	–	–	≈68 (5 years)	78 (5 years)
Yanada et al. [26]	1995–2004	43	Non ATO	Autologous	85	2.7	22 (4 years)	–	80 (4 years)
	2006–2012	141	ATO	Autologous	95	3.3	8.5 (4 years)	–	93 (4 years)

MR molecular remission
[a]Tested in 30 patients
[b]3 relapses

long-term remissions without HSCT, overall prognosis is far from satisfactory, and outcomes seem much better for those who receive autologous or allogeneic HSCT. Available data supports the use of a HSCT modality for all transplant candidates.

Impact of Pretransplant Molecular Status

Molecular remission is a prerequisite for long-term disease control in APL. In ATO-naïve patients, ATO can induce hematological remissions in roughly 90% of patients. In addition, the use of at least two cycles of ATO results in the achievement of a second molecular remission in nearly 80% of patients [6, 20]. Whether or not, these results will be obtained after salvage therapy in patients receiving ATO as front-line therapy is unknown and may challenge treatment in the future, since relapsed patients will be from a more selective and high-risk population.

The presence of MRD positivity with detectable PML-RARA rearrangement tested by RT-PCR in the bone marrow before HSCT has a major impact on outcome and should guide the choice of HSCT modality. For instance, MRD positivity in the bone marrow at the time of autologous HSCT was highly predictive of relapse in most [5, 6] but not all reports [12]. The impact of MRD positivity in the allogeneic setting is not so well established [6] and potentially may be counterbalanced by the graft-versus-leukemia (GVL) effect.

Another important issue is whether the presence of molecular disease in harvested hematopoietic cells hampers autologous HSCT. Long-term molecular remission has been reported in two patients transplanted in second hematologic and molecular remission immediately prior to conditioning and who received an PML/RAR positive autograft [21, 22]. It was subsequently described in four patients who had molecular evidence of disease in at least one of the harvested samples and remained RT-PCR negative after autologous HSCT [8]. Leukemic contamination of stem cell grafts in APL patients undergoing HSCT, while bone marrow is in molecular remission at time of transplant, does not necessarily lead to leukemic relapse or preclude long-term remission. This could be explained by still unclear mechanisms of surveillance and the control of low numbers of leukemic cells or by the non-clonogenic nature of the PML/RARA-positive cells present in the graft. The persistence of differentiating elements which carry this specific rearrangement and spontaneously cleared during follow-up is a common event in patients receiving ATRA. In addition, long-term hematopoiesis after autologous HSCT would be sustained by the subset of CD34+/CD38− progenitor cells administered, and these immature progenitors have been shown to lack the PML/RAR rearrangement in APL patients.

HSCT in Patients with CNS Relapse

Central nervous system (CNS) involvement at time of relapse is uncommon in low- and intermediate-risk patients (≈1%), but the risk is increased in patients with high WBC counts at diagnosis (≈5%) and those who have had a CNS hemorrhage during induction (≈20%) [23, 24]. Patients with CNS relapse have classically been associated with a poorer outcome than those with isolated bone marrow relapse [24]. The recommended approach for patients with CNS relapse, even for patients with isolated CNS relapse, consist of weekly triple intrathecal therapy (ITT) with methotrexate, hydrocortisone, and cytarabine until complete clearance of blasts in the cerebrospinal fluid, followed by six to ten more spaced out ITT treatments as consolidation [5]. Since CNS disease is almost invariably accompanied by hematologic or molecular relapse in the marrow, systemic treatment should also be given following the same rules as for patients in hematologic relapse. Chemotherapy agents with high CNS penetrance (e.g., high-dose cytarabine) have been used in this situation. In patients responding to treatment, the consolidation treatment of choice, including appropriate CNS irradiation, should be allogeneic or autologous HSCT. It appears that an ATO-based salvage therapy, an agent with good CNS penetration, may contribute to improved prognosis when consolidated with HSCT, with a reported OS of 90% [6].

Autologous or Allogeneic HSCT

There are no strict guidelines as regards the choice of autologous or allogeneic HSCT once achieving a second CR in relapsed APL patients. The relative efficacy of autologous and allogeneic HSCT in relapsed APL has not been compared in randomized controlled studies. Autologous HSCT offers antileukemic efficacy through high-dose chemo-/radiotherapy with subsequent stem cell support, while the effect of allogeneic HSCT is mainly based on the immunologic surveillance of donor cells to residual blasts, the so-called GVL effect. Autologous HSCT is obviously associated with a lower transplantation-related mortality (TRM) and is a reasonable option in patients without detectable MRD and prolonged duration of first CR (more than 1 year). In contrast, allogeneic HSCT involves a greater risk of nonrelapse mortality but offers a potentially greater antileukemic activity due to the GVL effect. Allogeneic HSCT could be, therefore, recommended in patients failing to achieve a second molecular remission and for those with a short first CR duration [25]. Large retrospective series of transplanted APL patients have been reported by the European Bone Marrow Transplantation (EBMT) Cooperative Group, before the availability of ATRA [9] and after the introduction of this drug [10], by other European [6, 7] and Japanese [20, 26] groups, as well as the Center for International Blood and Marrow Transplant Research (CIBMTR) in the USA [12]. Focusing on patients in second CR, all studies showed that the relapse rate was lower in patients who received an allogeneic HSCT as compared to patients who underwent autologous HSCT. However, TRM was higher in the allografted than in the autografted group. Overall, patients achieved better survival and leukemia-free survival after autologous HSCT. However, most studies could not estimate the relapse rate on the basis of the RT-PCR status at time of transplantation. Due to the high risk of relapse for patients with detectable MRD undergoing auto-HSCT, allogeneic HSCT is only recommended in patients failing to achieve a second molecular remission.

Allogeneic HSCT offers potent antileukemic efficacy through donor-derived and immune-mediated mechanisms. Evidence of GVL effect in APL was elegantly shown in two patients with persistent RT-PCR positivity after allogeneic HSCT that converted to sustained RT-PCR negativity 1 month after withdrawal of immunosuppression [27]. Cumulative incidence of relapse ranged from 17 to 39% in a selected population of high-risk patients with early relapse or persistent MRD after salvage therapy [6, 10, 12, 27]. Interestingly, allogeneic HSCT was able to overcome the negative impact of pretransplant PCR positivity on relapse [6, 7, 12, 27].

The high antileukemic efficacy has been counterbalanced by an elevated TRM that ranged from 24 to 80% [7–10, 12, 27]. It is unclear whether these results can be extrapolated to more recent and up-to-date transplant programs. The vast majority of the reported experience in allogeneic HSCT is from transplants performed over a decade ago, since the allogeneic HSCT activity has been decreasing overtime favoring autologous HSCT [10]. Most transplants used myeloablative conditionings with either TBI or oral busulfan-based regimens. The type of salvage treatment before HSCT is likely to have a major impact on toxicity. In fact, higher TRM was observed after more intensive salvage chemotherapy [7]. The use of reduced-intensity and reduced-toxicity conditioning regimens, improved supportive care, and optimized graft-versus-host disease prophylaxis have certainly contributed to reduce TRM in recent years. Another step forward in the HSCT field has been the universal donor availability with the use of alternative donors and stem cell sources. However, there is little data on unrelated-donor transplants and no reports on umbilical cord blood transplants or haploidentical HSCT in patients with APL.

Conclusions

The high cure rate currently obtained in patients with APL using modern treatments with ATRA plus chemotherapy or ATRA plus ATO indicates that there is no role for HSCT in front-line therapy. The HSCT in first complete remission has been relegated only to the very small fraction of patients with persistent MRD at the end of consolidation or relapsed patients. Relapsed patients with APL who achieve second CR after salvage therapy with ATRA and chemotherapy or ATRA plus ATO must be additionally treated with further post-remission therapy, including HSCT when possible. The selection of the most appropriate post-remission treatment option for patients in second CR, as well as the modality of HSCT when indicated, depends on a variety of prognostic and logistic variables, mainly pretransplant molecular status, duration of first remission, age, and donor availability. There are no strict guidelines as regards the choice of autologous or allogeneic HSCT. Autologous HSCT is associated with a lower TRM and is a reasonable option in patients without detectable MRD and prolonged duration of first CR (more than 1 year). In contrast, allogeneic HSCT involves a greater risk of nonrelapse mortality, but offers a potentially greater anti-leukemic activity due to the GVL effect. Allogeneic HSCT could be, therefore, recommended in patients failing to achieve a second molecular remission and for those with a short first CR duration.

References

1. Esteve J, Escoda L, Martin G, et al. Outcome of patients with acute promyelocytic leukemia failing to front-line treatment with all-trans retinoic acid and anthracycline-based chemotherapy (PETHEMA protocols LPA96 and LPA99): benefit of an early intervention. Leukemia. 2007;21(3):446–52.
2. Coco Lo F, Avvisati G, Vignetti M, et al. Retinoic acid and arsenic trioxide for acute promyelocytic leukemia. N Engl J Med. 2013;369(2):111–21.
3. Sanz MA, Montesinos P, Rayon C, et al. Risk-adapted treatment of acute promyelocytic leukemia based on all-trans retinoic acid and anthracycline with addition of cytarabine in consolidation therapy for high-risk patients: further improvements in treatment outcome. Blood. 2010;115(25):5137–46.
4. Ades L, Guerci A, Raffoux E, et al. Very long-term outcome of acute promyelocytic leukemia after treatment with all-trans retinoic acid and chemotherapy: the European APL Group experience. Blood. 2010;115(9):1690–6.
5. Sanz MA, Grimwade D, Tallman MS, et al. Management of acute promyelocytic leukemia: recommendations from an expert panel on behalf of the European LeukemiaNet. Blood. 2009;113(9):1875–91.
6. Lengfelder E, Lengfelder E, Lo-Coco F, et al. Arsenic trioxide-based therapy of relapsed acute promyelocytic leukemia: registry results from the European LeukemiaNet. Leukemia. 2015;29(5):1084–91.
7. de Botton S, Fawaz A, Chevret S, et al. Autologous and allogeneic stem-cell transplantation as salvage treatment of acute promyelocytic leukemia initially treated with all-trans-retinoic acid: a retrospective analysis of the European acute promyelocytic leukemia group. J Clin Oncol. 2005;23(1):120–6.
8. Thomas X, Dombret H, Cordonnier C, et al. Treatment of relapsing acute promyelocytic leukemia by all-trans retinoic acid therapy followed by timed sequential chemotherapy and stem cell transplantation. APL Study Group. Acute promyelocytic leukemia. Leukemia. 2000;14(6):1006–13.
9. Mandelli F, Labopin M, Granena A, et al. European survey of bone marrow transplantation in acute promyelocytic leukemia (M3). Working Party on Acute Leukemia of the European Cooperative Group for Bone Marrow Transplantation (EMBT). Bone Marrow Transplant. 1994;14(2):293–8.
10. Sanz MA, Labopin M, Gorin NC, et al. Hematopoietic stem cell transplantation for adults with acute promyelocytic leukemia in the ATRA era: a survey of the European Cooperative Group for Blood and Marrow Transplantation. Bone Marrow Transplant. 2007;39(8):461–9.
11. Ganzel C, Mathews V, Alimoghaddam K, et al. Autologous transplant remains the preferred therapy for relapsed APL in CR2. Bone Marrow Transplant. 2016;51(9):1180–3.
12. Holter Chakrabarty JL, Rubinger M, Le Rademacher J, et al. Autologous is superior to allogeneic hematopoietic cell transplantation for acute promyelocytic leukemia in second complete remission. Biol Blood Marrow Transplant. 2014;20(7):1021–5.
13. Sanz MA, Lo-Coco F, Martin G, et al. Definition of relapse risk and role of nonanthracycline drugs for consolidation in patients with acute promyelocytic leukemia: a joint study of the PETHEMA and GIMEMA cooperative groups. Blood. 2000;96(4):1247–53.
14. Breccia M, Diverio D, Noguera NI, et al. Clinico-biological features and outcome of acute promyelocytic leukemia patients with persistent polymerase chain reaction-detectable disease after the AIDA front-line induction and consolidation therapy. Haematologica. 2004;89(1):29–33.
15. Sanz MA, Martín G, Gonzalez M, et al. Risk-adapted treatment of acute promyelocytic leukemia with all-trans-retinoic acid and anthracycline monochemotherapy: a multicenter study by the PETHEMA group. Blood. 2004;103(4):1237–43.
16. Platzbecker U, Avvisati G, Cicconi L, et al. Improved outcomes with retinoic acid and arsenic trioxide compared with retinoic acid and chemotherapy in

non-high-risk acute promyelocytic leukemia: final results of the Randomized Italian-German APL0406 Trial. J Clin Oncol. 2017;35(6):605–12.
17. Estey EH. Treatment options for relapsed acute promyelocytic leukaemia. Best Pract Res Clin Haematol. 2003;16(3):521–34.
18. Castagnola C, Lunghi M, Corso A, et al. Management of acute promyelocytic leukemia relapse in the ATRA era. Haematologica. 1998;83(8):714–7.
19. Thirugnanam R, George B, Chendamarai E, et al. Comparison of clinical outcomes of patients with relapsed acute promyelocytic leukemia induced with arsenic trioxide and consolidated with either an autologous stem cell transplant or an arsenic trioxide-based regimen. Biol Blood Marrow Transplant. 2009;15(11):1479–84.
20. Yanada M, Tsuzuki M, Fujita H, et al. Phase 2 study of arsenic trioxide followed by autologous hematopoietic cell transplantation for relapsed acute promyelocytic leukemia. Blood. 2013;121(16): 3095–102.
21. Sanz MA, La Rubia de J, Bonanad S, et al. Prolonged molecular remission after PML/RAR alpha-positive autologous peripheral blood stem cell transplantation in acute promyelocytic leukemia: is relevant pretransplant minimal residual disease in the graft? Leukemia. 1998;12(6):992–5.
22. Ruiz-Arguelles GJ, Garces-Eisele J, Ruiz-Arguelles A. Continued complete remission after a PML/RAR-alpha+ autograft in acute promyelocytic leukaemia. Eur J Haematol. 1996;56(3):186–7.
23. Montesinos P, Diaz-Mediavilla J, Deben G, et al. Central nervous system involvement at first relapse in patients with acute promyelocytic leukemia treated with all-trans retinoic acid and anthracycline monochemotherapy without intrathecal prophylaxis. Haematologica. 2009;94(9):1242–9.
24. de Botton S, Sanz MA, Chevret S, et al. Extramedullary relapse in acute promyelocytic leukemia treated with all-trans retinoic acid and chemotherapy. Leukemia. 2006;20(1):35–41.
25. Tallman MS, Tallman MS. Treatment of relapsed or refractory acute promyelocytic leukemia. Best Pract Res Clin Haematol. 2007;20(1):57–65.
26. Yanada M, Yanada M, Yano S, et al. Autologous hematopoietic cell transplantation for acute promyelocytic leukemia in second complete remission: outcomes before and after the introduction of arsenic trioxide. Leuk Lymphoma. 2017;58(5):1061–7.
27. Lo-Coco F, Romano A, Mengarelli A, et al. Allogeneic stem cell transplantation for advanced acute promyelocytic leukemia: results in patients treated in second molecular remission or with molecularly persistent disease. Leukemia. 2003;17(10):1930–3.

14 Acute Promyelocytic Leukemia in Children

Matthew A. Kutny and Anna Maria Testi

Introduction

Acute promyelocytic leukemia (APL) is rare in children, but it is now one of the most curable forms of acute leukemia. Both children and adults with APL have shared in the great success of advances in treatment of this disease. While new cancer therapies in children frequently wait for safety demonstration in adult populations, current standard treatments for children with APL now include all-trans retinoic acid (ATRA) and arsenic trioxide (ATO). These treatments have demonstrated tolerability and excellent activity in children. Further advances in treatment of children with APL will come from regimens proven in adult patients, and currently under investigation in pediatric patients, that remove or reduce traditional chemotherapy through repeated cycles of ATRA and ATO.

M.A. Kutny, M.D. (✉)
Division of Hematology/Oncology, Department of Pediatrics, University of Alabama at Birmingham, Lowder 512, 1600 7th Avenue South, Birmingham, AL 35233-1711, USA
e-mail: mkutny@peds.uab.edu

A.M. Testi, M.D.
Department of Cellular Biotechnologies and Hematology, Sapienza, University of Rome, Roma RM, Italy

Epidemiology

While leukemia is the most common type of cancer in children, acute myeloid leukemia (AML) accounts for only 15% of childhood leukemia and acute promyelocytic leukemia accounts for approximately 10–15% of AML. Thus due to its rarity, larger cooperative group or multinational trials are required to study this disease. There does appear to be some variance in prevalence among different geographic areas. Some parts of Central and South America as well as Mediterranean countries have reported that APL comprises over 20% of AML cases in those regions [1–3]. It is unclear whether this is due to genetic factors among different ethnic groups or if environmental exposures play a role. In children, APL most often occur de novo without an identified predisposing cause. APL can more rarely occur as a secondary cancer following prior chemotherapy, and such cases have been reported in pediatric patients [4, 5].

Clinical Characteristics

Diagnosis

Children presenting with signs and symptoms concerning for leukemia are often first identified as potential cases of APL by the unique appear-

O. Abla et al. (eds.), *Acute Promyelocytic Leukemia*, https://doi.org/10.1007/978-3-319-64257-4_14

ance of the blasts either in peripheral blood or bone marrow. APL most often has a characteristic morphology with hypergranular promyelocytes which may contain Auer rods. This comprises the M3 morphologic category in the French-American-British (FAB) classification of AML. It is important to note that non-APL AML cases may also have Auer rods, and thus this should not be used as the sole diagnostic criteria. There is also a microgranular variant of APL designated M3v which may be more difficult for clinicians to initially distinguish from other AML cases due to the lack of the more classic APL granules and Auer rods. In children with APL, the M3v microgranular variant accounts for a minority of cases (up to 30%) but occurs at higher rates than among adults with APL [6, 7]. Flow cytometry markers are useful in diagnosis, but confirmation of an APL diagnosis is made by cytogenetic analysis including fluorescence in situ hybridization (FISH) and chromosome analysis. The 2008 WHO classification of AML includes APL due to t(15;17) as a distinct diagnosis under the category of AML with recurrent genetic changes. Recent pediatric cooperative group studies have further required confirmation of *PML-RARA* transcript by reverse transcriptase PCR (RT-PCR). This carries the advantage of high specificity for *PML-RARA* including cryptic lesions (those not demonstrable by standard chromosome analysis) and establishes the breakpoint-specific transcript for monitoring for persistent MRD or for surveillance to detect relapse. While t(15;17) accounts for most cases of APL, there are rare variant fusion gene partners [8]. Due to their rarity, the prevalence of these variants has not been adequately described in a pediatric population.

CNS Disease

Due to coagulopathy risk, lumbar puncture at diagnosis is not standard in the initial evaluation of APL. Thus, the true incidence of CNS disease in pediatric APL is difficult to estimate. However, there have been evaluations of the incidence of CNS relapse in pediatric APL. A review of trials including children with standard-risk APL found isolated CNS relapse in less than 1% of patients [9]. This is similar to data from adult patients with APL such as the LPA96 and LPA99 trials conducted by the Spanish PETHEMA group which demonstrated a 1.1% 3-year incidence of CNS relapse [10].

Risk Grouping

WBC at initial diagnosis is the most validated risk marker in both adult and pediatric APL. Pediatric trials have used Sanz modified criteria to identify high-risk patients as those with WBC $\geq$ 10,000/μL. Patients with WBC < 10,000/μL are considered standard risk (including Sanz low and intermediate risk). The AIDA 0493 trial demonstrated that pediatric patients with high-risk disease had a significantly worse EFS compared to those with standard-risk disease [11]. In the Children's Oncology Group (COG) Study AAML0631 and the European I-BFM study ICC-APL 01, patients with high-risk disease were treated with an extra cycle of consolidation compared to those with standard-risk disease. Early induction deaths due to differentiation syndrome and coagulopathy occur more frequently in patients with high-risk disease. The risk of relapse has also been higher in patients with high-risk disease, although recent data from the COG AAML0631 study suggests that with arsenic trioxide (ATO) consolidation, the risk of relapse is not significantly different between standard- and high-risk APL [personal communication, John Gregory, MD].

There are some studies suggesting that worse outcomes may be seen in other subsets of patients including those with M3v, certain immunophenotypes, or FLT3 mutant [6, 12]. These factors, however, are associated with higher WBC, and thus it has been unclear whether any of these represent independent risk criteria. Further, there is limited data on these risk factors specific to pediatric patients. A COG study did demonstrate an increased risk of early death in pediatric patients with APL who had mutations of the FLT3 gene [13].

The effect of age on APL outcomes within the pediatric population has been studied and there have been disparate results. Data from two consecutive trials conducted by the European APL group showed similar outcomes for children <13 years old compared to adolescents. Among children, however, those less than 5 years old had a higher risk of relapse compared to older children. For patients <5 years old (N = 12), the relapse rate was 52%, and for patients 5–12 years old (N = 16), the relapse rate was 17.6% [7]. In contrast, the COG analyzed pediatric patients treated on the North American Intergroup Trial CALGB 9710 and found no difference in outcomes between young children <5 years old (N = 16), older children 5–12 years old (N = 25), and adolescents 13–18 years old (N = 45) [14].

Disease Complications

Differentiation Syndrome

Differentiation syndrome is a constellation of symptoms including weight gain, pulmonary edema with respiratory distress, pleural and pericardial effusions, hypotension, and renal failure. This was initially described as "retinoic acid syndrome" or "ATRA syndrome" as it most often occurs following initiation of treatment with ATRA during induction therapy prior to achievement of remission [15]. Differentiation syndrome can occur without ATRA treatment due to effects of the APL blasts alone. Standard treatment includes use of steroids (most commonly dexamethasone) and holding doses of ATRA. Differentiation syndrome is associated with higher WBC including both high WBC at diagnosis and also high WBC (hyperleukocytosis) that develops due to the differentiating effect of ATRA and/or ATO treatment.

Children treated on the first North American Intergroup study (INT0129) were randomized to induction with ATRA 45 mg/m^2/day divided BID (N = 27) or chemotherapy with daunorubicin and cytarabine (N = 26). Per protocol, differentiation syndrome was managed with dexamethasone and temporary cessation of ATRA. Differentiation syndrome occurred in 19% of children receiving ATRA, and one patient died of this toxicity during induction [16]. In the Italian GIMEMA-AIEOP AIDA 0493 trial, children with APL were treated in induction with ATRA 25 mg/m^2/day divided BID and idarubicin. Differentiation syndrome was managed similar to INT0129 with dexamethasone and holding of ATRA. Among 107 patients, only three had differentiation syndrome, and no deaths were attributed to this toxicity [11]. It is difficult to know whether the lower rate of differentiation syndrome seen on AIDA0493 compared to INT0129 might be due to the lower ATRA dose, the use of idarubicin or other confounders including patient characteristics such as WBC.

Rates of differentiation syndrome in children with APL have been reported from several other multi-institutional studies (Table 14.1). Pediatric patients with APL from France,

Table 14.1 Differentiation syndrome (DS) in pediatric APL clinical trials

	INT0129	AIDA0493	APL93 + 2000	C9710	AAML0631
ATRA daily dose	45 mg/m^2	25 mg/m^2	45 mg/m^2	45 mg/m^2	25 mg/m^2
Other chemo	None	Idarubicin	+/−daunorubicin +/−cytarabine	Daunorubicin Cytarabine	Idarubicin
Treatment of DS	Dexamethasone	Dexamethasone	Dexamethasone	Dexamethasone	Dexamethasone
Prophylaxis against DS	None	None	None	None	None
Total # patients	27	107	26 children 58 adolescents	83	101
Rate of DS %	19%	2.8%	16% (children) 26.7% (adolescents)	37%	20%
Death due to DS # (%)	1 (3.7%)	0	0	0	2 (2%)

Belgium, Switzerland, Spain, and Germany treated on APL93 and APL 2000 all received ATRA at 45 mg/m^2/day divided BID during induction and randomizations (assigned by initial WBC) included addition of daunorubicin with or without cytarabine. Differentiation syndrome was managed with dexamethasone. Differentiation syndrome occurred in 16% of 26 children and in 26.7% of 58 adolescents treated on these trials, and there were no deaths due to differentiation syndrome [7]. The second North American Intergroup study C9710 induction therapy included ATRA 45 mg/m^2/day divided BID along with cytarabine and daunorubicin. Among 83 patients <18 years old treated on this study, the rate of differentiation syndrome was 37%, but there were no deaths due to differentiation syndrome. On the COG AAML0631 trial, patients received ATRA 25 mg/m^2/day divided BID along with idarubicin. Differentiation syndrome was managed with dexamethasone. Among 101 patients, differentiation syndrome occurred in 20% of patients and resulted in two deaths (personal communication, John Gregory, MD).

All the studies above utilized dexamethasone to treat differentiation syndrome once symptoms arose. More recently, some studies including predominantly adult APL patients have utilized prophylactic treatment with steroids to prevent differentiation syndrome. There are multiple variations in these strategies including choice of steroid (oral prednisone, IV methylprednisolone, or dexamethasone), the duration of prophylactic treatment, and the target population (selected based on WBC versus all patients). Since death due to differentiation syndrome occurs in <5% of patients, it has been impossible to conclude from these studies whether steroid prophylaxis impacts death rate due to differentiation syndrome [17].

Coagulopathy

In comparison to other types of leukemia, APL is associated with a unique propensity toward coagulopathy. This complication is associated with fatal bleeding and thrombotic events that occur early in the course, either at presentation or during induction therapy. The risk of coagulopathy is directly correlated with WBC, and patients with high-risk APL (WBC $\geq$ 10,000 at diagnosis) more commonly experience this deadly complication. An analysis of pediatric patients treated on the North American intergroup trial C9710 demonstrated that presence of a FLT3 mutation was associated with increased risk of early death due to coagulopathy. Patients with elevated WBC and FLT3 mutation had a 47% induction death rate compared to no deaths among patients with elevated WBC and no FLT3 mutation [13]. Other clinical characteristics including laboratory results of prothrombin time, platelets, and D-dimer have been used in computation of bleeding risk based upon the International Society on Thrombosis and Haemostasis (ISTH) DIC scoring system, and a report on adult APL patients suggested that a score $\geq$ 6 was correlated with risk of fatal coagulopathy events [18]. An analysis of pediatric APL patients treated on the COG AAML0631 also demonstrated that a ISTH DIC score $\geq$ 6 was significantly correlated with risk of both fatal and significant but nonfatal bleeding and thrombotic events [19].

Supportive care recommendations on pediatric APL trials have included correction of abnormal prothrombin time (PT), abnormal partial thromboplastin time (PTT), thrombocytopenia, and hypofibrinogenemia with aggressive blood product support. Specific thresholds for platelet support have varied but most often include maintenance of platelets above 50,000 during the initial risk period of coagulopathy (1–2 weeks). The role of fibrinolytic therapy has not been well studied in pediatric patients, but data in adult patients does not support their routine use [20–23]. Recent studies of recombinant thrombomodulin (rTM) suggest this is a very promising new therapy for coagulopathy arising from various etiologies including APL [24, 25]. Use of rTM remains investigational, and it is currently only approved for use in Japan. Further there has only been a few case reports of pediatric patients receiving rTM for coagulopathy due to leukemia [26, 27].

Treatment

ATRA Plus Chemotherapy Regimens

Prior to the discovery of ATRA as an effective APL treatment, pediatric APL was treated similarly to other types of AML with chemotherapy including combination of cytarabine and anthracyclines. Combination therapy with ATRA and chemotherapy still required high cumulative doses of anthracyclines to achieve high cure rates for this subtype of AML. The Italian AIDA0493 regimen demonstrated long-term survival near 90%, but therapy included 80 mg/m^2 of idarubicin and 50 mg/m^2 of mitoxantrone which is approximately 600 mg/m^2 daunorubicin equivalents (assuming a 5:1 conversion ratio for idarubicin:daunorubicin and a 4:1 conversion ratio for mitoxantrone:daunorubicin as used in the Children's Oncology Group, Long-Term Follow-up Guidelines, Version 4.0, Oct 2013, www.survivorshipguidleins.org) [11]. On the LPA96/99 trials, the PETHEMA group used dose intensification of anthracycline plus ATRA (without any cytarabine) to achieve an overall survival of 87%, but this therapy used a very high cumulative anthracycline dose of 600–735 mg/m^2 [28]. Treatment with anthracyclines places patients at significant risk for cardiac toxicity [29, 30]. The risk increases with higher cumulative doses (especially over 300 mg/m^2 daunorubicin equivalents), and the risk is higher when children are exposed at a young age [31]. There were 26 children and 58 adolescents on the European APL93 and APL2000 trials in which the treatments included a total of 495 mg/m^2 of daunorubicin. Three cases of severe cardiac toxicity occurred in these young patients including one patient with fatal heart failure while on treatment, one patient with heart failure occurring 6 years after therapy, and one patient with heart failure requiring heart transplant occurring after treatment for relapsed APL [7]. In the North American Intergroup C9710 trial, 56 children were treated with 400 mg/m^2 of daunorubicin, and there were two deaths due to cardiac toxicity (personal communication, James Feusner, MD) [32].

High-dose cytarabine consolidation has been reported to reduce relapse risk in APL when studied in cohorts including predominantly adult patients [33, 34]. A direct comparison of treatment with and without high cytarabine has not been studied in a larger group of pediatric APL patients. The AIDA0493 trial and AML-BFM 93/98/2004 series both included high-dose cytarabine treatment of pediatric patients and reported 82–89% overall survival at 10 years. The CI relapse at 5 years was 14% on the AML-BFM series and 19% on the ADIA0493 trial. In contrast, the C9710 trial did not include high-dose cytarabine and reported a relapse risk of 36% at 5 years [32].

Following discovery of ATRA as an effective medication to induce APL remission, the efficacy of this targeted therapy was evaluated in children treated on the first North American Intergroup trial (INT0129). Patients randomized to receive ATRA during induction, maintenance, or both had a superior 5-year disease-free survival of 48% compared to 0% for patients not receiving ATRA [16]. In addition to reducing relapse risk, treatment with ATRA during induction has resulted in reduction of early deaths in children with APL [35]. The rates of induction death on pediatric APL trials including ATRA in induction range from 3–8% (Table 14.2) [7, 11, 28, 32, 36, 37]. An analysis of multiple pediatric hospitals in the United States including 163 pediatric patients presenting with APL and treated with ATRA found a 7.4% early death rate. Resource utilization during the first week of treatment included vasopressors, steroids, and diuretics used in approximately 11%, 40%, and 50% of patients, respectively. Pediatric APL patients required significantly more blood product support (platelets, fresh frozen plasma, and cryoprecipitate) compared to non-APL AML patients treated during the same period [38].

A particular side effect of ATRA called pseudotumor cerebri (PTC) involves increased intracranial pressure causing headache and blurry vision. Children and adolescents treated with ATRA have higher rates of PTC compared to adults. Decreased doses of ATRA, however, result in lower rates of PTC. Thus, a number of

Table 14.2 Outcomes for pediatric APL on selected cooperative group trials with ATRA containing regimens

	AIDA0493	AML-BFM 93/98/04	C9710	PETHEMA LPA96/99	European APL 93/2000	ICC APL 01 [37]	AAML0631
Total # patients	107	81	83	66	Child: 26 Adolescent: 58	227	103
3–5-year OS	89% (5 year)	89% (5 year)	82% (5 year)	87% (5 year)	Child: 80% (5 year) Adolescent: 94% (5 year)	95% (3 year)	94% (3 year)
3–5-year EFS	76% (5 year)	73% (5 year)	54% (5 year)	82% (5 year)	NR	83% (3 year)	91% (3 year)
Induction death # (%)	4 (3.7%)	6 (7.4%)	7 (8.4%)	5 (7.5%)	Child: 1 (4%) Adolescent: 0 (0%)	7 (3.1%)	4 (4%)
Relapse # (CIR%)	21 (19%)	9 (11%)	23 (36%)	7 (17%)	Child: (28%) Adolescent: (20%)	14 (15%)	3 (4%)
Key treatment details[a]	Anthracycline 600 mg/m^2; intermediate-dose cytarabine	Anthracycline 350 mg/m^2; high-dose cytarabine	Anthracycline 400 mg/m^2; low-dose cytarabine	Anthracycline 600–735 mg/m^2; no cytarabine	Anthracycline 495 mg/m^2; high-dose cytarabine	Anthracycline 355–405 mg/m^2; intermediate-dose cytarabine	Anthracycline 355-405 mg/m^2; intermediate-dose cytarabine; ATO consolidation

[a]Anthracycline dose conversion assuming Daunorubicin:Idarubicin = 5:1 and Daunorubicin:Mitoxantrone = 4:1

pediatric trials (including the most recent cooperative group trials of the COG and I-BFM) have now adopted the standard pediatric dose of ATRA as 25 mg/m^2/day divided BID. The COG AAML0631 trial required sites to report detailed information on PTC during each course of therapy. With an ATRA dose of 25 mg/m^2/day, the incidence of PTC was ≤6% during each cycle (personal communication, John Gregory, MD).

Arsenic Trioxide

Arsenic trioxide (ATO) was initially used as a highly effective salvage therapy for relapsed APL. The North American Intergroup C9710 trial randomized patient's ≥15 years old to therapy with or without two cycles (5 weeks each) of ATO consolidation. Adult patients receiving ATO had significantly improved outcomes [39]. Among adolescents 15–18 years old ($N = 21$), 12 patients received ATO with 92% EFS and 0% relapse, while 9 patients received standard consolidation without ATO with 56% EFS and 44% relapse risk (personal communication, Jim Feusner, MD). In the COG AAML0631 trial, children received 10 weeks of ATO (given as two courses of 5 weeks each) similar to the C9710 ATO consolidation cycles. This trial demonstrated excellent outcomes with 3-year EFS and OS >90% and a low relapse risk of 4%. The European ICC APL 01 included chemotherapy but without ATO consolidation and the 3-year EFS was lower at 83% due to increased relapses. Overall survival on AIDA 0493 (no ATO), ICC APL 01 (no ATO but reduced anthracycline), and AAML0631 (ATO consolidation and reduced anthracycline) all demonstrate that pediatric APL is a highly curable disease with even relapsed patients having a good salvage rate using ATO therapy, but high-risk APL patients do have a worse survival than standard-risk APL patients due to increased incidence of early death events (Fig. 14.1).

ATO has also been given as monotherapy for newly diagnosed APL in trials conducted in Iran and India. These studies, including both children and adults, reported 5-year OS rates of 64–74% [40, 41]. Combination therapy of ATO and ATRA has been more effective achieving excellent results for adult patients with standard-risk disease on the Italian-German APL0406 trial [42]. Based upon those results, trials for pediatric APL are currently active in the COG (AAML1331) and the I-BFM (ICC APL 02) which include an ATO/ATRA regimen with the addition of either idarubicin (COG) or gemtuzumab ozogamicin (I-BFM) during induction therapy for high-risk APL patients.

Similar to ATRA, ATO can induce differentiation of APL blasts, and thus differentiation and hyperleukocytosis may occur during ATO therapy. ATO is also known to prolong the QT interval with risk for cardiac dysrhythmia. In the COG AAML0631 trial, children received 10 weeks of ATO (given as two courses of 5 weeks each), and QT interval prolongation was monitored closely on the trial. Twenty-four patients had prolonged QT interval during their ATO cycles, but all were Grade 1 or 2, were transient, and did not require dose adjustment [43].

Maintenance Therapy

The Italian AIDA 0493 trial included four arms for maintenance randomization. Patients could receive no maintenance (observation arm), oral chemotherapy including mercaptopurine and methotrexate, ATRA alone, or a combination of both ATRA and oral chemotherapy. The first two arms (without ATRA) were closed early, but an analysis of the ATRA arms in pediatric patients showed a superior disease-free survival in the combination ATRA plus chemotherapy arm versus ATRA alone (77% vs. 42%, $P = 0.018$) [11]. An evaluation with long-term follow-up of adult patients treated on AIDA0493, however, showed no significant difference in survival between the four maintenance arms [44]. The North American Intergroup C9710 study began with a maintenance randomization to ATRA alone versus observation. Only three pediatric patients were randomized before the maintenance randomization was amended to ATRA alone versus ATRA plus oral chemotherapy with mercaptopurine and methotrexate. There was a nonsignificant trend

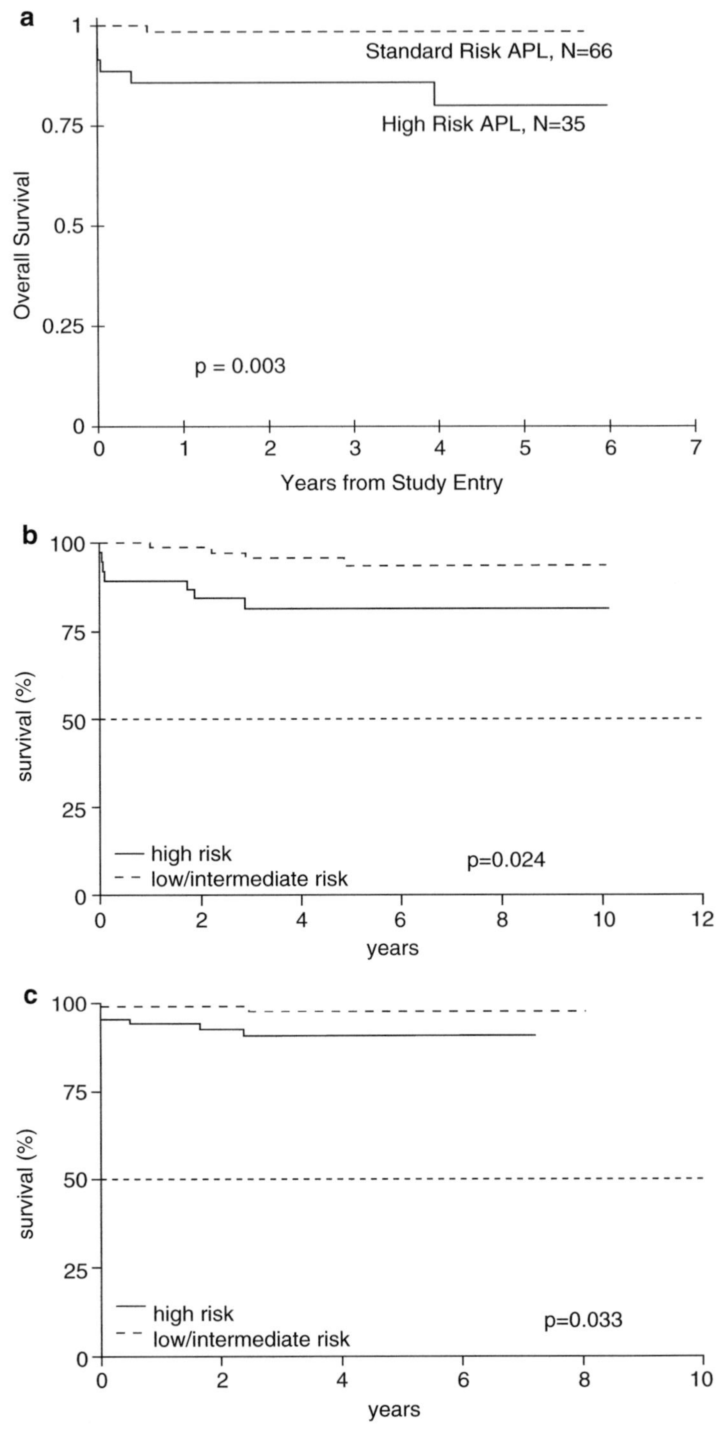

Fig. 14.1 Overall survival by Risk Group on COG AAML0631 (**a**), GIMEMA/AIEOP AIDA 0493 (**b**), and ICC APL 01 (**c**)

toward lower EFS in the ATRA only maintenance compared to ATRA plus chemotherapy maintenance (41% vs. 72%, $P = 0.12$) (personal communication, James Feusner, MD).

The benefit of maintenance therapy for patients who receive ATO consolidation is uncertain. Among adult patients enrolled on C9710, there was no difference in survival for the initial randomization to observation versus ATRA, and patients who received ATO consolidation had similar survival in both arms of the amended randomization to ATRA alone versus ATRA plus oral chemotherapy maintenance [45, 46]. Adult patients with standard-risk APL treated with ATO/ATRA on APL0406 had excellent outcomes without maintenance therapy [42]. The current COG AAML1331 and I-BFM ICC APL 02 trials include ATO/ATRA regimens without maintenance therapy and will thus determine if ATO treatment can allow maintenance-free regimens in pediatric patients with APL.

Novel Therapies

APL blasts have robust expression of CD33, and thus the anti-CD33 immunoconjugate gemtuzumab ozogamicin (GO) has been an agent of great interest in APL treatment. Following initial expedited approval by the FDA, this medication was later voluntarily withdrawn due to failure to achieve superiority in a confirmatory study. With these supply challenges, there has been limited experience with GO in pediatric APL. However, the current I-BFM ICC APL 02 is studying the efficacy of GO in conjunction with ATO/ATRA for treatment of children with high risk APL.

Disease Response

Reverse transcriptase PCR (RT-PCR) is a very sensitive assay to detect very low levels of residual *PML-RARA* transcript. Quantified RT-PCR (RQ-PCR) allows standardization to a housekeeping gene and ensures adequate RNA quality. Failure to enter molecular remission (persistent of PCR detectable *PML-RARA* transcripts) at the end of consolidation prior to maintenance therapy is correlated with high risk of relapse [47, 48]. In the COG study AAML0631, which included ATO consolidation, all patients tested PCR negative at end of consolidation (personal communication, John Gregory, MD). In the I-BFM ICC APL 01 trial (which did not include ATO consolidation) 4% of patients failed to enter molecular remission at end of consolidation, and these patients were eligible for treatment with ATO salvage therapy [37].

PCR monitoring is often employed during remission to monitor for disease recurrence. It is preferable to detect molecular relapse rather than awaiting an overt hematologic relapse in order to minimize the risk of coagulopathy or differentiation syndrome [49]. Molecular relapse as detected by PCR will invariably progress to hematologic relapse if left untreated [50, 51].

RQ-PCR testing should be performed on bone marrow samples every 3 months. With the assay's sensitivity of 1 in 10^4 cells in bone marrow and the kinetics of relapse disease progression at approximately 1.1 log fold increase in RQ-PCR transcript per month, testing every 3 months generally allows detection before frank hematologic disease [52]. However, in pediatric patients, bone marrow evaluations are frequently done with sedation. Thus, risks of these sedated procedures must be balanced with the benefit of such monitoring particularly as patients are treated with ATO consolidation, and the relapse risk is expected to be very low.

Management of APL Relapse

Incidence of Relapse and Risk Factors

In pediatric patients with APL, despite the improvement in survival rate after modern combination regimens including ATRA and anthracycline-based first-line therapy, 17–27% of children have been reported to relapse [11, 7, 16, 34, 36, 37]. Retrospective studies involving both adults and children have clearly demonstrated that high WBC count ($\geq 10 \times 10^9$/L) at diagnosis and persistence of *PML/RARA* positivity after first-line consolidation phase are associated with increased risk of disease recurrence [11, 53]. In adults, complex karyotype, expression of CD56, and *FLT3* mutation are other poor prognostic factors with ATRA and chemotherapy regimens [12, 54]. In APL, most relapses occur within 3 years from consolidation treatment, but rare very late relapses (>36 months from diagnosis) have also been described (incidence 4–6%). The majority of relapses occur in the bone marrow as hematological or molecular relapse. Hematological relapse is defined as the reappearance of >5% leukemic promyelocytes; molecular relapse is conventionally defined as two consecutive *PML/RARA* RT-PCR positive tests in marrow samples collected 2 weeks apart after previous negative results. Rarely, other sites such as CNS, the skin and the testis (extramedullary relapse) can be involved at disease recurrence [55, 56]. Interestingly, several reports in adults and children have suggested that the external auditory canal and the skin at sites of vascular access may be unique sites of extramedullary APL relapse and are mostly associated with concomitant bone marrow molecular relapse [57–59].

In APL, early identification of disease recurrence and preemptive therapy at the time of molecular relapse have clearly demonstrated benefits including better tolerated treatment, reduced hospitalization time, and decreased incidence of reinduction deaths [60–62]. Although MRD monitoring by sequential RT-PCR measurement of *PML/RARA* can predict overt relapse, some hematological relapses occur in patients, both adult and children, with previous PCR negativity. Recently, the quantitative RQ-PCR assays offer the possibility of measuring the kinetics of *PML/RARA* transcript and better monitoring for minimal residual disease (MRD) [63, 64]. This increases the opportunity to deliver early salvage treatment and consequently improve the outcome of patients who present with only MRD positive disease compared with those treated at the time of hematological relapse.

Reinduction Salvage Therapy

Current literature on the treatment of relapsed APL comes predominantly from adult studies and is mainly available for patients relapsing after ATRA and chemotherapy. During the past decades, the widely adopted strategy for the treatment of APL relapse included ATRA and cytotoxic chemotherapy as salvage reinduction therapy with autologous or allogeneic transplantation for consolidation after second or greater remission. These regimens applied in adults and only in small series of children induced high second remission rates (CR2) but had low cure rates. They were often associated with severe toxicity leading to fatal outcome or to a considerable rate of contraindications against subsequent stem cell transplantation [65, 66]. In particular, the high cumulative doses of anthracycline delivered in the front-line therapy could result in significant cardiac toxicity for which pediatric patients are at increased risk [30, 31]. Other drugs such as GO have also been successfully tested in relapsed APL. A number of preliminary reports have highlighted the sensitivity of APL to GO given alone or in combination with other agents. GO, as single agent, has demonstrated strong activity for the treatment of 16 patients with APL who had relapsed at the molecular level [67]. Quantitative RQ-PCR studies showed that responding patients experienced a dramatic decline of the *PML/RARA* transcript after the first GO dose. At high doses, GO can favor the occurrence of the hepatic sinusoidal obstructive syndrome (SOS); lower doses of GO have been employed in patients at high risk of complications, and comparable results have been reported with reduced treatment toxicity [68, 69].

Currently, the salvage strategy for relapsed APL includes the administration of ATO-based reinduction. The first experience with ATO in relapsed APL was reported by a group from China, and several subsequent studies, mainly in adults, demonstrated that approximately 80–90% of patients who relapse following initial ATRA and chemotherapy can achieve a CR2 with limited toxicity from ATO therapy [70]. Some reports suggest that remission duration is longer when ATO is combined with either ATRA or chemotherapy; a synergistic effect between ATO and ATRA accelerates the differentiation and apoptosis of abnormal promyelocytes. For this reason, the current adult guidelines support ATO ± ATRA as salvage therapy for relapsed APL. In 2008, a European registry of relapsed APL was established by the European LeukemiaNet; data of the outcome were available for 155 patients (141 adults and 14 children) treated, in first relapse, with ATO, after front-line therapy with ATRA and chemotherapy [59]. The results confirmed the efficacy of ATO in reinduction remission, with 91% CR2. The rate of molecular CR, after induction and consolidation therapy, did not differ significantly in patients with hematological or molecular relapse. However, induction deaths occurred only in patients with hematological relapse.

In pediatric APL patients, ATO-containing salvage therapy has been only sporadically described, but reports demonstrate that ATO as a single agent, or in combination with ATRA, can induce CR2 in 85% of relapse/refractory childhood APL and result in long-term molecular remission [71–73]. Based on reports in limited pediatric series and adult data, ATO has become the current preferred pediatric salvage treatment. In this age group, the formulation of oral ATO is particularly interesting; oral ATO in association with ATRA has demonstrated to be equally effective and better manageable [66]. Limited data are available on the efficacy of ATO treatment in relapsed patients who had prior ATO-containing therapy. These reports suggest that ATO-based reinduction regimens remain effective despite prior ATO therapy with a CR2 rate of approximately 80% [74–76].

Consolidation Salvage Therapy

Despite high remission rate with ATO ± ATRA in relapsed cases of APL, second or subsequent relapses are observed in a high proportion of these cases. Thus, post-remission treatment is very important to prolong remission and achieve a long-term cure. Hematopoietic stem cell transplant (HSCT) represents a widely adopted strategy as part of salvage therapy in relapsed APL. However, the optimal strategy for post-remission therapy remains controversial. Options for consolidation include repeated courses of ATO ± ATRA, conventional chemotherapy (with or without ATO), or HSCT. In retrospective studies, mostly performed during ATRA + chemotherapy era, autologous (auto)-HSCT showed a trend toward better outcomes compared with allogeneic (allo)-HSCT or consolidation chemotherapy [77, 78]. Allo-HSCT decreased the relapse risk, but this advantage was outweighed by higher treatment-related mortality compared with auto-HSCT and other treatments. However, the major limitation of these studies is their retrospective nature and missing data; in particular, the pre-transplant *PML/RARA* status was often lacking in these reports. More recently, the registry study of the European LeukemiaNet has clearly demonstrated the role of allogeneic HSCT as consolidation therapy for patients with relapse not achieving a molecular CR and suggested autologous HSCT as a suitable option for patients in molecular CR2 [59]. In this report, that included the largest cohort of APL patients in first relapse treated with ATO, the results of univariable and multivariable analyses demonstrated that first CR duration <18 months and persistent PCR positivity after consolidation are poor prognostic factors on overall survival (OS) and leukemia-free survival (LFS). Other studies have confirmed the unfavorable impact of first CR duration and failure to achieve molecular CR on OS after relapse. In the more recent studies including the administration of ATO-based reinduction, the long-term survival for those patients who received previous ATO-based regimens was inferior compared to those never treated with ATO (ATO-naïve) [74]. Prior ATO treatment has shown to be independently associated with worse relapse-free survival (RFS) [74].

Recommendations in Pediatric Age

In an attempt to develop therapy guidelines for children with relapsed APL, pediatric APL experts including members of the North American Children's Oncology Group (COG) and the International Berlin-Frankfurt-Munster Study Group (I-BFM SG), have recently published treatment recommendations that are based upon informative literature and personal experience with relapsed APL [79]. Prognostic factors such as time to relapse <18 months from diagnosis, prior ATO therapy, and failure to achieve a second molecular remission were used to predict the risk of further relapse and consequently to guide the salvage treatment. In summary, ATO-naïve children with late (>18 months from diagnosis) or very late relapse (≥36 months) can be reinduced with ATO-ATRA plus GO followed by ATO consolidation without HSCT if they demonstrate molecular remission after four salvage cycles. ATO-naïve children with early relapse or children with prior ATO exposure and early or late relapse who demonstrate molecular remission after four cycles can be consolidated with auto-HSCT. In selected children who are ATO- and GO-naïve with early relapse who rapidly reach molecular remission after four cycles, or not suitable for auto-HSCT, consolidation with ATO-based therapy could represent a reasonable alternative. Children with primary/refractory APL, those with previous ATO exposure and early relapse, those with ≥ second relapse, or those with persistence of *PML/RARA* after four cycles should be considered for consolidation with allo-HSCT. Relapsed APL patients, however, are a heterogeneous population and these schemas may require modifications based on individual patient characteristics as well as the resources that are available to the treating physician [79].

Very Late Relapse

Only sporadic reports of patients with very late APL relapses (>36 months from diagnosis) have been published [80, 81]. Late relapse seems to occur in less than 5% of APL patients. In these cases, bone marrow involvement is frequently associated with relapse in extramedullary sites as well. Most of the patients present at late relapse with the same immunophenotypic, cytogenetic, and molecular pattern as at diagnosis suggest that the relapse is due to reemergence of the initial disease clone. There are no systematic trials evaluating treatment of late relapses in adults and children. Given the long period of disease-free survival (DFS), drug resistance is unlikely in these patients. However, for patients who previously received intensive chemotherapy, the risk of cumulative toxicity must be weighed as a contraindication for the reemployment of these drugs in the salvage schemas. It has been reported that patients with late relapse can be salvaged with regimens similar to those used at initial diagnosis with CR2 achieved in a majority of patients [82]. As previously reported, in the recent years, ATO ± ATRA demonstrated high efficacy and low toxicity for the treatment of APL relapses; although very limited data are available on the use of ATO in very late relapse in children, the use of this agent should be considered. While the role of ATO in remission reinduction is now well established, the best consolidation therapy for patients with late relapses, is still controversial. The utility of transplant can be questioned for patients relapsing after very prolonged first CR since ATRA-ATO salvage alone might be curative. Though limited to a small number of patients, a prolonged molecular CR2 with ATO-based salvage therapy has been described in the literature. Eight out of nine Italian APL patients were salvaged with prolonged ATO-ATRA therapy without transplant procedures [83]; an 8-year-old boy with bone marrow relapse occurring at 7 years from initial diagnosis achieved a durable molecular CR2 with prolonged ATO as single treatment [72]. As previously reported, GO has also been demonstrated to be safe, tolerable, and particularly active in APL patients with molecular relapse. Thus, GO is an appealing therapeutic option for patients with very late relapse. A very late relapse occurring after more than 15 years of molecular remission has been recently described in a pediatric patient previously treated with ATRA + chemotherapy. In this case, molecular relapse was also associated with extramedullary involvement of the left mastoid [84]. The patient was rescued with an ATO-based protocol including GO without HSCT consolidation. Combinations of these new drugs, in repeated consolidation courses, together with *PML/RARA* quantitative monitoring may be used to avoid HSCT in patients with late relapse achieving a molecular CR2.

Extramedullary Relapse

Extramedullary relapse is an uncommon complication of APL occurring in about 3–5% of patients. Several factors that increase the risk of extramedullary relapse have been identified including WBC count at diagnosis ($\geq 10 \times 10^9$/L), expression of CD56, bcr3 isoform, and *FLT3* gene mutation. The most common site of extramedullary relapse is the CNS, and it is often accompanied by disease in the bone marrow [85]. The PETHEMA group has also identified elevated serum dehydrogenase (LDH) levels and previous CNS hemorrhage during induction as risk factors for subsequent CNS relapse [10]. The best management of such patients is still controversial. The European LeukemiaNet has recommended treating CNS relapse with intrathecal chemotherapy together with systemic therapy that should include drugs with high CNS penetrance [59]. In these patients, high-dose cytarabine has been used successfully. In patients who achieve CNS remission and molecular CR2, consolidation with auto- or allo-HSCT should be considered. It has also been shown that ATO and its metabolites are capable of crossing the blood-brain barrier and may be beneficial as a therapeutic agent for CNS disease. However, the concentration of ATO in cerebral spinal fluid (CSF) is probably not adequate to treat meningeal leukemia alone, and further studies are necessary to identify the exact role of ATO treatment in patients with CNS relapse [86]. APL extramedullary relapse can involve other sites such as the skin, the testis, or the external auditory canal. Infiltration of the ear is exceedingly infrequent in other types of leukemia, and the anatomical and biological reasons underlying this particular APL localization are unknown. Some authors suggested a role of ATRA during initial therapy as a predisposing factor. ATRA has been shown to influence the expression of adhesion molecules on leukemic cells; this could explain the pathophysiology of extramedullary involvement in APL patients treated with this agent. However, APL relapse in the ear was also observed before the advent of ATRA. Patients with extramedullary relapse frequently also have bone marrow molecular recurrence.

ATO accumulates well in epidermal tissue, and thus it could represent a therapeutic choice in cutaneous relapses. In patients with external auditory canal relapse, ATO ± ATRA demonstrated high efficacy and low toxicity [86]. These observations suggest that ATO is reasonable as single agent or in combination with ATRA, for the treatment of non-CNS extramedullary relapse. Local radiotherapy has also been used in extramedullary relapse with mixed results [87, 88]. The optimal therapeutic approach for these patients is still unknown especially for those with isolated and/or very late extramedullary relapse. Management of these patients should be individualized.

References

1. Gomez SM, Schuttenberg V, Armendariz H, Alba L, Martinez M, Fynn A, et al. Childhood acute leukemia: a single institution experience in La Plata, Argentina. Med Pediatr Oncol. 2001;36(3):383–5.
2. Malta Corea A, Pacheco Espinoza C, Cantu Rajnoldi A, Conter V, Lietti G, Masera G, et al. Childhood acute promyelocytic leukemia in Nicaragua. Ann Oncol. 1993;4(10):892–4.
3. Maule MM, Dama E, Mosso ML, Magnani C, Pastore G, Merletti F, et al. High incidence of acute promyelocytic leukemia in children in northwest Italy, 1980–2003: a report from the Childhood Cancer Registry of Piedmont. Leukemia. 2008;22(2):439–41.
4. Ogami A, Morimoto A, Hibi S, Todo S, Sugimoto T, Mori K, et al. Secondary acute promyelocytic leukemia following chemotherapy for non-Hodgkin's lymphoma in a child. J Pediatr Hematol Oncol. 2004;26(7):427–30.
5. Lopez-Andrew JA, Ferris J, Verdeguer A, Esquembre C, Senent ML, Castel V. Secondary acute promyelocytic leukemia in a child treated with epipodophyllotoxins. Am J Pediatr Hematol Oncol. 1994;16(4):384–6.
6. Guglielmi C, Martelli MP, Diverio D, Fenu S, Vegna ML, Cantu-Rajnoldi A, et al. Immunophenotype of adult and childhood acute promyelocytic leukaemia: correlation with morphology, type of PML gene breakpoint and clinical outcome. A cooperative Italian study on 196 cases. Br J Haematol. 1998;102(4):1035–41.
7. Bally C, Fadlallah J, Leverger G, Bertrand Y, Robert A, Baruchel A, et al. Outcome of acute promyelocytic leukemia (APL) in children and adolescents: an analysis in two consecutive trials of the European APL Group. J Clin Oncol. 2012;30(14):1641–6.
8. Grimwade D, Biondi A, Mozziconacci MJ, Hagemeijer A, Berger R, Neat M, et al. Characterization of acute promyelocytic leukemia cases lacking the classic t(15;17): results of the European Working Party. Groupe Francais de Cytogenetique Hematologique, Groupe de Francais d'Hematologie Cellulaire, UK Cancer Cytogenetics Group and BIOMED 1 European

Community-Concerted Action "Molecular Cytogenetic Diagnosis in Haematological Malignancies". Blood. 2000;96(4):1297–308.

9. Chow J, Feusner J. Isolated central nervous system recurrence of acute promyelocytic leukemia in children. Pediatr Blood Cancer. 2009;52(1):11–3.
10. Montesinos P, Diaz-Mediavilla J, Deben G, Prates V, Tormo M, Rubio V, et al. Central nervous system involvement at first relapse in patients with acute promyelocytic leukemia treated with all-trans retinoic acid and anthracycline monochemotherapy without intrathecal prophylaxis. Haematologica. 2009;94(9):1242–9.
11. Testi AM, Biondi A, Lo Coco F, Moleti ML, Giona F, Vignetti M, et al. GIMEMA-AIEOPAIDA protocol for the treatment of newly diagnosed acute promyelocytic leukemia (APL) in children. Blood. 2005;106(2):447–53.
12. Montesinos P, Rayon C, Vellenga E, Brunet S, Gonzalez J, Gonzalez M, et al. Clinical significance of CD56 expression in patients with acute promyelocytic leukemia treated with all-trans retinoic acid and anthracycline-based regimens. Blood. 2011;117(6):1799–805.
13. Kutny MA, Moser BK, Laumann K, Feusner JH, Gamis A, Gregory J, et al. FLT3 mutation status is a predictor of early death in pediatric acute promyelocytic leukemia: a report from the Children's Oncology Group. Pediatr Blood Cancer. 2012;59(4):662–7.
14. Kutny MA, Geyer S, Laumann KM, Gregory J, Willman CL, Stock W, et al. Effect of young age on outcomes in pediatric acute promyelocytic leukemia (APL): North American Intergroup Study CALGB 9710 (Alliance). Blood. 2014;124(21):2301.
15. Frankel SR, Eardley A, Lauwers G, Weiss M, Warrell RP Jr. The "retinoic acid syndrome" in acute promyelocytic leukemia. Ann Intern Med. 1992;117(4):292–6.
16. Gregory J, Kim H, Alonzo T, Gerbing R, Woods W, Weinstein H, et al. Treatment of children with acute promyelocytic leukemia: results of the first North American Intergroup trial INT0129. Pediatr Blood Cancer. 2009;53(6):1005–10.
17. Sanz MA, Montesinos P. How we prevent and treat differentiation syndrome in patients with acute promyelocytic leukemia. Blood. 2014;123(18):2777–82.
18. Mitrovic M, Suvajdzic N, Bogdanovic A, Kurtovic NK, Sretenovic A, Elezovic I, et al. International Society of Thrombosis and Hemostasis Scoring System for disseminated intravascular coagulation >/= 6: a new predictor of hemorrhagic early death in acute promyelocytic leukemia. Med Oncol. 2013;30(1):478.
19. Kutny MA, Rajpurkar M, Alonzo TA, Gerbing RB, Gamis AS, Feusner JH, et al. Evaluation of ISTH DIC score to predict significant bleeding and thrombosis events in pediatric acute promyelocytic leukemia; a report from the Children's Oncology Group AAML0631 Trial. Blood. 2014;124(21):3669.
20. Rodeghiero F, Avvisati G, Castaman G, Barbui T, Mandelli F. Early deaths and anti-hemorrhagic treatments in acute promyelocytic leukemia. A GIMEMA retrospective study in 268 consecutive patients. Blood. 1990;75(11):2112–7.
21. Hashimoto S, Koike T, Tatewaki W, Seki Y, Sato N, Azegami T, et al. Fatal thromboembolism in acute promyelocytic leukemia during all-trans retinoic acid therapy combined with antifibrinolytic therapy for prophylaxis of hemorrhage. Leukemia. 1994;8(7):1113–5.
22. Sanz MA, Martin G, Gonzalez M, Leon A, Rayon C, Rivas C, et al. Risk-adapted treatment of acute promyelocytic leukemia with all-trans-retinoic acid and anthracycline monochemotherapy: a multicenter study by the PETHEMA group. Blood. 2004;103(4):1237–43.
23. Brown JE, Olujohungbe A, Chang J, Ryder WD, Morganstern GR, Chopra R, et al. All-trans retinoic acid (ATRA) and tranexamic acid: a potentially fatal combination in acute promyelocytic leukaemia. Br J Haematol. 2000;110(4):1010–2.
24. Saito H, Maruyama I, Shimazaki S, Yamamoto Y, Aikawa N, Ohno R, et al. Efficacy and safety of recombinant human soluble thrombomodulin (ART-123) in disseminated intravascular coagulation: results of a phase III, randomized, double-blind clinical trial. J Thromb Haemost. 2007;5(1):31–41.
25. Kawano N, Kuriyama T, Yoshida S, Yamashita K, Ochiai H, Nakazaki S, et al. Clinical features and treatment outcomes of six patients with disseminated intravascular coagulation resulting from acute promyelocytic leukemia and treated with recombinant human soluble thrombomodulin at a single institution. Intern Med. 2013;52(1):55–62.
26. Ogawa E, Yagasaki H, Kato M, Shichino H, Chin M, Mugishima H. Successful treatment of disseminated intravascular coagulation in a child with acute myelogenous leukaemia using recombinant thrombomodulin. Br J Haematol. 2010;149(6):911–2.
27. Saito A, Okamoto Y, Seki Y, Matsunaga M, Nakagawa S, Kodama Y, et al. DIC Complicating APL Successfully Treated With Recombinant Thrombomodulin Alfa. J Pediatr Hematol Oncol. 2016;38(6):e189–90.
28. Ortega JJ, Madero L, Martin G, Verdeguer A, Garcia P, Parody R, et al. Treatment with all-trans retinoic acid and anthracycline monochemotherapy for children with acute promyelocytic leukemia: a multicenter study by the PETHEMA Group. J Clin Oncol. 2005;23(30):7632–40.
29. Aldouri MA, Lopes ME, Yacoub M, Mitchell AG, Fox K, Evans TR, et al. Cardiac transplantation for doxorubicin-induced cardiomyopathy in acute myeloid leukaemia. Br J Haematol. 1990;74(4):541.
30. Thomas X, Le QH, Fiere D. Anthracycline-related toxicity requiring cardiac transplantation in long-term disease-free survivors with acute promyelocytic leukemia. Ann Hematol. 2002;81(9):504–7.

31. Shankar SM, Marina N, Hudson MM, Hodgson DC, Adams MJ, Landier W, et al. Monitoring for cardiovascular disease in survivors of childhood cancer: report from the Cardiovascular Disease Task Force of the Children's Oncology Group. Pediatrics. 2008;121(2):e387–96.
32. Feusner JG, Gregory J, Moser B, Hars V, Willman C, Powell B, Larson R. Dose-intensified daunorubicin induction and consolidation plus combined modality maintenance therapy for children with newly diagnosed acute promyelocytic leukemia (APL): North American Intergroup Study C9710. J Clin Oncol. 2010;28(15s):abstr 9510.
33. Ades L, Chevret S, Raffoux E, de Botton S, Guerci A, Pigneux A, et al. Is cytarabine useful in the treatment of acute promyelocytic leukemia? Results of a randomized trial from the European Acute Promyelocytic Leukemia Group. J Clin Oncol. 2006;24(36):5703–10.
34. Sanz MA, Montesinos P, Rayon C, Holowiecka A, de la Serna J, Milone G, et al. Risk-adapted treatment of acute promyelocytic leukemia based on all-trans retinoic acid and anthracycline with addition of cytarabine in consolidation therapy for high-risk patients: further improvements in treatment outcome. Blood. 2010;115(25):5137–46.
35. Mann G, Reinhardt D, Ritter J, Hermann J, Schmitt K, Gadner H, et al. Treatment with all-trans retinoic acid in acute promyelocytic leukemia reduces early deaths in children. Ann Hematol. 2001;80(7):417–22.
36. Creutzig U, Zimmermann M, Dworzak M, Urban C, Henze G, Kremens B, et al. Favourable outcome of patients with childhood acute promyelocytic leukaemia after treatment with reduced cumulative anthracycline doses. Br J Haematol. 2010;149(3):399–409.
37. Testi AM, Pession A, Grimwade D, Diverio D, Ragu C, Elitzur S, et al. Risk-group stratified and minimal residual disease (MRD)-guided treatment with extended ATRA and reduced-anthracycline chemotherapy in childhood acute promyelocytic leukemia (APL): results from ICC APL Study 01. Blood. 2015;126(23):563.
38. Fisher BT, Singh S, Huang YS, Li Y, Gregory J, Walker D, et al. Induction mortality, ATRA administration, and resource utilization in a nationally representative cohort of children with acute promyelocytic leukemia in the United States from 1999 to 2009. Pediatr Blood Cancer. 2014;61(1):68–73.
39. Powell BL, Moser B, Stock W, Gallagher RE, Willman CL, Stone RM, et al. Arsenic trioxide improves event-free and overall survival for adults with acute promyelocytic leukemia: North American Leukemia Intergroup Study C9710. Blood. 2010;116(19):3751–7.
40. Mathews V, George B, Chendamarai E, Lakshmi KM, Desire S, Balasubramanian P, et al. Single-agent arsenic trioxide in the treatment of newly diagnosed acute promyelocytic leukemia: long-term follow-up data. J Clin Oncol. 2010;28(24):3866–71.
41. Ghavamzadeh A, Alimoghaddam K, Rostami S, Ghaffari SH, Jahani M, Iravani M, et al. Phase II study of single-agent arsenic trioxide for the front-line therapy of acute promyelocytic leukemia. J Clin Oncol. 2011;29(20):2753–7.
42. Lo-Coco F, Avvisati G, Vignetti M, Thiede C, Orlando SM, Iacobelli S, et al. Retinoic acid and arsenic trioxide for acute promyelocytic leukemia. N Engl J Med. 2013;369(2):111–21.
43. Kutny MA, Alonzo TA, Gerbing RB, Wang Y-C, Fu C, Meshinchi S, et al. Arsenic trioxide is a well tolerated consolidation regimen in children with newly diagnosed acute promyelocytic leukemia; toxicity results of the Children's Oncology Group AAML0631 Trial. Blood. 2014;124(21):985.
44. Avvisati G, Lo-Coco F, Paoloni FP, Petti MC, Diverio D, Vignetti M, et al. AIDA 0493 protocol for newly diagnosed acute promyelocytic leukemia: very long-term results and role of maintenance. Blood. 2011;117(18):4716–25.
45. Powell BL, Moser BK, Stock W, Gallagher RE, Willman CL, Stone RM, et al. Adding mercaptopurine and methotrexate to alternate week ATRA maintenance therapy does not improve the outcome for adults with acute promyelocytic leukemia (APL) in first remission: results from North American Leukemia Intergroup Trial C9710. ASH Annual Meeting Abstracts. Blood. 2011;118(21):258.
46. Coutre SE, Othus M, Powell B, Willman CL, Stock W, Paietta E, et al. Arsenic trioxide during consolidation for patients with previously untreated low/intermediate risk acute promyelocytic leukaemia may eliminate the need for maintenance therapy. Br J Haematol. 2014;165(4):497–503.
47. Grimwade D, Lo Coco F. Acute promyelocytic leukemia: a model for the role of molecular diagnosis and residual disease monitoring in directing treatment approach in acute myeloid leukemia. Leukemia. 2002;16(10):1959–73.
48. Lo Coco F, Diverio D, Falini B, Biondi A, Nervi C, Pelicci PG. Genetic diagnosis and molecular monitoring in the management of acute promyelocytic leukemia. Blood. 1999;94(1):12–22.
49. Esteve J, Escoda L, Martin G, Rubio V, Diaz-Mediavilla J, Gonzalez M, et al. Outcome of patients with acute promyelocytic leukemia failing to front-line treatment with all-trans retinoic acid and anthracycline-based chemotherapy (PETHEMA protocols LPA96 and LPA99): benefit of an early intervention. Leukemia. 2007;21(3):446–52.
50. Breccia M, Diverio D, Noguera NI, Visani G, Santoro A, Locatelli F, et al. Clinico-biological features and outcome of acute promyelocytic leukemia patients with persistent polymerase chain reaction-detectable disease after the AIDA front-line induction and consolidation therapy. Haematologica. 2004;89(1):29–33.
51. Diverio D, Rossi V, Avvisati G, De Santis S, Pistilli A, Pane F, et al. Early detection of relapse by prospective reverse transcriptase-polymerase chain

reaction analysis of the PML/RARalpha fusion gene in patients with acute promyelocytic leukemia enrolled in the GIMEMA-AIEOP multicenter "AIDA" trial. GIMEMA-AIEOP Multicenter "AIDA" Trial. Blood. 1998;92(3):784–9.
52. Grimwade D, Jovanovic JV, Hills RK, Nugent EA, Patel Y, Flora R, et al. Prospective minimal residual disease monitoring to predict relapse of acute promyelocytic leukemia and to direct pre-emptive arsenic trioxide therapy. J Clin Oncol. 2009;27(22):3650–8.
53. Tallman M, Douer D, Gore S, Powell BL, Ravandi F, Rowe J, et al. Treatment of patients with acute promyelocytic leukemia: a consensus statement on risk-adapted approaches to therapy. Clin Lymphoma Myeloma Leuk. 2010;10(Suppl 3):S122–6.
54. Cicconi L, Divona M, Ciardi C, Ottone T, Ferrantini A, Lavorgna S, et al. PML-RARα kinetics and impact of FLT3-ITD mutations in newly diagnosed acute promyelocytic leukaemia treated with ATRA and ATO or ATRA and chemotherapy. Leukemia. 2016;30(10):1987–92.
55. Kaspers G, Gibson B, Grimwade D, pession A, Smith O, Testi AM. Central nervous system involvement in relapsed acute promyelocytic leukemia. Pediatr Blood Cancer. 2009;53(2):235–6.
56. Vega-Ruiz A, Faderl S, Estrov Z, Pierce S, Cortes J, Kantarjian H, Ravandi F. Incidence of extramedullary disease in patients with acute promyelocytic leukemia: a single-institution experience. Int J Hematol. 2009;89(4):489–96.
57. Albano F, Specchia G. Extramedullary disease in acute promyelocytic leukemia: two-in-one disease. Mediterr J Hematol Infect Dis. 2011;3(1).
58. Igarashi K, Hori T, Yamamoto M, Inazawa N, Noguchi H, Suzuki N. Extramedullary relapse in RARA rearrangement-negative acute promyelocytic leukemiasuccessfully treated in combination with chemotherapy, local radiotherapy, and cord blood transplantation. J Pediatr Hematol Oncol. 2015;37(4).
59. Lengfelder E, Lo-Coco F, Ades L, Montesinos P, Grimwade D, Kishore B, et al. Arsenic trioxide-based therapy of relapsed acute promyelocytic leukemia: registry results from the European LeukemiaNet. Leukemia. 2015;29(5):1084–91.
60. Lo Coco F, Diverio D, Avvisati G, Petti MC, Meloni G, Pogliani EM, et al. Therapy of molecular relapse in acute promyelocytic leukemia. Blood. 1999;94(7):2225–9.
61. Mandelli F, Avvisati G, Lo Coco F. Advances in the understanding and management of acute promyelocytic leukemia. Rev Clin Exp Hematol. 2002;6(1):60–71.
62. Sanz MA, Grimwade D, Tallman MS, Lowenberg B, Fenaux P, Estey EH, et al. Management of acute promyelocytic leukemia: recommendations from an expert panel on behalf of the European LeukemiaNet. Blood. 2009;113(9):1875–91.
63. De Angelis F, Breccia M. Molecular monitoring as a path to cure acute promyelocytic leukemia. Rare Cancers Ther. 2015;3:119–32.
64. Zhang L, Cao Z, Zou Y, Ruan M, Li Q, Wang J, Zhu X. Quantification of PML/RARa transcript after induction predicts outcome in children with acute promyelocytic leukemia. Int J Hematol. 2012;95(5):500–8.
65. Thomas X, Dombret H, Cordonnier C, Pigneux A, Gardin C, Guerci A, et al. Treatment of relapsing acute promyelocytic leukemia by all-trans retinoic acid therapy followed by timed sequential chemotherapy and stem cell transplantation. Leukemia. 2000;14:1006–13.
66. Castagnola C, Lunghi M, Corso A, Tajana M, Zappasodi P, Dabusti M, et al. Management of acute promyelocytic leukemia relapse in the ATRA era. Haematologica. 1998;83:714–7.
67. Lo Coco F, Cimino G, Breccia M, Noguera NI, Diverio D, Finolezzi E, et al. Gentuzumab ozogamicin (Mylotarg) as a single agent for molecularly relapsed acute promyelocytic leukemia. Blood. 2004;104(7):1995–9.
68. Lo Coco F, Latagliata R, Breccia M. Management of acute promyelocytic leukemia in the elderly. Mediterr J Hematol Infect Dis. 2013;5(1).
69. Aplenc R, Alonzo TA, Gerbing RB, Lange BJ, Hurwitz CA, Wells RJ, et al. Safety and efficacy of gemtuzumab ozogamicin in combination with chemotherapy for pediatric acute myeloid leukemia: a report from the Children's Oncology Group. J Clin Oncol. 2008;26:2390–3295.
70. Yanada M, Tsuzuki M, Fujita H, Fujimaki K, Fujisawa S, Sunami K, et al. Phase 2 study of arsenic trioxide followed by autologous hematopoietic cell transplantation for relapsed acute promyelocytic leukemia. Blood. 2013;121(16):3095–102.
71. Fox E, Razzouk BI, Widemann BC, Xiao S, O'Brien M, Goodspeed W, et al. Phase I trial and pharmacokinetic study of arsenic trioxide in children and adolescents with refractory or relapsed acute leukemia, including acute promyelocytic leukemia or lymphoma. Blood. 2008;111:566–73.
72. Ebinger M, Schwarze CP, Feuchtinger T, Scheel-Walter HG, Lang P, Hildenbrand S, et al. Long-term remission after first-line single-agent treatment with arsenic trioxide of relapsed acute promyelocytic leukemia in an 8-year-old boy. Pediatr Hematol Oncol. 2011;28:334–7.
73. Au WY, Li CK, Lee V, Yuen HL, Yau J, Chan GC, et al. Oral arsenic trioxide for relapsed acute promyelocytic leukemia in pediatric patients. Pediatr Blood Cancer. 2012;58(4):630–2.
74. Lou Y, Suo S, Tong Y, Tong H, Qian W, Meng H, et al. Outcomes and prognostic factors of first relapsed acute promyelocytic leukemia patients undergoing salvage therapy with intravenous arsenic trioxide and chemotherapy. Ann Hematol. 2014;93(6):941–8.
75. Thirugnanam R, George B, Chendamarai E, Lakshmi KM, Balasubramanian P, Viswabandya A, et al. Comparison of clinical outcomes of patients with relapsed acute promyelocytic leukemia induced with arsenic trioxide and consolidated with either an autologous stem cell transplant or an

arsenic trioxide-based regimen. Biol Blood Marrow Transplant. 2009;15(11):1479–84.
76. Au WY, Chim CS, Lie AK, Liang R, Kwong YL. Combined arsenic trioxide and all-trans retinoic acid treatment for acute promyelocytic leukemia recurring from previous relapses successfully treated using arsenic trioxide. Br J Haematol. 2002;117(1):130–2.
77. Ganzel C, Mathews V, Alimoghaddam K, Ghavamzadeh A, Kuk D, Devlin S, et al. Autologous transplant remains the preferred therapy for relapsed APL in CR2. Bone Marrow Transplant. 2016;51(9):1180–3.
78. De Botton S, Fawaz A, Chevret S, Dombret H, Thomas X, Sanz M, et al. Autologous and allogeneic stem-cell transplantation as salvage treatment of acute promyelocytic leukemia initially treated with all-trans-retinoic acid: a retrospective analysis of the European acute promyelocytic leukemia group. J Clin Oncol. 2005;23:120–6.
79. Abla O, Kutny MA, Testi AM, Feusner JH, Creutzig U, Gregory J Jr, et al. Management of relapsed and refractory childhood acute promyelocytic leukemia: recommendations from an international expert panel. Br J Haematol. 2016;175:588–601.
80. Au WY, Chan GC, Chim CS, Shek TW, Ooi GC, Ho WK, et al. Unusual sites of involvement by hematologic malignancies. Case 3. External auditory canal tumor: a rare chloroma in acute promyelocytic leukemia with a complete response to arsenic trioxide. J Clin Oncol. 2001;19:3993–5.
81. Cicconi L, Divona M, Ciardi C, Ottone T, Ferrantini A, Lavorgna S, et al. PML-RARα kinetics and impact of FLT3-ITD mutations in newly diagnosed acute promyelocytic leukaemia treated with ATRA and ATO or ATRA and chemotherapy. Leukemia. 2016;30(10):1987–92.
82. Ades L, Guerci A, Raffoux E, Sanz M, Chevallier P, Lapusan S, et al. Very long-term outcome of acute promyelocytic leukemia after treatment with all-trans retinoic acid and chemotherapy: the European APL group experience. Blood. 2010;115:1690–6.
83. Breccia M, Cicconi L, Minotti C, Latagliata R, Gianni L, Lo Coco F. Efficacy of prolonged therapy with combined arsenic trioxide and ATRA for relapse of acute promyelocytic leukemia. Haematologica. 2011;96:1390–1.
84. Testi AM, Moleti ML, Canichella M, Mohamed S, Diverio D, De Propris MS, et al. Very late relapse in a patient with acute promyelocytic leukemia (APL) rescued with a chemotherapy-free protocol. Leuk Lymphoma. 2016;23:1–3. [Epub ahead of print].
85. Sahin DG, Gunduz E, Akay OM, Gulbas Z. Central nervous system relapse in a patient with acute promyelocytic leukaemia: does the risk stratification matter? BMJ Case Rep. 2013;6:2013.
86. Au WY, Tam S, Fong BM, Kwong YL. Determinants of cerebrospinal fluid arsenic concentration in patients with acute promyelocytic leukemia on oral arsenic trioxide therapy. Blood. 2008;112(9):3587–90.
87. He Z, Tao S, Deng Y, Chen Y, Song L, Ding B, et al. Extramedullary relapse in lumbar spine of patient with acute promyelocytic leukemia after remission for 16 years: a case report and literature review. Int J Clin Exp Med. 2015;8(12):22430–4.
88. Kai T, Kimura H, Shiga Y, Ogawa K, Sato H, Maruyama Y, et al. Recurrent extramedullary relapse of acute promyelocytic leukemia after allogeneic stem cell transplantation: successful treatment by arsenic trioxide in combination with local radiotherapy. Int J Hematol. 2006;83(4):337–40.

Management of Acute Promyelocytic Leukemia in the Elderly

15

Ramy Rahmé, Lionel Adès, and Pierre Fenaux

Introduction

Despite considerable improvement in the management of APL over the last two decades, the outcome of inpatients >60 years of age has remained poorer than in younger patients with conventional therapy combining *all-trans*-retinoic acid (ATRA) and chemotherapy [1–3]. This poorer outcome is mainly due to a higher rate of early death during induction therapy and a higher death rate during consolidation and maintenance (due to sepsis) in elderly patients, as opposed to disease resistance like in other AML subtypes [4, 5]. Recent treatment approaches incorporating arsenic trioxide (ATO) and reducing or avoiding chemotherapy especially anthracyclines are less myelosuppressive and more promising in the elderly.

R. Rahmé, M.D. (✉)
Service Hématologie Séniors, Hôpital Saint-Louis, Assistance Publique—Hôpitaux de Paris, Paris, France

Université Paris Diderot, Paris, France

Université Paris Diderot, Sorbonne Paris Cité, Institut Universitaire d'Hématologie, Hôpital St. Louis, Paris, France

INSERM UMR 944, Equipe Labellisée par la Ligue Nationale contre le Cancer, Hôpital St. Louis, Paris, France

CNRS UMR 7212, Hôpital St. Louis, Paris, France

Assistance Publique des Hôpitaux de Paris, Oncologie Moléculaire, Hôpital St. Louis, Paris, France
e-mail: ramy.rahme@gmail.com

L. Adès, M.D., Ph.D. • P. Fenaux, M.D., Ph.D.
Service Hématologie Séniors, Hôpital Saint-Louis, Assistance Publique—Hôpitaux de Paris, Paris, France

Université Paris Diderot, Paris, France

Epidemiology of APL in the Elderly

In multicenter APL clinical trials, the median age at presentation is between 40 and 45 years, and the rate of patients older than 60 and 70 years ranged from 6% to 26% and from 3% to 9%, respectively [6–14]. However, recently published population-based studies support a higher proportion of older patients among APL cases [15–18]. Therefore, the frequency of APL in the elderly may be underestimated because many patients are not enrolled on clinical trials, mostly due to poorer performance status at presentation [19–21]. In a French retrospective multicenter study, patients not included in an APL clinical trial (APL 2006 trial) were mainly characterized by their older age (median 62 vs. 47 years, $p = 0.0001$) [22].

Specific Characteristics of APL in the Elderly

The proportion of high-risk APL, defined by a baseline white blood cell (WBC) count $>10 \times 10^9$/L according to Sanz classification, is generally similar in older and younger patients [23], although some studies reported a slightly lower proportion of high-risk patients in the elderly [24]. Therapy-related APL (tAPL), mainly reported after the use of topoisomerase II inhibitors for the treatment of cancers (or multiple sclerosis in the case of mitoxantrone), also tends to be more frequent in elderly than in younger adults, probably reflecting the fact

O. Abla et al. (eds.), *Acute Promyelocytic Leukemia*, https://doi.org/10.1007/978-3-319-64257-4_15

that cancer treatment is mainly administered to elderly people [19–21]. Other APL characteristics are similar in elderly and younger adults, except for a possible increase in the frequency of additional chromosomal abnormalities in the former, without any impact on prognosis [25].

Outcome of Elderly APL Patients with Frontline Conventional ATRA-Chemotherapy Regimens

All published studies using ATRA-chemotherapy regimens showed poorer outcome in elderly patients, compared to younger adults: this poorer outcome resulted from lower complete remission (CR) rates and higher rates of deaths in CR in the elderly, without differences in relapse rates according to age. Poorer CR rates in the elderly are the consequence of a higher incidence of early death rather than of resistant leukemia, which is almost nonexistent in APL irrespective of age. While CR rates in patients older than 60 are high (around 85%), they are significantly lower than those reported in younger patients (around 95%) [1–3, 26–28]. Early death (ED) is the main cause of failure, observed in 10–18% of patients enrolled on clinical trials (Table 15.1). ED rates are even greater in population-based reports (Table 15.2) and in patients >70 years of age (Table 15.3). In addition, the rates of death in CR are uniformly higher in elderly patients, ranging from 8 to 22% (Table 15.1) and occurring mainly during consolidation cycles, but also during maintenance treatment with 6-mercaptopurine and methotrexate [4, 5, 14, 23, 24, 26, 29].

Reducing the intensity of chemotherapy may improve outcome in elderly APL patients, at least those with standard-risk APL. The Italian GIMEMA group reported an improvement in survival when elderly patients received a single consolidation course instead of three, with a reduction in the rate of death in CR from 13 to 7.4% and with a similar relapse rate [29]. The Spanish

Table 15.1 Outcome in elderly APL patients treated with ATRA and chemotherapy in clinical trials

Author	Number of patients	Follow-up (years)	ED (%)	Death in CR (%)	OS (%)	DFS (%)	CIR (%)
Mandelli et al. (2003) [4]	134	–	12	12	56	59	–
Sanz et al. (2004) [24]	104	6	15	8	–	79	9
Adès et al. (2005) [5]	129	4	14	18.6	58	–	16
Latagliata et al. (2011) [29]	60	5	10	8	69	65	27
Ono et al. (2012) [26]	46	10	11	22	63	65	15
Lengfelder et al. (2013) [14]	56	7	18	19.6	45	48	24

ED early death, *OS* overall survival, *DFS* disease-free survival, *CIR* cumulative incidence of relapse

Table 15.2 Results of population-based studies

Author	Age groups (years)	Number of patients	Incidence per 100,000	ED rate (%)	Outcome
Lehmann et al. (2011) [15]	<40 40–59 ≥60	28 37 40	–	19.0 16.0 50.0	5-year OS 82.0% 74.0% 24.0%
Park et al. (2011) [16]	<35 35–54 ≥54	433 463 502	0.13 0.26 0.42	12.3 16.0 24.2	3-year OS 76.3% 72.0% 46.4%
Chen et al. (2012) [17]	<20 20–39 40–59 ≥60	149 372 427 449	0.06 0.19 0.22 0.36	–	5-year relative survival 0.52 0.57 0.57 0.24

Early death (ED) rates are higher and long-term outcome worse in older patients

Table 15.3 Outcome in advanced age APL patients (>70 years) treated with ATRA and chemotherapy

Author	Number of patients	Follow-up (years)	ED (%)	Death in CR (%)	OS (%)
Adès et al. (2005) [5]	34	4	15	–	–
Disperati et al. (2007) [27]	13	2	8	10	76
Lengfelder et al. (2013) [14]	18	7	33	–	25
Finsinger et al. (2015) [28]	13	5	0	–	64.5

PETHEMA group showed that ATRA plus anthracycline monochemotherapy treatment (avoiding cytarabine) improved long-term disease-free survival (DFS) in elderly APL, by reducing the rate of deaths in CR without increasing the relapse rate [24]. Reducing the intensity of chemotherapy, and in particular avoiding cytarabine, may however increase relapse in higher-risk APL as shown by a French-Spanish joint study [30].

Treatment with Arsenic Trioxide (ATO) in Elderly

Recently, ATRA-ATO combinations (without chemotherapy) have demonstrated, at least in standard-risk APL, that such regimens were at least equivalent and probably superior to ATRA-chemotherapy combinations in terms of CR and relapse rates, because they combined both a superior antileukemic effect with fewer relapses and less myelosuppression reducing the frequency of early deaths and deaths in CR [31–33].

In the British AML17 trial, the 4-year survival of patients older than 60 years (37 low-risk and 12 high-risk patients) was 80% in the ATRA and ATO group, compared with 74% in patients receiving ATRA and chemotherapy [33]. Ravandi et al., in 23 APL patients aged >60 years treated with ATRA-ATO during induction, reported a CR rate of 83%. With a median follow-up of more than 2 years, event-free survival (EFS) and overall survival (OS) in the older population were 69.5% and 74%, respectively [34]. Adès et al. reported in standard-risk APL aged >70 years, treated with ATRA-ATO and reduced chemotherapy, a CR rate of 92% and a 5-year EFS of 80% [35]. Interestingly, reduction of mortality in CR with this regimen was only seen when consolidation chemotherapy was reduced from 3 days to 1 single day of idarubicin [35].

Conclusions

Given the excellent results reported with ATRA and ATO regimens without chemotherapy in standard-risk APL patients (irrespective of age, with very high CR rates, very few relapses, and very limited mortality in CR), those regimens should be favored in elderly patients. This less toxic therapeutic strategy is currently tested in high-risk younger patients, in combination with very limited chemotherapy, for example, 2 days of anthracycline or reduced-dose gemtuzumab ozogamicin during induction treatment. Whether this strategy is also feasible in elderly patients will have to be confirmed.

References

1. Forghieri F, Luppi M, Morselli M, et al. Acute promyelocytic leukemia in very elderly patients: stilla clinical challenge. Leuk Lymphoma. 2009;50:119–21.
2. Tallman MS. Treatment of elderly adults with acute promyelocytic leukemia: put the pedal to metal. Leuk Lymphoma. 2009;50:12–3.
3. Tallman MS, Altman JK. Curative strategies in acute promyelocytic leukemia. Hematology Am Soc Hematol Educ Program. 2008:391–9.
4. Mandelli F, Latagliata R, Avvisati G, et al. Treatment of elderly patients (> or =60 years) with newly diagnosed acute promyelocytic leukemia. Results of the Italian multicenter group GIMEMA with ATRA and idarubicin (AIDA) protocols. Leukemia. 2003;17:1085–90.
5. Ades L, Chevret S, De Botton S, Thomas X, Dombret H, Beve B, et al. Outcome of acute promyelocytic leukemia treated with all trans retinoic acid and chemotherapy in elderly patients: the European group experience. Leukemia. 2005;19:230–3.
6. Kanamaru A, Takemoto Y, Tanimoto M, Murakami H, Asou N, Kobayashi T, et al. All-trans retinoic acid for the treatment of newly diagnosed acute promyelocytic leukemiaJapan Adult Leukemia Study Group. Blood. 1995;85:1202–6.

7. Burnett AK, Grimwade D, Solomon E, Wheatley K, Goldstone A. Presenting white blood cell counts and kinetics of molecular remission predict prognosis in acute promyelocytic leukemia treated with all-trans retinoic acid: results of the randomized MRC trial. Blood. 1999;93:4131–43.
8. Mandelli F, Diviero D, Avvisati G, Luciano A, Barbui T, Bernasconi C, et al. Molecular remission in PML/RARα-positive acute promyelocytic leukemia by combined all-trans retinoic acid and idarubicin (AIDA) therapy. Blood. 1997;90:1014–21.
9. Tallman MS, Andersen JW, Schiffer CA, Appelbaum FR, Feusner JH, Woods WG, et al. All-trans retinoic acid in acute promyelocytic leukemia: long-term outcome and prognostic factor analysis from the North American Intergroup protocol. Blood. 2002;100:4298–302.
10. Fenaux P, Chastang C, Chevret S, Sanz M, Dombret H, Archimbaud E, et al. A randomized comparison of all transretinoic acid (ATRA) followed by chemotherapy and ATRA plus chemotherapy and the role of maintenance therapy in newly diagnosed acute promyelocytic leukemia. The European APL Group. Blood. 1999;94:1192–200.
11. Sanz MA, Montesinos P, Rayón C, Holowiecka A, de la Serna J, Milone G, et al. Risk-adapted treatment of acute promyelocytic leukemia based on all-trans retinoic acid and anthracycline with addition of cytarabine in consolidation therapy for high-risk patients: further improvements in treatment outcome. Blood. 2010;115:5137–46.
12. Burnett AK, Hills RK, Grimwade D, Jovanovic JV, Craig J, McMullin MF, et al. Inclusion of chemotherapy in addition to anthracycline in the treatment of acute promyelocytic leukaemia does not improve outcomes: results of the MRC AML15 Trial. Leukemia. 2013;27:843–51.
13. Lengfelder E, Haferlach C, Saussele S, Haferlach T, Schultheis B, Schnittger S, et al. High dose ara-C in the treatment of newly diagnosed acute promyelocytic leukemia: long-term results of the German AMLCG. Leukemia. 2009;23:2248–58.
14. Lengfelder E, Hanfstein B, Haferlach C, Braess J, Krug U, Spiekermann K, et al. Outcome of elderly patients with acute promyelocytic leukemia: results of the German Acute Myeloid Leukemia Cooperative Group. Ann Hematol. 2013;92:41–52.
15. Lehmann S, Ravn A, Carlsson L, Antunovic P, Deneberg S, Möllgård L, et al. Continuing high early death rate in acute promyelocytic leukemia: a population-based report from the Swedish Adult Acute Leukemia Registry. Leukemia. 2011;25:1128–34.
16. Park JH, Qiao B, Panageas KS, Schymura MJ, Jurcic JG, Rosenblat TL, et al. Early death in acute promyelocytic leukemia remains high despite all-trans retinoic acid. Blood. 2011;118:1248–54.
17. Chen Y, Kantarjian H, Wang H, Cortes J, Ravandi F. Acute promyelocytic leukemia: a population-based study on incidence and survival in the United States, 1975–2008. Cancer. 2012;118:5811–8.
18. Dores GM, Devesa SS, Curtis RE, Linet MS, Morton LM. Acute leukemia incidence and patient survival among children and adults in the United States, 2001–2007. Blood. 2012;119:34–43.
19. Mengis C, Aebi S, Tobler A, et al. Assessment of differences in patient populations selected for excluded from participation in clinical phase III acute myelogenous leukemia trials. J Clin Oncol. 2003;21:3933–9.
20. de la Serna J, Montesinos P, Vellenga E, et al. Causes and prognostic factors of remission induction failure in patients with acute promyelocytic leukemia treated with all-trans retinoic acid and idarubicin. Blood. 2008;111:3395–402.
21. Ferrara F, Finizio O, D'Arco A, et al. Acute promyelocytic leukemia in patients aged over 60 years: multicenter experience of 34 consecutive unselected patients. Anticancer Res. 2010;30:967–71.
22. Rahmé R, Thomas X, Recher C, Vey N, Delaunay J, Deconinck E, et al. Early death in acute promyelocytic leukemia (APL) in French centers: a multicenter study in 399 patients. Leukemia. 2014;28(12):2422–4.
23. Ades L, Guerci A, Raffoux E, et al. Very long-term outcome of acute promyelocytic leukemia after treatment with all-trans retinoic acid and chemotherapy: the European APL Group experience. Blood. 2010;115:1690–6.
24. Sanz MA, Vellenga E, Rayon C, et al. All-trans retinoic acid and anthracycline monochemotherapy for the treatment of elderly patients with acute promyelocytic leukemia. Blood. 2004;104:3490–3.
25. De Botton S, Chevret S, Sanz M, Dombret H, Thomas X, Guerci A, et al. Additional chromosomal abnormalities in patients with acute promyelocytic leukaemia (APL) do not confer poor prognosis: results of APL 93 trial. Br J Haematol. 2000;111(3):801–6.
26. Ono T, Takeshita A, Kishimoto Y, Kiyoi H, Okada M, Yamauchi T, et al. Long-term outcome and prognostic factors of elderly patients with acute promyelocytic leukemia. Cancer Sci. 2012;103:1974–8.
27. Disperati P, Minden MD, Gupta V, Schimmer AD, Schuh AC, Yee KW, et al. Acute promyelocytic leukemia in patients aged 70 years and over—a single center experience of unselected patients. Leuk Lymphoma. 2007;48:1654–8.
28. Finsinger P, Breccia M, Minotti C, Carmosino I, Girmenia C, Chisini M, et al. Acute promyelocytic leukemia in patients aged > 70 years: the cure beyond age. Ann Hematol. 2015;94(2):195–200.
29. Latagliata R, Breccia M, Fazi P, Vignetti M, Di Raimondo F, Sborgio M, et al. GIMEMA AIDA 0493 amended protocol for elderly patients with acute promyelocytic leukaemia. Long-term results and prognostic factors. Br J Haematol. 2011;154(5):564–8.
30. Adès L, Sanz MA, Chevret S, Montesinos P, Chevallier P, Raffoux E, et al. Treatment of newly diagnosed acute promyelocytic leukemia (APL): a

comparison of French-Belgian-Swiss and PETHEMA results. Blood. 2008;111(3):1078–84.
31. Lo-Coco F, Avvisati G, Vignetti M, Thiede C, Orlando SM, Lacobelli S, et al. Retinoic acid and arsenic trioxide for acute promyelocytic leukemia. N Engl J Med. 2013;369(2):111–21.
32. Platzbecker U, Avvisati G, Cicconi L, Thiede C, Paoloni F, Vignetti M, et al. Improved outcomes with retinoic acid and arsenic trioxide compared with retinoic acid and chemotherapy in non-high-risk acute promyelocytic leukemia: final results of the randomized Italian-German APL0406 Trial. J Clin Oncol. 2016. pii: JCO671982.
33. Burnett AK, Russell NH, Hills RK, Bowen D, Kell J, Knapper S, et al. Arsenic trioxide and all-trans retinoic acid treatment for acute promyelocytic leukaemia in all risk groups (AML17): results of a randomised, controlled, phase 3 trial. Lancet Oncol. 2015;16(13):1295–305.
34. Ravandi F, Estey E, Jones D, Faderl S, O'Brien S, Fiorentino J, et al. Effective treatment of acute promyelocytic leukemia with all-trans-retinoic acid, arsenic trioxide, and gemtuzumab ozogamicin. J Clin Oncol. 2009;27(4):504–10.
35. Ades L, Thomas X, Guerci A, Pigneux A, Vey N, Raffoux E, et al. Arsenic trioxide (ATO) and ATRA with limited chemotherapy (CT) in newly diagnosed standard risk APL in the elderly: a report by the French Belgian Swiss APL Group (APL 2006 trial). Abstract ASH. Blood. 2016;128:898.

16 Special Situations in Acute Promyelocytic Leukemia

Massimo Breccia, Gloria Iacoboni,
and Miguel A. Sanz

Introduction

Therapeutic strategies in acute promyelocytic leukemia (APL) have changed greatly since the introduction of all-*trans*-retinoic acid (ATRA) and, more recently, arsenic trioxide (ATO) in the treatment of this disease, improving enormously the outcome of these patients. Several treatment strategies using these agents, alone or usually in combination with chemotherapy, have provided excellent therapeutic results, in fit patients whose clinical situation does not generate special difficulty for the administration of conventional therapy. However, there are conditions that prevent partially or completely the administration of ATRA, ATO, or chemotherapy, complicating the management of these patients. In this chapter, we review some of these peculiar clinical situations which, differently from the standard of care, require more careful attention. Thus, we will discuss the management of APL in older and other frail patients, children and pregnant women, as well as those with therapy-related leukemia, extramedullary relapse and the extremely rare situation of the genetic variants of APL.

M. Breccia, M.D., Ph.D.
Department of Cellular Biotechnologies and Hematology, Sapienza University, Rome, Italy

G. Iacoboni, Ph.D.
Department of Hematology, Hospital Universitari i Politècnic La Fe, Valencia, Spain

M.A. Sanz, M.D. (✉)
Department of Medicine, Hospital Universitari i Politecnic La Fe, University of Valencia, Valencia, Spain

Centro de Investigacion Biomedica en Red de Cancer, Instituto Carlos III, Madrid, Spain
e-mail: msanz@uv.es

Management of Special Situations

Older and Other Fragile Patients

APL is uncommon in older patients. This group tends to have a worse outcome, even if stratified as lower risk at baseline, due to a higher therapy-related toxicity leading to an increased treatment-related mortality, not only during induction but also during consolidation, maintenance, and even off therapy. The reported mortality rate in complete remission (CR) ranges from less than 1% in patients younger than 60 to 19% in patients older than 70 years [1]. It should be noted, however, that lower rates of relapse are observed in patients over 70 years of age receiving ATRA and moderately reduced anthracycline-based chemotherapy [1–4]. Therefore, it is reasonable to design less intensive therapeutic strategies aiming to reduce morbidity and mortality in this group. With the aim of decreasing the rate of treatment-related deaths, the Gruppo Italiano Malattie Ematologiche Maligne dell'Adulto (GIMEMA) group amended the AIDA protocol

O. Abla et al. (eds.), *Acute Promyelocytic Leukemia*, https://doi.org/10.1007/978-3-319-64257-4_16

and reduced the number of consolidation courses from three to only one, which resulted in an improved overall survival (OS) [5]. The outcome with ATO-based treatments in elderly patients has not specifically been reported, except for a small series of 33 patients aged 60 years or older [6]. This study showed 88% CR rate and a 10-year cumulative incidence of relapse, OS, and disease-free survival (DFS) of 10.3%, 69.3%, and 64.8%, respectively, which are comparable to those reported in younger APL patients. The main reported side effect was leukocytosis, and no increased rate of secondary malignancies was reported after long-term follow-up. Based on these results, ATO could be considered as a first-line treatment option for elderly patients with APL, but more data is needed to really turn it into the standard of care for patients unfit for conventional therapy in this age group. The APL0406 trial reported similar efficacy in patients aged 60–70 years when compared to younger patients, with an improved EFS and toxicity rate [7]. Gemtuzumab ozogamicin (GO) has also been tested in the elderly, with efficacy reported also at lower doses [8, 9]. Unfortunately, the drug was temporarily withdrawn from the market in 2010 and reapplied for US and EU approval in early 2017. Therefore, we can conclude that an ATRA-ATO regimen may be appropriate in the elderly setting, but further data are still required to validate its use. See Chap. 15, "APL in the Elderly," for more details.

Similar to the outlined approach for older patients, in younger patients who are not candidates for first-line intensive chemotherapy due to certain comorbidities (in particular, severe cardiac impairment or other organ dysfunctions), there are alternative treatment approaches which minimize the use of cytotoxic agents. These would be based on the use of ATRA in combination with ATO, with minimal or no chemotherapy. The outcome in this particular setting is not sufficiently documented. It should be noted that any therapeutic strategy used in these patients should aim to achieve molecular remission and guide the need for additional therapy with minimal residual disease (MRD) monitoring.

Children

APL is a rare disease in children, with a reported median age of 9–12 years and a female prevalence. At presentation, there is a reported higher rate of hyperleukocytosis (40% versus 20–25% in adults) and of the variant morphologic hypogranular (M3v) subtype, with an increased incidence of the bcr2/bcr3 transcript type [10]. It has been suggested that the difference in the WBC count is mainly observed in children under the age of 12 years old [10]. Apart from two relatively small pediatric series from the German-Austrian-Swiss group [11] and the European APL group [12], as well as two larger series from the GIMEMA [13] and PETHEMA [14] groups, there is a recent analysis from the European APL group [15] that reports the outcome in different age groups of children and adolescents. In this analysis, children under 4 years old presented the highest relapse rate (52% versus 18% in children age 5–12 years old), a new finding owing to the lack of studies with different age groups in children. This observation was not attributed to a higher WBC count or other high-risk features. The treatment strategy with the simultaneous combination of ATRA and chemotherapy derives from adult trials. The GIMEMA and PETHEMA groups reported the larger cohorts of patients, with a CR rate higher than 90% and OS ranging between 71 and 89% [13, 14]. In children with APL, a reduction in the dose of ATRA, from 45 to 25 mg/m^2/day, is recommended to reduce the incidence of severe headache and pseudotumor cerebri (PTC), still maintaining excellent therapeutic results [16]. The study by Castaigne et al. [17] showed no difference in terms of pharmacokinetics, therapeutic efficacy, triggering of hyperleukocytosis, or differentiation syndrome with ATRA at the reduced dose as compared to the standard dose. Headache is a relatively common complication during ATRA therapy in children, but it is always necessary to rule out PTC, CNS leukemia, and bleeding. PTC diagnosis is based on increased intracranial pressure with normal cerebrospinal fluid (CSF) composition and negative cerebral imaging studies, usually accompanied by papilledema at the fundoscopic exam.

This latter evidence is not a requirement for the diagnosis of PTC but is helpful in the differential diagnosis [18]. Sometimes, the symptoms of PTC resolve with the initial "diagnostic" lumbar puncture. If this occurs, no further medical treatment is required. If symptoms persist, temporary discontinuation or dose reduction of ATRA and analgesics and administration of steroids and acetazolamide are the mainstays of the medical treatment of this neurological complication. Acetazolamide is administered in an initial dose of 25 mg/kg/day and progressively increased until clinical response is attained (maximum dose 100 mg/kg/day). Electrolytes must be monitored for an early detection of hypokalemia and acidosis, common side effects during acetazolamide treatment. If this diuretic treatment is ineffective, then prednisone can be given at a dose of 2 mg/kg/day for 2 weeks followed by a 2-week taper.

Given the long life span in children cured from this disease, there is a wide concern about the potential long-term cardiac toxicity that high-dose anthracyclines can produce. Therefore, there have been some attempts to simply reduce the exposure to these agents without any additional treatment modifications, which has resulted in worse outcomes in the past [19]. The Japanese group tried to minimize anthracycline exposure with a single administration in second induction and consolidation courses: only two deaths were reported, but no cardiac adverse events or treatment-related deaths were observed in subsequent phases [20]. Similarly to older patients, other therapeutic options are being studied in order to reduce the dose of cytotoxic agents, with ATO being one of the most promising alternatives. Indeed, ATO appears to be effective in pediatric APL [21, 22], similarly to adults, but there is still very limited data. See Chap. 14, "APL in Children," for more details.

Pregnancy

The diagnosis of APL during pregnancy is uncommon, and most reports are based on individual cases or very small series. The risk of thrombohemorrhagic complications and infections may be higher during pregnancy, whereas identification of differentiation syndrome (DS) could be more difficult. This is a challenging situation in which decision-making must be carried out with a multidisciplinary perspective, involving the patient, hematologist, obstetrician, and neonatologist. With this approach, there is a higher chance for a successful outcome for both mother and baby, as was highlighted in the guidelines on the management of AML in the United Kingdom [23]. A recent systematic analysis showed 43 articles with 71 patients with new-onset APL during pregnancy [24]. The results suggested that in case of pregnancy, the start of treatment should not be delayed, or it could compromise the chance for a successful remission: pregnancy in APL must be considered a medical emergency. The key problem in this special situation is the teratogenic potential of chemotherapy, ATRA, and ATO on the fetus. Therefore, the gestational age is key in this situation, and management should be adapted accordingly.

Management of APL During the First Trimester of Pregnancy

A conventional therapeutic approach is not possible during the first trimester of pregnancy, due to the highly teratogenic side effects of ATRA [25]. Five out of the nine reported APL cases diagnosed in early pregnancy ended in abortion (four induced and one spontaneous). The remaining four pregnant women delivered two healthy infants, one with transient dilated cardiomyopathy and one with low birthweight, jaundice, and respiratory distress syndrome at birth [24, 26]. In a Spanish series, all early pregnancies terminated in abortion (four induced and one spontaneous) [26]. During the first trimester, the only option is anthracycline-based chemotherapy. The use of daunorubicin is usually preferred over idarubicin, probably due to a wider experience with the former drug and because idarubicin is more lipophilic and can favor an increased placental transfer [27]. Even with chemotherapy, there is an increased risk of fetal malformations, abortion, and low birthweight [28]. Therefore, the first decision that should take place when APL is diagnosed in the first trimester is whether or not to continue with the pregnancy. Women who, after receiving all the accurate information, wish to continue with their pregnancy should receive anthracycline chemotherapy alone; in case of pregnancy interruption, they can receive conventional treatment with ATRA and cytotoxic agents. It should be taken into account that chemotherapy alone can increase the risk of hemorrhage due to release of procoagulants and plasminogen activators from malignant promyelocytes. If remission is achieved with chemotherapy and the pregnancy is progressing normally, ATRA could be safely administered during the second and third trimesters. Although ATO is an alternative treatment in other groups of patients, it is not an option during pregnancy due to a high potential for teratogenicity; in fact, this drug cannot be recommended at any stage of pregnancy. Human data are very limited and restricted to people exposed to arsenic from drinking water, working in, or living near metal smelters. Low birthweight, spontaneous abortion, and stillbirth were reported in this population [29]. Taking the above into account, female APL patients who are receiving conventional treatment should be advised against becoming pregnant during exposure to ATRA and/or ATO. On the other hand, it appears that fertility is maintained after ATO treatment is finalized [30].

Management of APL During the Second and Third Trimesters of Pregnancy

During the second and third trimesters of pregnancy, conventional treatment with ATRA and chemotherapy is a reasonable option, even though the literature on this subject is extremely scarce. The maternal outcome seems to be the same as in nonpregnant women when conventional therapy is used. ATRA does not seem to be teratogenic past the first trimester [24, 26, 28]. This agent can be safely administered, preferably monitoring the cardiac function, due to some reports of reversible fetal arrhythmias and other cardiac complications at birth. On the other hand, although chemotherapy does not seem to cause congenital malformation, it increases in some cases the risk of abortion, premature delivery, low birthweight, neonatal neutropenia, and sepsis. Two different possible approaches could be adopted:

(a) *Sequential use of ATRA and chemotherapy*. This approach implies the administration of ATRA alone until CR, delaying the administration of chemotherapy until elective delivery is possible. A gestational age of at least 32 weeks is considered relatively safe when appropriate neonatal care is provided [31]. For deliveries before 36 weeks of gestation, antenatal corticosteroids are recommended to reduce the risk of respiratory distress syndrome [32]. ATRA alone induces similar CR rates as compared to ATRA plus chemotherapy, but it can have an unfavorable impact on the risk of relapse and a possible increased rate of DS (approximately 25%) [33, 34]. If this strategy is followed, the administration of chemotherapy should not be delayed excessively to avoid resistance and disease recurrence, and post-remission therapy should be reinforced.

(b) *Simultaneous administration of ATRA and chemotherapy*. This approach provides the best chances of cure for the pregnant women and is a reasonable option for high-risk patients with hyperleukocytosis and for those in which appropriate RQ-PCR monitoring is not possible. Daunorubicin is preferred to idarubicin, as mentioned previously. Vaginal delivery is preferred, due to its association with a reduced risk of bleeding. Caesarean section should only take place if it is required for other reasons [28]. After delivery, breastfeeding is contraindicated if chemotherapy or ATO is needed. The rest of management does not differ from nonpregnant women with APL.

Therapy-Related APL

The true incidence of therapy-related APL (tAPL) is still a matter of discussion since these patients are less likely to be enrolled into clinical trials. Available data is based on retrospective series [35, 36] or experience of single referral centers [37, 38]. The incidence reported in these studies ranges from less than 5–22% of all APL cases. The incidence of tAPL has increased over the last few years due to the use of topoisomerase II-targeted drugs in both malignant and nonmalignant diseases. Breast carcinoma is the most frequent previous cancer, followed by lymphoma, with a large predominance of non-Hodgkin lymphoma, whereas other tumor types have a lower incidence [35]. Epirubicin and mitoxantrone are the most common implicated drugs in tAPL, but a number of cases have been reported after exposure to radiotherapy alone [39–42]. Cases of secondary APL occurring in patients whose primary tumor was treated only by surgery, without chemotherapy or radiotherapy, have also been reported [35, 36]. The latency period between chemotherapy exposure and onset of tAPL is usually relatively short (less than 3 years) and occurs without a previous myelodysplastic phase. Hematologic findings are similar to de novo APL, as also previously reported for other tAML with a specific karyotype [43, 44]. Cases of tAPL are increasingly reported in patients treated for nonmalignant diseases, in particular in patients affected by aggressive forms of multiple sclerosis treated with mitoxantrone [45]. The risk of developing this complication has been estimated at approximately 1 in 400 patients with multiple sclerosis treated with this topoisomerase II inhibitor [45]. In these patients, specific genomic loci were identified, such as PML intron 6 and RUNX1 intron 5, containing preferential sites of topoisomerase II-mediated DNA cleavage [46, 47].

In the past, a higher incidence of early death during treatment was reported [35, 48]. However, a more precise knowledge on the outcome of patients with tAPL treated with state-of-the-art therapy should be prospectively established. At present, there is no specific reason to manage these patients differently from those with de novo APL. However, in a significant number of patients with tAPL, the use of anthracycline-based regimens is limited by previous exposure to topoisomerase II inhibitors. In such situations, ATO in combination with ATRA provides an option for consolidation following standard induction therapy or as first-line treatment using schedules such as those published by the MD Anderson and GIMEMA groups [49]. See Chap. 19, "Therapy-Related APL," for more details.

Genetic Variants of APL

Less than 1% of APL cases are due to rare variant translocations, which typically involve *RARA* [50]. No APL variants with *PML* involvement alone have been identified to date; thus, *RARA* is assumed to have a key role in the pathogenesis of APL. Several variant translocations have been identified, including *ZBTB16/RARA* (previously named *PLZF-RARA*), *NMP/RARA*, *NUMA/RARA*, *STAT5B/RARA*, *PRKAR1a/RARA*, *BCOR/RARA*, and *FIP1L1/RARA* [51]. APL with complex, cryptic, or variant translocations usually present with the same clinical features of typical APL. There are no specific guidelines for rare genetic variants of APL, because the available evidence is mostly based on single case reports. Nevertheless, it is a general rule that patients with ATRA-sensitive variants (*NUMA-RARA*, *NPM1-RARA*, *BCOR/RARA*, *PRKAR1a/RARA*, and *FIP1L1-RARA*) should be treated with standard protocols involving ATRA combined with anthracycline-based chemotherapy, while those with ATRA-resistant variants (*ZBTB16/RARA*, *STAT5b-RARA*) should be managed with AML-like approaches [51]. For those relatively ATRA resistant (*PLZF-RARA*), it is reasonable to combine ATRA with AML-like chemotherapy. Sensitivity to ATO has not been documented outside *PML-RARA*-positive APL, except for *PLZF-RARA*-positive APL that has been shown to be resistant [52]. See Chap. 20, "Rare APL Variants," for more details.

Central Nervous System and Other Extramedullary Relapses

Central nervous system (CNS) and other extramedullary relapses are uncommon in APL. In particular, CNS involvement can occur as an isolated event or associated with bone marrow involvement at first relapse or, more frequently, after two or more hematological relapses. The reported incidence of CNS relapses in APL ranges from 0.6 to 2% [53, 54]. Hyperleukocytosis at presentation is a predisposing factor, and the optimal management of such patients is still controversial [55].

The literature on this subject is scarce, but it seems pragmatic to manage these cases just like an extramedullary relapse of acute lymphoblastic leukemia or non-APL AML. In this regard, treatment of CNS relapse should consist of weekly triple intrathecal therapy (ITT) with methotrexate, hydrocortisone, and cytarabine until complete clearance of blasts in the CSF, followed by six to ten more spaced-out ITT treatments as consolidation [56]. Since CNS disease is almost invariably accompanied by hematologic or molecular relapse in the marrow, systemic treatment should also be given. Chemotherapy regimens with high CNS penetrance (e.g., high-dose cytarabine) have been used in this situation, and, in patients responding to treatment, allogeneic or autologous transplant should be the consolidation approach of choice with appropriate craniospinal irradiation. In case of any extramedullary localization (peculiar localizations include the ear, scalp, and skin [53, 54, 57]), local radiation and intensive systemic therapy should be considered. See Chap. 12, "Treatment of Refractory and Relapsed APL," for more details.

References

1. Sanz MA, Vellenga E, Rayon C, Diaz-Mediavilla J, Rivas C, Amutio E, et al. All-trans retinoic acid and anthracycline monochemotherapy for the treatment of elderly patients with acute promyelocytic leukemia. Blood. 2004;104(12):3490–3.
2. Mandelli F, Latagliata R, Avvisati G, Fazi P, Rodeghiero F, Leoni F, et al. Treatment of elderly patients (> or =60 years) with newly diagnosed acute promyelocytic leukemia. Results of the Italian multicenter group GIMEMA with ATRA and idarubicin (AIDA) protocols. Leukemia. 2003;17(6):1085–90.
3. Lengfelder E, Hofmann WK, Nolte F. Management of elderly patients with acute promyelocytic leukemia: progress and problems. Ann Hematol. 2013;92(9):1181–8.
4. Ades L, Chevret S, De Botton S, Thomas X, Dombret H, Beve B, et al. Outcome of acute promyelocytic leukemia treated with all trans retinoic acid and chemotherapy in elderly patients: the European group experience. Leukemia. 2005;19(2):230–3.
5. Latagliata R, Breccia M, Fazi P, Vignetti M, Di Raimondo F, Sborgia M, et al. GIMEMA AIDA 0493 amended protocol for elderly patients with acute promyelocytic leukemia. Long-term results and prognostic factors. Br J Haematol. 2011;154(5):564–8.
6. Zhang Y, Zhang Z, Li J, Li L, Han X, Han L, et al. Long-term efficacy and safety of arsenic trioxide for first-line treatment of elderly patients with newly diagnosed acute promyelocytic leukemia. Cancer. 2013;119(1):115–25.
7. Lo Coco F, Avvisati G, Vignetti M, Thiede C, Orlando SM, Iacobelli S, et al. Retinoic acid and arsenic trioxide for acute promyelocytic leukemia. N Engl J Med. 2013;369(2):111–21.
8. Lo Coco F, Cimino G, Breccia M, Noguera NI, Diverio D, Finolezzi E, et al. Gemtuzumab ozogamicin (Mylotarg) as a single agent for molecularly relapsed acute promyelocytic leukemia. Blood. 2004;104(7):1995–9.
9. Breccia M, Cimino G, Diverio D, Gentilini F, Mandelli F, Lo Coco F. Sustained molecular remission after low dose gemtuzumab-ozogamicin in elderly patients with advanced acute promyelocytic leukemia. Haematologica. 2007;92(9):1273–4.
10. Testi AM, D'Angiò M, Locatelli F, Pession A, Lo Coco F. Acute promyelocytic leukemia (APL): comparison between children and adults. Mediterr J Hematol Infect Dis. 2014;6(1):e2014032.
11. Mann G, Reinhardt D, Ritter J, et al. Treatment with all-trans retinoic acid in acute promyelocytic leukemia reduces early deaths in children. Ann Hematol. 2001;80(7):417–22.
12. de Botton S, Coiteux V, Chevret S, et al. Outcome of childhood acute promyelocytic leukemia with all-trans-retinoic acid and chemotherapy. J Clin Oncol. 2004;22(8):1404–12.
13. Testi AM, Biondi A, Lo Coco F, et al. GIMEMA-AIEOPAIDA protocol for the treatment of newly diagnosed acute promyelocytic leukemia (APL) in children. Blood. 2005;106(2):447–53.
14. Ortega JJ, Madero L, Martin G, et al. Treatment with all-trans retinoic acid and anthracycline monochemotherapy for children with acute promyelocytic leukemia: a multicenter study by the PETHEMA Group. J Clin Oncol. 2005;23(30):7632–40.
15. Bally C, Fadlallah J, Leverger G, et al. Outcome of acute promyelocytic leukemia (APL) in children and adolescents: an analysis in two consecutive trials of the European APL Group. J Clin Oncol. 2012;30(14):1641–6.
16. Abla O, Ribeiro RC. How I treat children and adolescents with acute promyelocytic leukemia. Br J Haematol. 2014;164(1):24–38.
17. Castaigne S, Lefebvre P, Chomienne C, et al. Effectiveness and pharmacokinetics of low-dose all-trans retinoic acid (25 mg/m2) in acute promyelocytic leukemia. Blood. 1993;82(12):3560–3.
18. Wang SJ, Silberstein SD, Patterson S, Young WB. Idiopathic intracranial hypertension without papilledema: a case-control study in a headache center. Neurology. 1998;51(1):245–9.
19. Powell BL, Moser B, Stock W, et al. Arsenic trioxide improves event-free and overall survival for adults with acute promyelocytic leukemia: North American Leukemia Intergroup Study C971. Blood 2010; 116(19): 3751–3757.

20. Takahashi H, Watanabe T, Kinoshita A, et al. High event-free survival rate with minimum-dose-anthracycline treatment in childhood acute promyelocytic leukaemia: a nationwide prospective study by the Japanese Paediatric Leukaemia/Lymphoma Study Group. Br J Haematol. 2016;174(3):437–43.
21. Fox E, Razzouk BI, Widemann BC, et al. Phase 1 trial and pharmacokinetic study of arsenic trioxide in children and adolescents with refractory or relapsed acute leukemia, including acute promyelocytic leukemia or lymphoma. Blood. 2008;111(2):566–73.
22. George B, Mathews V, Poonkuzhali B, Shaji RV, Srivastava A, Chandy M. Treatment of children with newly diagnosed acute promyelocytic leukemia with arsenic trioxide: a single center experience. Leukemia. 2004;18(10):1587–90.
23. Milligan DW, Grimwade D, Cullis JO, et al. Guidelines on the management of acute myeloid leukaemia in adults. Br J Haematol. 2006;135(4):450–74.
24. Verma V, Giri S, Manandhar S, Pathak R, Bhatt VR. Acute promyelocytic leukemia during pregnancy: a systematic analysis of outcome. Leuk Lymphoma. 2016;57(3):616–22.
25. Lammer EJ, Chen DT, Hoar RM, et al. Retinoic acid embryopathy. N Engl J Med. 1985;313(14):837–41.
26. Sanz MA, Montesinos P, Casale MF, et al. Maternal and fetal outcomes in pregnant women with acute promyelocytic leukemia. Ann Hematol. 2015;94(8):1357–61.
27. Cardonick E, Iacobucci A. Use of chemotherapy during human pregnancy. Lancet Oncol. 2004;5(5):283–91.
28. Culligan DJ, Merriman L, Kell J, et al. The management of acute promyelocytic leukemia presenting during pregnancy. Clin Leuk. 2007;1:183–91.
29. U.S. Environmental Protection Agency. Arsenic compounds. http://www.epa.gov. Accessed 8 Jan 2008.
30. Breccia M, Molica M, Efficace F, et al. Pregnancy in acute promyelocytic leukemia after frontline therapy with arsenic trioxide and all-trans retinoic acid. Br J Haematol. 2014;167(3):428–30.
31. Slattery MM, Morrison JJ. Preterm delivery. Lancet. 2002;360(9344):1489–97.
32. Royal College of Obstetricians and Gynecologists. Antenatal corticosteroids to reduce respiratory distress syndrome. Guideline No. 7. http://www.rcog.org.uk/resources/Public/pdf/Antenatal_corticosteroids_No7.pdf. Accessed 1 Apr 2007.
33. Fenaux P, Chastang C, Chevret S, et al. A randomized comparison of all transretinoic acid (ATRA) followed by chemotherapy and ATRA plus chemotherapy and the role of maintenance therapy in newly diagnosed acute promyelocytic leukemia. The European APL Group. Blood. 1999;94(4):1192–200.
34. Tallman MS, Andersen JW, Schiffer CA, et al. All-trans-retinoic acid in acute promyelocytic leukemia. N Engl J Med. 1997;337(15):1021–8.
35. Pulsoni A, Pagano L, Lo Coco F, et al. Clinicobiological features and outcome of acute promyelocytic leukemia occurring as a second tumor: the GIMEMA experience. Blood. 2002;100(6):1972–6.
36. Beaumont M, Sanz M, Carli PM, et al. Therapy-related acute promyelocytic leukemia. J Clin Oncol. 2003;21(11):2123–37.
37. Mattson JC. Acute promyelocytic leukemia. From morphology to molecular lesions. Clin Lab Med. 2000;20(1):83–103, ix.
38. Pollicardo N, O'Brien S, Estey EH, et al. Secondary acute promyelocytic leukemia. Characteristics and prognosis of 14 patients from a single institution. Leukemia. 1996;10(1):27–31.
39. Mistry AR, Felix CA, Whitmarsh RJ, et al. DNA topoisomerase II in therapy-related acute promyelocytic leukemia. N Engl J Med. 2005;352(15):1529–38.
40. Andersen MK, Pedersen-Bjergaard J. Therapy-related MDS and AML in acute promyelocytic leukemia. Blood. 2002;100(5):1928–9; author reply 1929.
41. Pedersen-Bjergaard J. Insights into leukemogenesis from therapy-related leukemia. N Engl J Med. 2005;352(15):1591–4.
42. Smith SM, Le Beau MM, Huo D, et al. Clinical-cytogenetic associations in 306 patients with therapy-related myelodysplasia and myeloid leukemia: the University of Chicago series. Blood. 2003;102(1):43–52.
43. Pedersen-Bjergaard J, Philip P, Larsen SO, Jensen G, Byrsting K. Chromosome aberrations and prognostic factors in therapy-related myelodysplasia and acute non-lymphocytic leukemia. Blood. 1990;76(6):1083–91.
44. Quesnel B, Kantarjian H, Bjergaard JP, et al. Therapy-related acute myeloid leukemia with t(8;21), inv(16), and t(8;16): a report on 25 cases and review of the literature. J Clin Oncol. 1993;11(12):2370–9.
45. Ledda A, Caocci G, Spinicci G, Cocco E, Mamusa E, La Nasa G. Two new cases of acute promyelocytic leukemia following mitoxantrone treatment in patients with multiple sclerosis. Leukemia. 2006;20(12):2217–8.
46. Hasan SK, Mays AN, Ottone T, et al. Molecular analysis of t(15;17) genomic breakpoints in secondary acute promyelocytic leukemia arising after treatment of multiple sclerosis. Blood. 2008;112:3383–90.
47. Ottone T, Hasan SK, Montefusco E, et al. Identification of a potential "hotspot" DNA region in the RUNX1 gene targeted by mitoxantrone in therapy-related acute myeloid leukemia with t(16;21) translocation. Genes Chromosomes Cancer. 2009;48:213–21.
48. Ghalie RG, Mauch E, Edan G, et al. A study of therapy-related acute leukaemia after mitoxantrone therapy for multiple sclerosis. Mult Scler. 2002;8(5):441–5.
49. Lo-Coco F, Avvisati G, Vignetti M, et al. Retinoic acid and arsenic trioxide for acute promyelocytic leukemia. N Engl J Med. 2013;369(2):111–21.
50. Wang ZY, Chen Z. Acute promyelocytic leukemia: from highly fatal to highly curable. Blood. 2008;111(5):2505–15.
51. Adams J, Nassiri M. Acute promyelocytic leukemia: a review and discussion of variant translocations. Arch Pathol Lab Med. 2015;139(10):1308–13.
52. Koken MH, Daniel MT, Gianni M, et al. Retinoic acid, but not arsenic trioxide, degrades the PLZF/RARalpha fusion protein, without inducing terminal differentiation

or apoptosis, in a RA-therapy resistant t(11;17)(q23;q21) APL patient. Oncogene. 1999;18(4):1113–8.
53. Specchia G, Lo Coco F, Vignetti M, et al. Extramedullary involvement at relapse in acute promyelocytic leukemia patients treated or not with all-trans retinoic acid: a report by the Gruppo Italiano Malattie Ematologiche dell'adulto. J Clin Oncol. 2001;19:4023–8.
54. De Botton S, Sanz M, Chevret S, et al. Extramedullary relapse in acute promyelocytic leukemia treated with all-trans retinoic acid and chemotherapy. European APL group; PETHEMA Group. Leukemia. 2006;20:35–41.
55. Breccia M, Carmosino I, Diverio D, et al. Early detection of meningeal localization in acute promyelocytic leukemia patients with high presenting leukocyte count. Br J Haematol. 2003;120:266–70.
56. Sanz MA, Grimwade D, Tallmann MS, et al. Guidelines on the management of acute promyelocytic leukemia: recommendations from an expert panel on behalf of the European LeukemiaNet. Blood. 2009;113:1875–91.
57. Breccia M, Petti MC, Testi AM, et al. Ear involvement in acute promyelocytic leukemia at relapse: a disease-associated sanctuary? Leukemia. 2002;16(6): 1127–30.

Acute Promyelocytic Leukemia in Developing Countries: A Chemotherapy-Based Approach

17

Luisa Corrêa de Araújo Koury, Raul Ribeiro, and Eduardo M. Rego

Geographical Differences in APL Frequency Among AML Subtypes

Although the actual incidence of acute promyelocytic leukemia (APL) is not known, studies show that it can vary by ethnic group. Large cooperative groups in the United States and Europe have reported that APL comprises 5–13% of acute myeloid leukemia (AML) in Caucasian patients [1–4]. A population-based report from the Swedish Adult Acute Leukemia Registry that included 98% of all cases of acute leukemias found that APL constituted 3.2% of all AML cases [5]. In contrast, several studies reported an APL frequency of more than 20% among patients with AML in Latin American countries [6–11].

In 1996, Douer et al. reported a significantly higher frequency of APL (37.5% in those with AML) in patients of Latino origin than in those of non-Latino origin (6.5%) at the Los Angeles County—University of Southern California Medical Center [4]. Although this study suggested a genetic predisposition to APL, it was limited by the absence of a clear definition of the genetic background of Latinos. However, these findings were corroborated by studies reporting that APL represents 20% or more of all patients with AML in Brazil (28.2%) [6, 7], Mexico (20%) [8], Venezuela (27.8%) [9], Peru (22%) [10], and Costa Rica (34%) [11]. It is important to note that all these studies were based on hospital registries, and it was therefore not possible to estimate the actual incidence and prevalence of APL in patients from these countries. In a study data from 709 patients with APL in the Surveillance, Epidemiology, and End Results (SEER) Program, Matasar et al. [12] found that Hispanics did not have greater lifetime incidence rates than did whites. However, the age distribution for Hispanics was significantly different from that for non-Hispanic whites, with children aged 1–19 years and adults aged 20–44 years having a higher incidence of APL.

Challenges in the Diagnosis and Treatment of APL in Developing Countries

In an analysis of 157 patients with APL treated from January 2003 to March 2006 at 12 Brazilian institutions, Jácomo et al. reported a death rate of 32% during induction and 10.5% during

L.C. de Araújo Koury, M.D. • E.M. Rego, M.D., Ph.D. (✉)
Department of Internal Medicine, Medical School of Ribeirão Preto and Centre for Cell-Based Therapy, University of São Paulo, São Paulo, SP, Brazil
e-mail: rego.eduardousp@gmail.com

R. Ribeiro, M.D.
Division of Leukemia/Lymphoma, Department of Oncology, St. Jude Children's Research Hospital, Memphis, TN, USA

O. Abla et al. (eds.), *Acute Promyelocytic Leukemia*, https://doi.org/10.1007/978-3-319-64257-4_17

consolidation and a 2-year overall survival (OS) rate of less than 60% [13]. In contrast, long-term disease-free survival (DFS) rates of approximately 85% have been reported by European and North American groups [14].

The poor outcomes of patients with APL at Brazilian institutions were attributed to a combination of factors such as high frequency of patients with severe bleeding and infectious complications at presentation, difficulties in accessing healthcare services, and delay in establishing a diagnosis and initiating specific treatment. Another important barrier in the management of patients with APL was the high cost of mandatory tests required for genetic confirmation of APL, shipping of bone marrow samples to central reference laboratories for diagnosis, and the availability of medications [13, 15].

In 2004, the International Consortium on Acute Promyelocytic Leukemia (IC-APL), an initiative of the International Members Committee of the American Society of Hematology, was created with the objective of improving the outcomes of patients with APL. The consortium published guidelines for the management of patients with APL, including diagnosis, supportive care, and specific treatment adapted to the local or regional capacities [16].

Diagnostic Tests for APL

APL is considered a medical emergency, and therefore a method for rapid diagnosis needs to be readily available. Although the morphologic and immunophenotypic features of leukemia cells are usually suggestive of the diagnosis, it is necessary to identify the APL-specific translocation t(15;17), which results in the *PML–RARA* fusion in leukemic cells, at the chromosome, DNA, RNA, or protein levels. The most common diagnostic tests are karyotyping, fluorescence in situ hybridization (FISH), and reverse transcription polymerase chain reaction (RT-PCR). Although all these methods have high specificity, some considerations need to be made when selecting an assay suited for local healthcare settings. FISH is a rapid test, but its use is limited in developing countries due to high costs. Karyotyping is expensive and time-consuming and needs specialized laboratories and personnel. RT-PCR is the gold standard to confirm the diagnosis of APL with high specificity and sensitivity and is less expensive than FISH and karyotyping; however, it takes approximately 2 days to obtain the results.

The anti-PML immunofluorescence assay is an alternative to the more sophisticated and expensive assays for confirming the diagnosis of APL. The anti-PML antibody is directed against the amino-terminal region of the human PML gene product and produces a characteristic speckled nuclear pattern that reflects the localization of the protein into discrete structures (5–20 per nucleus) called PML nuclear bodies. The architecture of PML nuclear bodies appears to be disrupted in APL cells that harbor the t(15;17), thus resulting in a change in the nuclear staining pattern from speckled (wild-type PML protein) to microgranular (PML–RARA fusion protein) (Fig. 17.1). This assay is a simple, rapid (<6 h), and inexpensive method to diagnose APL and has been essential for the success of the collaborative protocol of IC-APL [17–19].

In an interim analysis of 130 patients in the IC-APL protocol, the anti-PML assay showed excellent concordance with RT-PCR and/or karyotyping. In 15 patients, diagnosis of APL was suspected on the basis of morphologic analysis, but results of the anti-PML assay were negative. Further, RT-PCR did not reveal the *PML/RARA* rearrangement, and cytogenetic analysis did not detect t(15;17) in any of these patients. Further, of 115 patients in whom the anti-PML assay was positive, *PML/RARA* transcripts were confirmed by RT-PCR in 59, by cytogenetics in 5, and by both methods in 51 patients [19]. These findings support the agreement between the anti-PML assay and RT-PCR and cytogenetic analysis. However, although the anti-PML test is very specific, it has low sensitivity and is not reliable to monitor minimal residual disease (MRD).

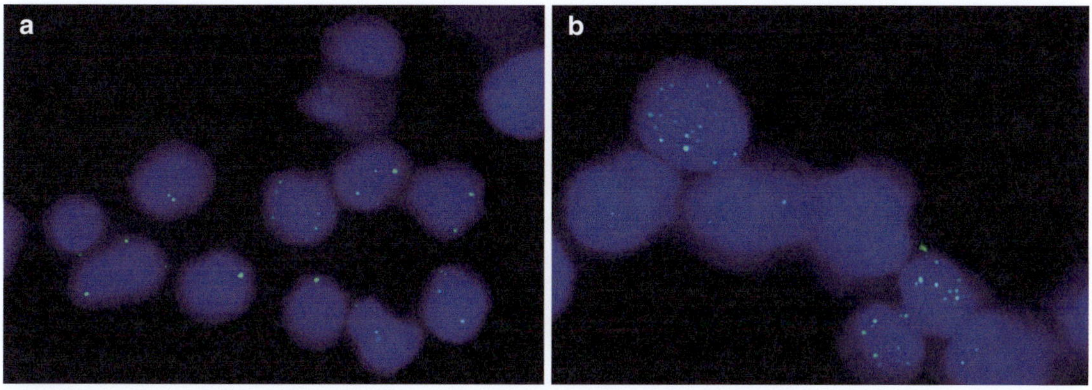

Fig. 17.1 Anti-PML immunofluorescence assay. (**a**) Negative: a characteristic nuclear speckled pattern showing the localization of the protein into discrete structures (PML nuclear bodies). (**b**) Positive: architecture of PML nuclear bodies appears to be disrupted in APL cells that harbor the t(15;17), thus resulting in a nuclear microgranular pattern (PML–RARA fusion protein)

Supportive Care Measures

The prompt initiation of all-*trans*-retinoic acid (ATRA) treatment is key to determining patient outcome, because it reduces the risk of fatal bleedings and early mortality. In the IC-APL protocol, the timely administration of ATRA was ensured by making it available in satellite pharmacies at the emergency rooms of participant institutions. ATRA treatment was initiated on the basis of suspicion of APL before genetic confirmation. In addition, aggressive transfusion support was immediately initiated to maintain platelet counts above 30,000–50,000/μL and the fibrinogen level above 150 mg/dL, and levels were monitored at least once daily [16, 19, 20].

IC-APL 2006 Treatment Regimen

The IC-APL 2006 treatment regimen consisted of the combination of ATRA and anthracycline-based chemotherapy, which was previously used in the Programa Español de Tratamiento en Hematologia/Dutch–Belgian Hemato-Oncology Cooperative Group (PETHEMA/HOVON) LPA2005 trial. However, idarubicin was replaced by daunorubicin because of its lower cost and easier availability in participating countries. Idarubicin was replaced by daunorubicin at a ratio of 1:5 (Fig. 17.2) [19].

After the genetic confirmation of APL, induction treatment was initiated with daunorubicin (60 mg/m^2/day given as an intravenous (IV) bolus on days 2, 4, 6, and 8 (except for patients aged >70 years, who received only three doses)). Oral ATRA (45 mg/m^2 divided in two daily doses or at 25 mg/m^2/day for patients aged ≤20 years) was administered until complete hematological response (CHR) was achieved. Patients with white blood cell (WBC) counts higher than 5000/μL at presentation or during the first 2 weeks of ATRA therapy received prophylaxis against differentiation syndrome (DS) with IV dexamethasone (2.5 mg/m^2/12 h for 15 days).

Patients who achieved CHR received three monthly consolidation courses with ATRA (45 mg/m^2/day divided into two daily doses for 2 weeks) and anthracycline-based chemotherapy, with the dose and duration adapted to the assessed risk of relapse, as outlined by the PETHEMA and Gruppo Italiano per le Malattie Ematologiche dell'Adulto (GIMEMA). This regimen was chosen to provide more intensive treatment for high-risk patients and minimize toxicities in low-risk patients [20, 21].

Low-risk patients received ATRA in combination with daunorubicin (25 mg/m^2 on days 1–4) in cycle 1, mitoxantrone (10 mg/m^2 on days 1–3) in cycle 2, and daunorubicin (60 mg/m^2 on day 1) in cycle 3. Intermediate-risk patients received intensified consolidation by increasing the dose

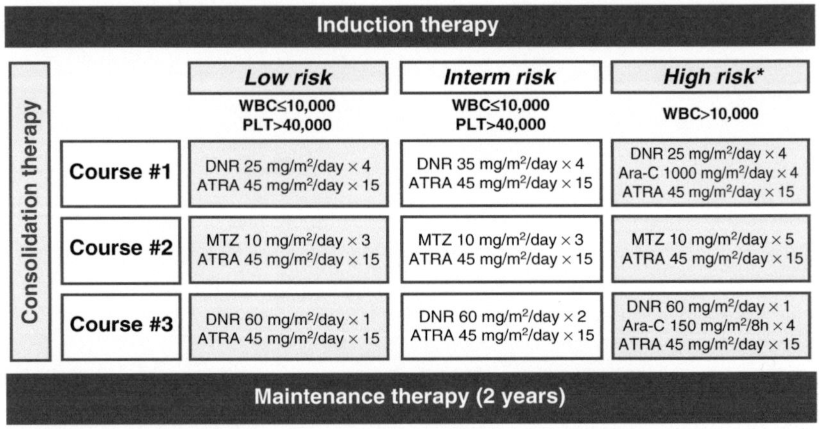

Fig. 17.2 The IC-APL 2006 treatment regimen

of daunorubicin to 35 mg/m^2 in cycle 1 and repeating the infusion at 60 mg/m^2 for 2 days in the third cycle. For high-risk patients, consolidation was further intensified by adding cytarabine in cycle 1 (1000 mg/m^2 on days 1–4) and cycle 3 (150 mg/m^2 every 8 h on days 1–4). In addition, mitoxantrone (10 mg/m^2/day) was administered for 5 days in cycle 2; the dosage of anthracyclines in cycles 1 and 3 was similar to that for low-risk patients. High-risk patients older than 60 years were treated as intermediate-risk patients.

At the end of the third consolidation, the presence of the *PML/RARA* rearrangement was assessed by RT-PCR. Patients in molecular remission received maintenance treatment for 2 years with ATRA (45 mg/m^2/day divided into two doses for 2 weeks each every 3 months) along with intramuscular or oral methotrexate (15 mg/m^2/week) and oral mercaptopurine (50 mg/m^2/day) during the ATRA pause. Central nervous system prophylaxis was not given. MRD was evaluated every 3 months for 2 years after the end of maintenance by RT-PCR for *PML/RARA*.

The IC-APL 2006 trial resulted in improved treatment outcomes for patients with APL in developing countries. The CHR rate was of 85%, and the mortality rate during induction was 15%. The main causes of early death were hemorrhage (48.1%), infection (25.9%), and DS (18.5%) [19]. Compared with the results reported by Jácomo et al. [13], there was a reduction in the mortality rate (~50%) during induction and an improvement in the 2-year OS of approximately 30% over historical controls. The DFS was 91%, and the 2-year cumulative incidence of relapse was 4.5%.

Because of the similarity in the design of the IC-APL 2006 trial and PETHEMA/HOVON LPA2005 trials [19, 21], a matched-pair analysis was performed to compare the efficacies of daunorubicin and idarubicin. Eligibility criteria for both trials were as follows: a diagnosis of de novo APL with demonstration of the t(15;17) and/or of the *PML/RARA* rearrangement in leukemic blasts, normal hepatic and renal function, no cardiac contraindication to anthracyclines, and an Eastern Cooperative Oncology Group performance status of less than 4. The study matched 175 patients in the IC-APL trial with 350 patients from the PETHEMA/HOVON LPA2005 trial [21]. Daunorubicin and idarubicin had similar antileukemic efficacy in terms of primary resistance, molecular persistence, and molecular and hematologic relapse. There were no significant differences in the number of deaths due to hemorrhage, infection, and DS between both cohorts [21].

The complete remission (CR) rate was significantly higher in the PETHEMA/HOVON (94%) cohort than in the IC-APL cohort (85%) (P = 0.002), but all induction failures in both cohorts were due to death during induction. There was also a significantly higher non-relapse mortality rate during consolidation in the IC-APL cohort than the PETHEMA/HOVON cohort (4.8% vs. 1.2%, respectively; P = 0.04), likely due to suboptimal prevention and treatment of infections during consolidation. Another important finding was a significantly higher DS-associated mortality among those with moderate or severe DS in the IC-APL cohort than in the PETHEMA/HOVON cohort (12% vs. 3%, respectively; $P = 0.01$), possibly due to differences in supportive care and management of DS [21]. Nonetheless, the IC-APL trial is ongoing, because it has already demonstrated that global networking and the use of protocols adapted to local resources can help reduce the gap between developed and developing countries with regard to the quality of care and treatment outcomes.

A chemotherapy-free ATRA and arsenic trioxide (ATO) regimen has recently emerged as the new standard care for patients with APL. Patients with the most curable form of AML who receive this regimen have higher cure rates than those given the standard ATRA plus chemotherapy regimen [22, 23]. Unfortunately, the high cost of ATO limits the access of this treatment for Latin American patients with APL. The results obtained for ATO by hematologists in India, where the drug is affordable, are very promising [24]. The future challenge for hematologists working in developing countries is to overcome the hurdle of ATO availability and compare the results obtained with ATRA plus chemotherapy versus ATRA plus ATO.

Lessons Learned and Recommendations

- A suspected diagnosis of APL is considered a medical emergency. ATRA and aggressive supportive care need to be initiated even before the molecular confirmation of APL.
- Anti-PML antibody test is a simple, rapid, and inexpensive method to diagnose APL.
- When used in combination with ATRA, daunorubicin and idarubicin have comparable efficacy.
- DS prophylaxis with dexamethasone (2.5 mg/m^2/12 h IV for 15 days) is indicated in patients with WBC counts higher than 5000/μL at presentation or during the first 2 weeks of ATRA.
- Risk-adapted consolidation courses provide more intensive treatment in high-risk patients and minimize toxicities in those with low-risk disease.
- Cure rates seen for patients with APL in developed countries can be achieved in developing countries by collaborative networking and using protocols adapted to local resources.

References

1. Cassileth PA, Lynch E, Hines JD, Oken MM, Mazza JJ, Bennett JM, et al. Varying intensity of postremission therapy in acute myeloid leukemia. Blood. 1992;79(8):1924–30.
2. Mayer RJ, Davis RB, Schiffer CA, Berg DT, Powell BL, Schulman P, et al. Intensive postremission chemotherapy in adults with acute myeloid leukemia. N Engl J Med. 1994;331:896–903.
3. Head D, Kopecky KJ, Weick J, Files JC, Ryan D, Foucar K, et al. Effect of aggressive daunomycin therapy on survival in acute promyelocytic leukemia. Blood. 1995;86:1717–28.
4. Douer D, Preston-Martin S, Chang E, Nichols PW, Watkins KJ, Levine AM. High frequency of acute promyelocytic leukemia among Latinos with acute myeloid leukemia. Blood. 1996;87(1):308–13.
5. Lehmann A, Ravin A, Carlsson L, Antunovic P, Deneberg S, Mollagard L, et al. Continuing high early death rate in acute promyelocytic leukemia: a population-based report from the Swedish Adult Acute Leukemia Registry. Leukemia. 2011;25:1128–34.
6. Rego EM, Jácomo RH. Epidemiology and treatment of acute promyelocytic leukemia in Latin America. Mediterr J Hematol Infect Dis. 2011;3(1):e2011049.
7. Melo RA, de Vasconcellos JF, Melo FC, Machado CG, Lacerda TM, Souto FR. PML-RARalpha fusion gene transcripts and biological features in acute promyelocytic leukemia patients. Clin Lab Haematol. 2006;28:126–9.
8. Ruiz-Arguelles GJ. Promyelocytic leukaemia in Mexican mestizos [letter]. Blood. 1997;89:348–9.
9. De Salvo L, Weir Medina J, Gómez Sánchez O, de Baena ES, de Ramos BU, Guevara J, et al. Acute promyelocytic leukemia in the west of Venezuela. Sangre (Barc). 1989;34:329–31.
10. Otero JC, Santillana S, Fereyros G. High frequency of acute promyelocytic leukemia among Latinos with acute myeloid leukemia. Blood. 1996;88:377.
11. Boza WB, Cruz GJ, Saenz MP, Umaña CM. High incidence of acute promyelocytic leukemia in the Caucasian population: the Costa Rica experience. Am J Hematol. 2004;76(1):96–7.
12. Matasar MJ, Ritchie EK, Consedine N, Magai C, Neugut AI. Incidence rates of acute promyelocytic

leukemia among Hispanics, blacks, Asians, and non-Hispanic whites in the United States. Eur J Cancer Prev. 2006;15(4):367–70.
13. Jácomo RH, Melo RA, Souto FR, de Mattos ER, de Oliveira CT, Fagundes EM, et al. Clinical features and outcomes of 134 Brazilians with acute promyelocytic leukemia who received ATRA and anthracyclines. Haematologica. 2007;92(10):1431–2.
14. Wang ZY, Chen Z. Acute promyelocytic leukemia: from highly fatal to highly curable. Blood. 2008;111(5):2505–15.
15. Koury LCA, Ganser A, Berliner N, Rego EM. Treating acute promyelocytic leukaemia in Latin America: lessons from the International Consortium on Acute Leukaemia experience. Br J Haematol. 2017;177(6):979–83.
16. Pagnano KBB, Rego EM, Rohr C, Chauffaille ML, Jacomo RH, Bittencourt R, et al. Guidelines on the diagnosis and treatment for acute promyelocytic leukemia: Associação Brasileira de Hematologia, Hemoterapia e Terapia Celular Guidelines Project: Associação Médica Brasileira – 2013. Rev Bras Hematol Hemoter. 2014;36(1):71–92.
17. Falini B, Flenghi L, Fagioli M, Lo Coco F, Cordone I, Diverio D, et al. Immunocytochemical diagnosis of acute promyelocytic leukemia (M3) with the monoclonal antibody PG-M3 (anti-PML). Blood. 1997;90(10):4046–53.
18. Dimov ND, Medeiros LJ, Kantarjian HM, Cortes JE, Chang KS, Bueso-Ramos CE, Ravandi F. Rapid and reliable confirmation of acute promyelocytic leukemia by immunofluorescence staining with an antipromyelocytic leukemia antibody: the M.D. Anderson Cancer Center experience of 349 patients. Cancer. 2010;116(2):369–76.
19. Rego EM, Kim HT, Ruiz-Argüelles GJ, Undurraga MS, Uriarte MR, Jácomo RH, et al. Improving acute promyelocytic leukemia (APL) outcome in developing countries through networking: results of the International Consortium on APL. Blood. 2013;121(11):1935–43.
20. Sanz MA, Grimwade D, Tallman MS, Lowenberg B, Fenaux P, Estey EH, et al. Management of acute promyelocytic leukemia: recommendations from an Expert Panel on behalf of the European LeukemiaNet. Blood. 2009;113:1875–91.
21. Sanz MA, Montesinos P, Kim HT, Ruiz-Argüelles GJ, Undurraga MS, Uriarte MR, et al. All-trans retinoic acid with daunorubicin or idarubicin for risk-adapted treatment of acute promyelocytic leukaemia: a matched-pair analysis of the PETHEMA LPA-2005 and IC-APL studies. Ann Hematol. 2015;94:1347–56.
22. Lo-Coco F, Avvisati G, Vignetti M, Thiede C, Orlando SM, Iacobelli S, et al. Retinoic acid and arsenic trioxide for acute promyelocytic leukemia. N Engl J Med. 2013;369(2):111–21.
23. Burnett AK, Russell NH, Hills RK, Bowen D, Kell J, Knapper S, et al. Arsenic trioxide and all-trans retinoic acid treatment for acute promyelocytic leukemia in all risk groups (AML17): results of a randomised, controlled, phase 3 trial. Lancet Oncol. 2015;16:1295–305.
24. Mathews V, George B, Chendamarai E, Lakshmi KM, Desire S, Balasubramanian P, et al. Single-agent arsenic trioxide in the treatment of newly diagnosed acute promyelocytic leukemia: long-term follow-up data. J Clin Oncol. 2010;28:3866–71.

Acute Promyelocytic Leukemia in Developing Countries: ATO-Based Approach

18

Vikram Mathews

Introduction

Significant and rapid advances in the management of acute promyelocytic leukemia (APL) over the last few decades have transformed it from a leukemia with the worst to one with the best prognosis [1]. With current diagnostic and treatment strategies, it is reasonable to expect greater than 90–95% remission rates along with long-term survival and possible cure exceeding 80%, even in high-risk APL [1]. Remarkably, most of these improvements in clinical outcome occurred without intensification of conventional chemotherapy but with the combination of non-myelotoxic differentiating agents such as *all-trans* retinoic acid (ATRA) and arsenic trioxide (ATO). This in turn was facilitated and paralleled by the detailed understanding of the cellular and molecular pathogenesis of this leukemia, and as a result APL has become a model of bench to bedside and back scientific progress. In the developed world, challenges remain in the management of patients with high-risk APL and a small subset of patients with relapsed APL. There also remain significant challenges with early mortality in newly diagnosed patients. In developing countries, there are even more fundamental challenges related to access to proper diagnosis and therapy primarily dictated by the high cost of treating acute myeloid leukemia (AML) and APL with conventional myelosuppressive regimens. However, an advantage in developing countries is the ease of access to low-cost generics which can offset the high costs of conventional therapy.

V. Mathews, M.B.B.S., M.D., D.M.
Department of Haematology, Christian Medical College and Hospital, Vellore 632004, India
e-mail: vikram@cmcvellore.ac.in

Challenges in Treating Myeloid Leukemia in a Developing Country

That the financial cost of treating AML is very high is a well-recognized fact [2]. However, there is limited data that has systematically addressed this issue [2–4]. Available data would suggest that the cost of treating AML in a developed country varies from US$ 80,000 to >100,000/patient [2–5]. With conventional treatment of AML, it is recognized that most of this cost is not related to the individual chemotherapeutic drugs used to treat this condition, but rather from the high cost of supportive care measures during repeated cycles of prolonged neutropenia induced by conventional chemotherapy. In contrast, with ATO-based regimens in APL, when the so-called expensive patented and innovator ATO was used, the 3-year direct pharmacy cost of drugs was higher with an ATO + ATRA

O. Abla et al. (eds.), *Acute Promyelocytic Leukemia*, https://doi.org/10.1007/978-3-319-64257-4_18

regimen compared with a conventional ATRA + chemotherapy regimen (Euro 46,700 vs. 6700), though the cost of supportive care was a third of conventional therapy [6]. In spite of these costs, the combination of ATO + ATRA was found to be cost-effective compared to conventional ATRA + chemotherapy in an analysis done in the United States (US) [7].

It is important to place all the above cost analysis in the context that 70% of the countries in the world, contributing >70% of the world's population, have a gross national income (GNI)/capita of less than US$10,000 [8] and that in many of these countries in the absence of universal health-care insurance, for most patients, these expenses are "out-of-pocket" self-paid expenses. As a result, it is estimated that approximately 39 million people in India alone (a figure which is greater than the entire population of Australia) will fall below the poverty line every year [9, 10].

Even in developed countries with well-established cancer registries, such as the US "Surveillance, Epidemiology, and End Results (SEER)-Medicare database," there is up to 50% underreporting of the diagnosis of AML [11]. In developing countries, in the absence of such registries, there are limited available records of the actual incidence or prevalence of patients with myeloid leukemia. However, it is recognized that outside the major metropolis in many of these countries, the access to even basic diagnostic tests such as flow cytometry and molecular studies is not available [12, 13].

While significant advances have been made in the management of APL, the majority of these advances are based on well-controlled clinical trials from countries with universal health-care access which tend to have a significant bias in the patients enrolled being younger and having better performance scores and less comorbidities than the average patient with this diagnosis. There is limited real-world data of clinical outcomes with conventional ATRA + chemotherapy. In AML and in APL, when such data is available, the observations and conclusions often seem at odds with published clinical trial data [14].

Advantage and Access to Generic Pharmaceutical Agents in a Developing Country

The importance of access to generic pharmaceutical agents in reducing the cost of medical therapy is well recognized, even in developed countries [15, 16]. This is even more relevant in developing economies and countries due to the combination of the absence of health insurance and a predominantly self-pay system. In India, a country which fulfills the above criteria, data suggests that the use of generic chemotherapy drugs results in an annual savings of approximately US$ 843 million [17]. Whether ATO should have been patented or not has been a controversy that has been extensively debated in the past [18, 19]. Regardless of which side of the argument one favors, the reality is that there is a significant difference in the cost of ATO depending on whether the patent applies in a particular country or not. At the author's center in 1998, the actual costing of in-house manufacturing of 10 mg of ATO was approximately 20 Indian rupees, which at that time was the equivalent of US50 cents. Subsequently, the manufacturing was transferred to a local pharmaceutical company (INTAS Ltd., Ahmedabad, India), and the current cost for a 10 mg vial is 450 Indian rupees (~US$ 7). Currently the cost of ATO in North America and Europe is US$676 and 393 Euros/vial, respectively. As a result, the use of ATO is considered very expensive in many developed countries, while it is considered the least expensive option in many developing countries, when costing analysis is limited to drug costs.

Experience with Arsenic Trioxide in Treating Acute Promyelocytic Leukemia

Arsenical compounds were used as a medicine as early as 2000 BC [20] and were familiar to the early physicians (Hippocrates (460–377 BC) and Aristotle (384–322 BC)). Paracelsus (1493–1541 AD) used arsenical compounds extensively and was quoted saying what we now consider a universal truth for most therapeutic drugs, "All substances are poisons; the right dose differentiates a poison from a remedy" [20].

The prominence of ATO in the treatment of APL historically followed the studies with a traditional Chinese recipe called "Ailing 1." These early studies were conducted by Chinese investigators at Harbin Medical University, and they labeled this native preparation 713 (for the year and month that the study was initiated). Using this agent, more than 1000 patients with various malignancies were evaluated [21]. They soon noted that this agent worked best in the treatment of patients with APL. Two subsequent Chinese studies confirmed the benefit of this agent in APL [22, 23].

It was subsequently reported that a dual effect of ATO was seen on promyelocytic cell lines. At low doses (0.1–0.5 μmol/L), there was partial differentiation, and at higher doses, there was preferential apoptosis (0.5–2 μmol/L) [24]. This has been subsequently demonstrated by a number of other groups independently [25, 26]. The differentiation with ATO is incomplete and usually proceeds only until the myelocyte stage, following which it appears that apoptosis is the predominant mode of action [24]. More recent data suggests that ATO, and not ATRA, can eliminate the leukemia-initiating compartment in APL [27, 28]. This could partly explain why single agent ATO, but not ATRA, is able to induce durable remissions in the clinic. Since then, numerous reports on the use of ATO in the treatment of relapsed and newly diagnosed cases of APL have been published and summarized in a recent review [29].

Pharmacokinetics, Pharmacogenomics, Dose, and Schedule of Arsenic Trioxide

The lethal dose recorded in the literature is a single dose of more than 100 mg [11]. The dose of arsenic trioxide in the initial published study by Zhi-Xiang et al. [30] was 10 mg/day for adults until complete hematological remission (CR) was achieved. Subsequently a break of 30 days was given and a second course of 28 days administered. It is important to recognize that this dosing was based on earlier experience with doses used in native Chinese medicine and not on conventional phase I clinical trials addressing dose-limiting toxicity. The study reported by Soignet et al. [31] used a similar dose for adults but used a dose of 0.15 mg/kg/day for children with a maximum dose of 10 mg. From their experience, they noted that ATO is active in APL at a dose ranging from 0.06 to 0.2 mg/kg. Within this range, no difference in efficacy was noted. Subsequent studies have used similar dosages of ATO. Pharmacokinetic studies done at this dosage demonstrated that mean peak plasma levels of 6.85 μmol/L (range, 5.54–7.30) were achieved. The plasma half-life was 12.13 ± 3.31 h. Importantly, these parameters did not change with continuous administration [30]. Reports of daily urinary excretion in the literature vary from 1–8% to 32–65% of the daily administered dose and more importantly are continued even after the drug administration had been stopped [30, 32]. There is limited data on the dose and scheduling of ATO in the event of significant renal failure or for patients on dialysis [33]. While the cumulative level of arsenic increases in the body (as demonstrated in hair and nail analysis) with continuous administration, the urinary excretion continues even after the ATO administration has stopped leading to a gradual decrease in the cumulative amount of the drug in the body. In our own experience, there was no significant difference in the ATO content from patients and normal control hair and nail samples during long-term follow-up [34]. This was the rationale for giving the 4-week intervals between the courses of ATO in our regimen [35], since these intervals were intended to reduce the cumulative dose significantly.

This pattern of ATO exposure is very different from that seen with environmental exposure where there is a slow but constant accumulation of arsenic leading to a toxicity profile that is different from that seen when ATO is used in therapy at the currently recommended doses and schedules. Extrapolating and anticipating the toxicity profile seen with chronic environmental exposure to the potential toxicity with currently used dosage schedules of ATO are unfair, unwarranted, and without any scientific basis. In the absence of a dose-finding phase I clinical trial, there is insufficient data on the upper limit of a safe therapeutic dose. It is of interest to note that in our initial cohort we noted a decreased risk of relapse among patients who had hepatotoxicity versus those who did not follow treatment with ATO [36]. This would suggest that there is either a significant interindividual variation in biotransformation of this agent, and as a result some patients were receiving less than an optimal dose, or that there were yet unknown variables that resulted in this association [36]. There is a need to revisit what is the optimal dose of ATO to treat APL in a large clinical trial. Furthermore, there is very limited data on the optimal duration of administration of ATO as a single agent in the management of APL. Based on the general consensus that maintenance was required in the management of APL, at our center, we arbitrarily opted for a 6-month duration of maintenance [35]. Recently published data from Iran suggests that four courses of ATO were significantly better than two [37]. Zhou et al. reported treating children with ATO for prolonged periods of up to 3 years with very good efficacy and without significant toxicity [38]. However, the optimal schedule and cumulative dose of ATO remain to be defined.

It has been noted that there is considerable interindividual variation in susceptibility to ATO-induced toxicity, which is probably related to differences in the in vivo biotransformation of arsenic. This in turn could be a result of age, nutritional status, comorbid conditions, environmental factors, and genetic polymorphisms [39]. In addition to a poorly characterized arsenic methyltransferase, a number of other enzyme systems and polymorphisms have been shown to have an effect on arsenic methylation [39, 40]. Among these, polymorphism in the methylenetetrahydrofolate reductase (MTHFR) gene, which results in MTHFR deficiency in 10–20% of the Caucasian population, has been reported to be associated with increased arsenic-related neurotoxicity [41]. The glutathione S-transferases (GST) are a family of proteins that conjugate glutathione (GSH) to various electrophiles [42]. Chiou et al. reported that genetic polymorphisms of GST M1 and GST T1 altered the methylation of arsenic [43]. GSTs catalyze the GSH-dependent reduction of hydroperoxides to their corresponding alcohols and help prevent propagation of free radicals. It is conceivable that genetic polymorphisms in these genes could alter the biotransformation of ATO, which in turn could have an impact on the efficacy and toxicity profile of this drug. We had earlier reported that the hepatotoxicity profile in a cohort of patients with newly diagnosed APL treated at our center with a single agent ATO regimen was significantly associated with the homozygous mutant of MTHFR 1298 (C/C) ($RR = 8.75$, $P = 0.004$), and there was a trend toward an increased risk of hepatotoxicity associated with the GST M1 null genotype ($RR = 3.28$, $P = 0.06$) [36]. We had hypothesized then that alteration in biotransformation possibly leads to quantitative and qualitative differences in the methylated intermediaries that are generated; these differences could have an effect on the efficacy and toxicity profile of ATO. A recent study, in part, validates this hypothesis by suggesting that dimethylarsinous acid is more toxic than inorganic ATO and monomethylarsinic acid [44], which are some of the methylated intermediaries produced in vivo in humans and animals. It is possible to consider in future the use of pure or combination of methylated ATO derivatives with optimal therapeutic and toxicity profiles.

Clinical Experience with the Use of ATO in APL

The earliest clinical data available on the use of ATO in the treatment of APL was from two Chinese publications [45, 46]. In these studies, the CR rates varied from 65.6 to 84%, and long-term survival (>10 years) was seen in 9/32 patients in one of these studies [30]. Most of the early trials involved relapsed cases of APL. There is limited data on the use of this as a single agent in the management of newly diagnosed cases of APL. Even when used as a single agent for induction chemotherapy, the subsequent consolidation therapy varies making comparisons between the published data difficult to interpret.

Our early experience with ATO consisted of two patients who were treated in the early 1990s with what was then considered standard of care regimens, one with ATRA and one without. Both these patients relapsed and were sent on palliative care considering that therapeutic options were limited, very expensive, and associated with poor clinical outcome. These patients subsequently took treatment from an "Ayurvedic" (indigenous Indian medicine) practitioner and went into durable remissions. We were aware that the agent used by the practitioner contained ATO, but we were not sure of the dose used. The therapeutic "Ayurvedic" mix was administered continuously in these cases and for more than 5 years in one case. One of these patients developed severe arsenic keratosis and died of a secondary squamous epithelial carcinoma [47].

It was only after the publication in 1997 by Shen et al. that we had a sense of the dose of pure ATO that could be used in humans [30]. In 1998, we initiated a study using single agent ATO to treat APL, with intravenous ATO being manufactured in-house in our hospital pharmacy with appropriate quality control measures. Due to legal-related issues, we transferred this manufacturing process to the industry in 2001 (INTAS Pharmaceuticals Ltd., Matoda, Gujarat, India). Our observation was that there was no significant difference with the agent prepared by us or that subsequently manufactured by industry in terms of infusion-related toxicity or efficacy (unpublished data).

From January 1998 to December 2004, 72 newly diagnosed cases of APL were treated with a regimen of single agent ATO at our center. The details of the regimen were as previously reported [34, 35]. Overall 62 (86.1%) achieved a hematological remission, and a total of 13 patients relapsed. As previously reported by us, at a median follow-up of 60 months, the 5-year estimate of event-free survival (EFS), disease-free survival (DFS), and overall survival (OS) were 69 ± 5.5%, 80 ± 5.2%, and 74.2 ± 5.2%, respectively (Fig. 18.1) [35]. This data has since been validated by a subsequent multicenter trial in India involving seven centers across the country [48].

However, until very recently, large multicenter randomized controlled clinical trials (RCT) to validate such low toxicity ATO-based regimes were not available to challenge the conventional ATRA plus chemotherapy regimens. The first large multicenter phase II study that reported such an approach and relied predominantly on the synergistic effect of ATRA and ATO combination with a conventional anthracycline administration being limited to induction therapy came from the Australasian Leukaemia and Lymphoma Group (ALLG) APML4 study.

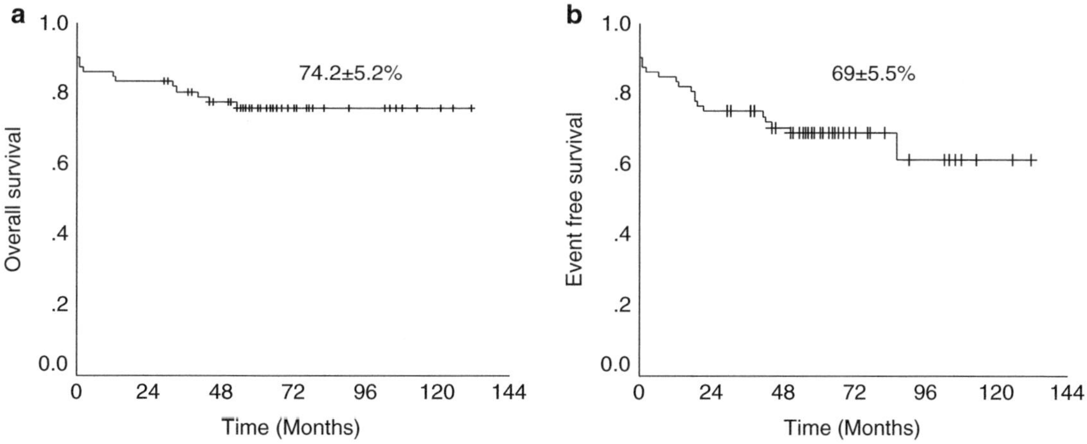

Fig. 18.1 Five-year Kaplan-Meier product limit estimate of (**a**) overall survival (n = 72) and (**b**) event-free survival (n = 72)

This was initially published in 2012 and was followed up with long-term data in 2016 [49]. Along with a similar approach but in a RCT design and with a regimen structure that was completely eliminated, all anthracyclines and other chemotherapeutic agents were reported by the combined Gruppo Italiano Malattie Ematologiche dell'Adulto, German-Austrian Acute Myeloid Leukaemia Study Group, and Study Alliance Leukaemia (GIMEMA-AMLSG-SAL) APL 0406 study in 2013 [50]. The APL 0406 study was limited to low- and intermediate-risk patients which account for two third to three quarters of patients with APL. This study demonstrated for the first time that the combination of ATRA and ATO without chemotherapy in induction and consolidation (four courses) and without maintenance therapy was superior to a conventional ATRA plus chemotherapy induction with repeated cycles of myelotoxic chemotherapy and 2 years of maintenance therapy. A similar RCT was reported by the UKMRC AML-17 trial which again demonstrated the superiority of ATO + ATRA over conventional chemotherapy in all risk groups [51]. A significant difference in the MRC-AML17 trial was the addition of gemtuzumab ozagomycin (GO) in the treatment of high-risk cases.

Based on the published literature [34, 52, 53] and experience, the data would suggest that it would be possible to cure APL in about 40–60% of patients with single agent ATO alone, and for the remaining low- and intermediate-risk patients, probably a combination of ATRA and ATO would suffice as demonstrated in the GIMEMA-AMLSG-SAL-APL 0406 study, without maintenance therapy in either of these hypothetical subsets. This approach would be truly beneficial for patients with APL in developing countries since with generic ATO, the cost of treatment would be very low in the absence of significant cytopenias and requirement of supportive care, especially post induction therapy. For the truly high-risk patients, the addition of an anthracycline, at least, in induction is probably warranted, and the role of maintenance therapy remains to be further evaluated. The data from major studies using either single agent ATO or ATO as a major component in frontline therapy [37, 38, 49–51, 54–56] is summarized in Table 18.1.

Table 18.1 Summary of studies using arsenic trioxide in frontline therapy in the treatment of APL

	N	CR	EFS/DFS
Mathews et al. [34]	72	86%	5-year EFS 69%
			5-year OS 74%
Ghavamzadeh et al. [37]	197	86%	5-year OS 64%
			5-year DFS 67%
Hu et al. [56] (+ATRA[a]+chemo)	85	94%	5-year EFS 89% 5-year OS 92%
Ravandi et al. [54] (+ATRA, +GO[b])	82	91%	3-year OS 85%
Niu et al. [60]	11	73%	1-year OS 73%
Powell et al. [80]	244	NA[c]	3-year EFS 80%
	(RCT[d] ATO post induction)		3-year OS 86%
Gore et al. [55]	45	NA	3-year EFS 76%
	(ATO post induction)		3-year OS 88%
Iland et al. [49]	124	95%	2-year OS 93.2%
Lo-Coco et al. [50]	*RCT: only low- and intermediate-risk groups*		
ATO + ATRA	77	100%	2-year EFS 97%
Conventional	79	95%	2-year EFS 86%
AK Burnett et al. [51]	*RCT: all risk groups. High-risk group also received GO*		
ATO + ATRA	119	94%	4-year EFS 91%
Conventional	116	89%	4-year EFS 70%

[a]*ATRA* all-trans retinoic acid
[b]*GO* gemtuzumab
[c]*NA* not applicable
[d]*RCT* randomized controlled trial

Toxicity Profile of Arsenic Trioxide

The toxicity profile in most studies reported to date was mild as illustrated in a publication from our center [35]. Our experience with single agent ATO was that there were no infusion-related toxicities, alopecia, or evidence of exacerbation of coagulopathy. Post induction, almost all patients for the rest of the duration of treatment had ECOG performance scores of 0 or 1. The non-hematological toxicities in most studies were mild, were frequently reverted on continuing ATO, and in the rest were reversible on discontinuing the drug for an interval of 1–2 weeks [35]. There were no sudden deaths attributable to a cardiac event in this series of patients, and during long-term follow-up, there were no cases with clinical cardiac dysfunction. There were no documented second malignancies in any of the long-term follow-up cohorts to date that could be attributed to the use of ATO. With the exception of some early reports of increased hepatic and cardiac toxicity [57–60], the majority of subsequent reports using ATO in newly diagnosed cases is similar to our experience [37, 38, 54–56].

There have been periodical major concerns raised about the administration of ATO. Very early there was a concern about cardiac arrhythmia-related sudden deaths in patients with APL who were treated with ATO. Almost all these deaths occurred during induction in previously heavily treated patients [57–59]. There have been no such deaths reported when ATO was used for treating a number of other malignancies, albeit in stable patients. Similarly, sudden death does not seem to occur when ATO is administered to APL patients who are in remission (none reported in the literature). The role of QTc interval prolongation and limitations of the corrected QTc interval value generated with tachycardia due to any cause such as infection have been reviewed previously, and it is increasingly recognized and accepted that QTc prolongation is an electrocardiographic phenomenon with little clinical significance in the majority of patients [61]. This does not mean we should not monitor it or ignore it, though response should be judicious and clinically appropriate. It has been reported that in more than 2900 cases treated by US FDA-approved ATO, there have been no arrhythmia-related deaths [61]. Secondly, there was a suggestion that acute hepatic failure and death from hepatotoxicity occurred with ATO [60]. There have been no other major reports since this initial publication about two decades ago. This has definitely not been our experience with more than 250 newly diagnosed and relapsed APL patients treated to date at our center.

There has always been a concern of second malignancies with the use of ATO. This is based on in vitro experiments suggesting oxidative DNA damage [62] and clinical observations from cases with long-term environmental exposure. This theoretical concern is in contrast to the available clinical data. In early reports of investigators from China, it was noted that there was no increase in second malignancies in patients followed up for 10 years [30]. A similar observation was made in 1982, in a cohort of 479 patients who had been treated with Fowler's solution [potassium arsenite] for duration varying from 2 weeks to 12 years during the period 1945–1969. The median cumulative dose in this cohort was 448 mg. There was a marginal increase in fatal and nonfatal skin cancers but no increase in the incidence of internal malignancies [63].

There have been concerns raised about embryo toxicity based on animal models and some data from cases with environmental exposure [64]. Again, this is not based on data in humans exposed to what is currently defined as a therapeutic dose of ATO, and for obvious ethical reasons, this data is unlikely to be ever generated. However, in our series, seven of the patients (four women and three men) have had eight normal babies delivered after completing treatment with ATO [34], though all happened after completion of therapy. In this relatively young cohort, there were no reports of abortions, fetal abnormalities, or stillbirths in any couple. While we did not actively evaluate fertility, there were no reports of couples requesting evaluation for sterility [34].

In studies looking at long-term accumulation of ATO in the body by studying hair and nail levels, there was no significant difference in the ATO retention in controls and patients who had completed therapy at least 2 years earlier [34]. The median levels, even among the patients who had just completed therapy, were below the lower limit of the normal range described for normal controls by the Agency for Toxic Substances and Disease Registry (ATSDR based in Atlanta, Georgia, USA) (http://www.atsdr.cdc.gov/) [34].

Pattern and Timing of Hematopoietic Recovery Following Treatment with Single Agent ATO

In our initial series, the median time to achieve CR was 42 days (range, 24–70) [35]. However, this figure does not reflect the entire details of the kinetics of leukemia clearance and pattern of normal hematopoietic recovery. As reported initially by us, about two thirds of patients have a leukocytosis response after initiation of single agent ATO, while in about a third, there is prolonged leucopenia prior to gradual normalization [65]. The leukocytosis can at times be very rapid and alarming, and based on our early observations, we had introduced hydroxyurea to control it with a recommended sliding scale to adjust the dose depending on the WBC count [35]. We also noted that this was at times not adequate; thus, we allowed the use of an anthracycline in induction if there was rapid rise in the WBC counts after initiation of therapy at predefined levels and time points [35]. Some cases of leukocytosis were followed by a second leukopenic phase (variable duration) and then recovery to normal values [65] (a triphasic response; Fig. 18.2). Unlike ATRA plus chemotherapy schedules, the WBC count remains high (in two thirds) or very low (in one third), with a low platelet count and significant circulating promyelocytes for the first 2 weeks as illustrated in Fig. 18.3. At this time point, there is often a concern raised, among those not familiar with this agent, as to whether ATO is doing anything at all to the disease, and a consideration to change protocol or add on additional drugs is discussed. However, if the diagnosis is correct, with adequate support during this period and continuing ATO, all patients will go on to achieve CR. Another common observation in some cases is a clinically stable patient in the fourth week of

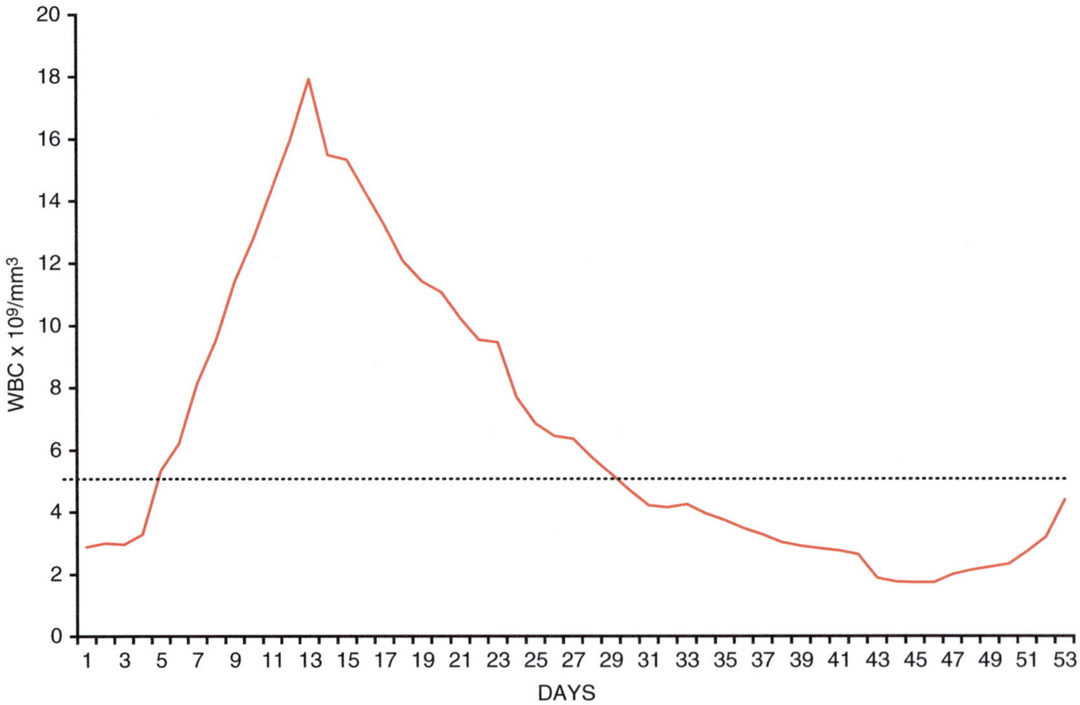

Fig. 18.2 Average WBC count among patients with a leukocytic response and who achieved complete remission ($n = 6$), illustrating the triphasic response

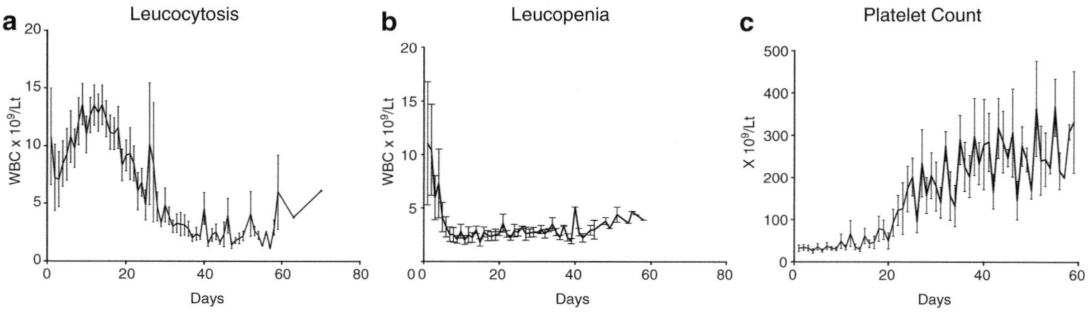

Fig. 18.3 The mean WBC and platelet count ± 1SE over time among patients treated on single agent ATO regimen. (**a**) WBC response among those with leukocytosis ($n = 40$). (**b**) WBC response among those without leukocytosis ($n = 18$). (**c**) Platelet count recovery ($n = 60$)

therapy, with a normal platelet count but very low WBC count, and a consideration to stop ATO is made based on the argument that the ATO is causing a myelosuppressive effect. Our experience would suggest that ATO can be safely continued for the intended duration, and one would probably be compromising treatment efficacy by prematurely stopping therapy at this time point.

Impact of Additional Cytogenetic and Molecular Markers Such as FLT3 Mutations on Clinical Response Following Treatment with ATO

The presence of cytogenetic abnormalities at diagnosis remains an important prognostic variable in patients with newly diagnosed AML [66]. Secondary cytogenetic changes have been reported to have an adverse impact in some subsets of AML, though in patients with APL treated with conventional chemotherapy, a similar adverse effect was not reported [67, 68]. At our center, we initially reported a small series of newly diagnosed patients with APL treated with single agent ATO in which there was no significant adverse impact of the presence of an additional karyotypic abnormality at diagnosis [69]. However, more recent analysis of our data (larger cohort) does suggest that there may be an adverse impact of an additional cytogenetic finding at diagnosis in newly diagnosed patients, though it was not significant in a multivariate analysis (unpublished data).

Fms-like tyrosine kinase 3 (FLT3) is a member of the class III receptor tyrosine kinase family and is expressed on hematopoietic progenitors [70, 71]. Mutations in the FLT3 receptors have been reported to be associated with a poor prognosis in both adult and pediatric patients with AML [70]. Mutations in the FLT3 receptor are commonly seen in patients with APL [70]. The common activating mutations of FLT3 in leukemia include the FLT3 internal tandem duplication (FLT3-ITD) and a point mutation in the activation loop (D835V) [70]. A recent gene expression profiling study reported that patients with APL could be segregated into those with and without a FLT3-ITD mutation, suggesting that these groups were biologically different [72]. A retrospective analysis of the impact of FLT3 mutations in patients with APL, treated with conventional ATRA plus chemotherapy regimens, reported a higher incidence of induction deaths in one study [73], while another study reported a trend toward a shorter OS [74]. More recently Chillon et al. [75] analyzed the Spanish cooperative group data and showed that patients with increased ITD mutant/wild-type ratio or longer ITD size displayed shorter 5-year relapse-free survival (RFS) ($P = 0.048$ and $P < 0.0001$, respectively), though patients with D835 mutations did not show differences in RFS or OS. In our series, we found that FLT3-ITD mutation in 21% and its presence did not impact the clinical outcome of patients treated with ATO [69]. We did however note a longer time to achieve molecular remission among those who were FLT3 mutation positive [69].

ATO for the Treatment of Relapsed APL

Patients who relapse following an ATRA/chemotherapy-based regimen can achieve a second CR in 60–95% of cases with chemotherapy, although the toxicity with such a regimen in this population approaches that seen with high-dose chemotherapy for AML [61]. There is a high incidence of ATRA resistance in this population especially if the relapse occurred within a year of completing an ATRA/chemotherapy protocol. In this setting, ATO is extremely effective in inducing molecular remissions in the majority of patients without the toxicity profile of combination chemotherapy and does not have cross-resistance with ATRA [61]. This is the only indication for which it is approved by the US Food and Drug Administration (FDA). Achieving molecular remission prior to a consolidation with an autologous hematopoietic stem cell transplant (HSCT), the preferred option in this setting, has a significant effect on long-term outcome. The use of single agent ATO as consolidation therapy after achieving molecular remission was less effective in this population with a 2-year OS of 41% in one series [61] and an EFS of 33% in another [60]. In our own series, we reported a significantly better clinical outcome in patients who were consolidated with an autologous HSCT versus those consolidated with ATO or ATO + ATRA following treatment of a frank hematological relapse of APL [76]. Based on the available data, it would be reasonable in patients with a hematological relapse to induce molecular remission with ATO and consolidate with an autologous HSCT in those who achieve molecular remission and consider an allogeneic HSCT for those who fail to achieve a molecular remission. We recently demonstrated the considerable synergy between ATO and a proteasome inhibitor. With in vitro studies, in vivo animal models, and preliminary clinical data, we have shown that the combination of bortezomib with ATO and ATRA is comparable to the effect of anthracycline with ATRA and ATO on malignant promyelocytes [77, 78]. In the evolving strategy of de-escalation of therapy in APL [79], the addition of bortezomib with ATO along with ATRA has the potential to further de-escalate the therapy in high-risk and relapsed APL by replacing the myelotoxic anthracycline with a relatively non-myelotoxic proteasome inhibitor.

Conclusions

There is no doubt as to the efficacy of ATO in the management of APL, and its position in the treatment algorithm of this condition has been recently re-defined as it can be considered standard of care for newly diagnosed cases. Based on the available data, it is clear that as a single agent, it is the most effective drug in the management of APL. For patients who have relapsed following conventional ATRA plus chemotherapy regimens, ATO is the established agent of choice to induce a second molecular remission. Preliminary concerns of fatal toxicity profile appear to be related more to the associated comorbid conditions than the drug itself, as noted by their absence when used in patients with newly diagnosed APL without comorbid conditions and in other malignant conditions. The ongoing concerns about potential long-term toxicity are not based on significant data. Better understanding of its in vivo biotransformation and the effect of the different methylated derivatives that are generated in this process might help further reduce its toxicity profile while enhancing its efficacy. This could be achieved by better methods to predict toxicity or efficacy, based on genetic polymorphisms that have an impact on biotransformation pathways, or by the use of specific methylated derivatives for therapy rather than the native compound. More research may potentially demonstrate that these derivatives have a more favorable therapeutic profile. In the developing world where the cost of generic ATO is low, the absence of grade III/IV neutropenia and mucositis along with the ability to administer the regimen in the outpatient setting post remission induction significantly reduces the cost of treating this condition in comparison to a standard ATRA plus chemotherapy regimen.

References

1. Wang ZY, Chen Z. Acute promyelocytic leukemia: from highly fatal to highly curable. Blood. 2008;111(5):2505–15.
2. Redaelli A, Botteman MF, Stephens JM, Brandt S, Pashos CL. Economic burden of acute myeloid leukemia: a literature review. Cancer Treat Rev. 2004;30(3):237–47.
3. Uyl-de Groot CA, Gelderblom-den Hartog J, Huijgens PC, Willemze R, van Ineveld BM. Costs of diagnosis, treatment, and follow up of patients with acute myeloid leukemia in the Netherlands. J Hematother Stem Cell Res. 2001;10(1):187–92.
4. Leunis A, Blommestein HM, Huijgens PC, Blijlevens NM, Jongen-Lavrencic M, Uyl-de Groot CA. The costs of initial treatment for patients with acute myeloid leukemia in the Netherlands. Leuk Res. 2012;37(3):245–50.
5. Stalfelt AM, Brodin H. Costs over time in conventional treatment of acute myeloid leukaemia. A study exploring changes in treatment strategies over two decades. J Intern Med. 1994;236(4):401–9.
6. Kruse M, Wildner R, Barnes G, Martin M, Mueller U, Lo-Coco F, et al. Budgetary impact of treating acute promyelocytic leukemia patients with first-line arsenic trioxide and retinoic acid from an Italian payer perspective. PLoS One. 2015;10(8):e0134587.
7. Tallman M, Lo-Coco F, Barnes G, Kruse M, Wildner R, Martin M, et al. Cost-effectiveness analysis of treating acute promyelocytic leukemia patients with arsenic trioxide and retinoic acid in the United States. Clin Lymphoma Myeloma Leuk. 2015;15(12):771–7.
8. Wikipedia. List of countries by GNI (nominal, Atlas method) per capita: http://en.wikipedia.org/wiki/List_of_countries_by_GNI_(nominal,_Atlas_method)_per_capita; 2014 [updated 10/06/201410/15/2014]. http://en.wikipedia.org/wiki/List_of_countries_by_GNI_(nominal,_Atlas_method)_per_capita.
9. Balarajan Y, Selvaraj S, Subramanian SV. Health care and equity in India. Lancet. 2011;377(9764):505–15.
10. Garg CC, Karan AK. Reducing out-of-pocket expenditures to reduce poverty: a disaggregated analysis at rural-urban and state level in India. Health Policy Plan. 2009;24(2):116–28.
11. Craig BM, Rollison DE, List AF, Cogle CR. Underreporting of myeloid malignancies by United States cancer registries. Cancer Epidemiol Biomark Prev. 2012;21(3):474–81.
12. Philip C, George B, Korula A, Srivastava A, Balasubramanian P, Mathews V. Treatment rates of paediatric acute myeloid leukaemia: a view from three tertiary centres in India—response to Gupta et al. Br J Haematol. 2016;175(2):347–9.
13. Philip C, George B, Ganapule A, Korula A, Jain P, Alex AA, et al. Acute myeloid leukaemia: challenges and real world data from India. Br J Haematol. 2015;170(1):110–7.
14. Juliusson G, Lazarevic V, Horstedt AS, Hagberg O, Hoglund M. Acute myeloid leukemia in the real world: why population-based registries are needed. Blood. 2012;119(17):3890–9.
15. Kerr D. Generic drugs: their role in better value cancer care. Ann Oncol. 2013;24(Suppl 5):v5. https://doi.org/10.1093/annonc/mdt321.
16. Experts in Chronic Myeloid Leukemia. The price of drugs for chronic myeloid leukemia (CML) is a reflection of the unsustainable prices of cancer drugs: from the perspective of a large group of CML experts. Blood. 2013;121(22):4439–42.
17. Lopes GL. Cost comparison and economic implications of commonly used originator and generic chemotherapy drugs in India. Ann Oncol. 2013;24(Suppl 5):v13–v6.
18. Cyranoski D. Arsenic patent keeps drug for rare cancer out of reach of many. Nat Med. 2007;13(9):1005.
19. Warrell RP Jr. Reply to 'Arsenic patent keeps drug for rare cancer out of reach for many'. Nat Med. 2007;13(11):1278.
20. Jolliffe DM. A history of the use of arsenicals in man. J R Soc Med. 1993;86(5):287–9.
21. Zhang TD. Treatment of acute granulocytic leukemia with "Ai ling No. 1"—clinical analysis and experimental research. Zhong Xi Yi Jie He Za Zhi. 1984;4(1):19–20.
22. Zhang PWS, Hu LH, Shi FD, Giu FQ, Hong GJ, et al. Treatment of acute promyelocytic leukemia with arsenic trioxide injection (713): clinical observations and study of action mode. Chin J Hematol. 1996;17:58–60.
23. Sun HDML, Hu XC, Zhang TD. Thirty two cases of treating acute promyelocytic leukemia by Ailing I therapy combined with syndrome differentiation treatment of traditional Chinese medicine. Chin J Comb Trad Chin Med West Med. 1992;1996(12):170–1.
24. Chen GQ, Shi XG, Tang W, Xiong SM, Zhu J, Cai X, et al. Use of arsenic trioxide (As2O3) in the treatment of acute promyelocytic leukemia (APL): I. As2O3 exerts dose-dependent dual effects on APL cells. Blood. 1997;89(9):3345–53.
25. Tang W, Chen G, Shi G. Double effects of arsenic trioxide (As2O3) on acute promyelocytic leukemic cell line. Zhonghua Yi Xue Za Zhi. 1997;77(7):509–12.
26. Chen Z, Wang ZY, Chen SJ. Acute promyelocytic leukemia: cellular and molecular basis of differentiation and apoptosis. Pharmacol Ther. 1997;76(1–3):141–9.
27. Zheng X, Seshire A, Ruster B, Bug G, Beissert T, Puccetti E, et al. Arsenic but not all-trans retinoic acid overcomes the aberrant stem cell capacity of PML/RARalpha-positive leukemic stem cells. Haematologica. 2007;92(3):323–31.
28. Ablain J, de The H. Revisiting the differentiation paradigm in acute promyelocytic leukemia. Blood. 2011;117(22):5795–802.
29. Mathews V, Chendamarai E, George B, Viswabandya A, Srivastava A. Treatment of acute promyelocytic leukemia with single-agent arsenic trioxide. Mediterr J Hematol Infect Dis. 2012;3(1):e2011056.
30. Shen ZX, Chen GQ, Ni JH, Li XS, Xiong SM, Qiu QY, et al. Use of arsenic trioxide (As2O3) in the

treatment of acute promyelocytic leukemia (APL): II. Clinical efficacy and pharmacokinetics in relapsed patients. Blood. 1997;89(9):3354–60.
31. Soignet SL, Maslak P, Wang ZG, Jhanwar S, Calleja E, Dardashti LJ, et al. Complete remission after treatment of acute promyelocytic leukemia with arsenic trioxide. N Engl J Med. 1998;339(19):1341–8.
32. Wang Z, Zhou J, Lu X, Gong Z, Le XC. Arsenic speciation in urine from acute promyelocytic leukemia patients undergoing arsenic trioxide treatment. Chem Res Toxicol. 2004;17(1):95–103.
33. Sweeney CJ, Takimoto C, Wood L, Porter JM, Tracewell WG, Darwish M, et al. A pharmacokinetic and safety study of intravenous arsenic trioxide in adult cancer patients with renal impairment. Cancer Chemother Pharmacol. 2010;66(2):345–56.
34. Mathews V, George B, Chendamarai E, Lakshmi KM, Desire S, Balasubramanian P, et al. Single-agent arsenic trioxide in the treatment of newly diagnosed acute promyelocytic leukemia: long-term follow-up data. J Clin Oncol. 2010;28(24):3866–71.
35. Mathews V, George B, Lakshmi KM, Viswabandya A, Bajel A, Balasubramanian P, et al. Single-agent arsenic trioxide in the treatment of newly diagnosed acute promyelocytic leukemia: durable remissions with minimal toxicity. Blood. 2006;107(7):2627–32.
36. Mathews V, Desire S, George B, Lakshmi KM, Rao JG, Viswabandya A, et al. Hepatotoxicity profile of single agent arsenic trioxide in the treatment of newly diagnosed acute promyelocytic leukemia, its impact on clinical outcome and the effect of genetic polymorphisms on the incidence of hepatotoxicity. Leukemia. 2006;20(5):881–3.
37. Ghavamzadeh A, Alimoghaddam K, Rostami S, Ghaffari SH, Jahani M, Iravani M, et al. Phase II study of single-agent arsenic trioxide for the front-line therapy of acute promyelocytic leukemia. J Clin Oncol. 2011;29(20):2753–7.
38. Zhou J, Zhang Y, Li J, Li X, Hou J, Zhao Y, et al. Single-agent arsenic trioxide in the treatment of children with newly diagnosed acute promyelocytic leukemia. Blood. 2010;115(9):1697–702.
39. Vahter M. Genetic polymorphism in the biotransformation of inorganic arsenic and its role in toxicity. Toxicol Lett. 2000;112–113:209–17.
40. Goering PLAH, Mass MJ, et al. The enigma of arsenic carcinogenesis: role of metabolism. Toxicol Sci. 1999;49:5–14.
41. Brouwer OF, Onkenhout W, Edelbroek PM, et al. Increased neurotoxicity of arsenic in MTHFR deficiency. Clin Neurol Neurosurg. 1992;94:307–10.
42. Pickett CB. Glutathione S-transferases: gene structure, regulation and biological function. Annu Rev Biochem. 1989;58:743–64.
43. Chiou HY, Hsueh YM, Hseih LL, et al. Arsenic methylation capacity, body retention and null genotypes of glutathione S-transferases M1 and T1 among current arsenic exposed residents of Taiwan. Mutat Res. 1997;386(3):197–207.
44. Naranmandura H, Carew MW, Xu S, Lee J, Leslie EM, Weinfeld M, et al. Comparative toxicity of arsenic metabolites in human bladder cancer EJ-1 cells. Chem Res Toxicol. 2011;24(9):1586–96.
45. Zhang PWS, Hu LH, Shi FD, Giu FQ, Hong GJ, et al. Arsenic trioxide treated 72 cases of acute promyelocytic leukemia. Chin J Hematol. 1996;2:58.
46. Sun HDML, Hu XC, Zhang TD. Ai-Lin I treated 32 cases of acute promyelocytic leukemia. Chin J Integrat Chin West Med. 1992;12:170.
47. Treleaven J, Meller S, Farmer P, Birchall D, Goldman J, Piller G. Arsenic and ayurveda. Leuk Lymphoma. 1993;10(4–5):343–5.
48. Mathews V, George B, Jijina F, Ross C, Nair R, Apte S, et al. Final analysis of a multi-center randomized controlled trial (IAPLSG04) to study the optimal duration of arsenic trioxide maintenance therapy in the treatment of newly diagnosed acute promyelocytic leukemia. ASH Annual Meeting Abstracts. 2011;118(21):426.
49. Iland HJ, Bradstock K, Supple SG, Catalano A, Collins M, Hertzberg M, et al. All-trans-retinoic acid, idarubicin, and IV arsenic trioxide as initial therapy in acute promyelocytic leukemia (APML4). Blood. 2012;120(8):1570–80; quiz 752.
50. Lo-Coco F, Avvisati G, Vignetti M, Thiede C, Orlando SM, Iacobelli S, et al. Retinoic acid and arsenic trioxide for acute promyelocytic leukemia. N Engl J Med. 2013;369(2):111–21.
51. Burnett AK, Russell NH, Hills RK, Bowen D, Kell J, Knapper S, et al. Arsenic trioxide and all-trans retinoic acid treatment for acute promyelocytic leukaemia in all risk groups (AML17): results of a randomised, controlled, phase 3 trial. Lancet Oncol. 2015;16(13):1295–305.
52. Ghavamzadeh A, Alimoghaddam K, Rostami S, Ghaffari SH, Jahani M, Iravani M, et al. Phase II study of single-agent arsenic trioxide for the front-line therapy of acute promyelocytic leukemia. J Clin Oncol. 2011;29(20):2753–7.
53. Estey E, Koller C, Cortes J, Reed P, Freireich E, Giles F, et al. Treatment of newly-diagnosed acute promyelocytic leukemia with liposomal all-trans retinoic acid. Leuk Lymphoma. 2001;42(3):309–16.
54. Ravandi F, Estey E, Jones D, Faderl S, O'Brien S, Fiorentino J, et al. Effective treatment of acute promyelocytic leukemia with all-trans-retinoic acid, arsenic trioxide, and gemtuzumab ozogamicin. J Clin Oncol. 2009;27(4):504–10.
55. Gore SD, Gojo I, Sekeres MA, Morris L, Devetten M, Jamieson K, et al. Single cycle of arsenic trioxide-based consolidation chemotherapy spares anthracycline exposure in the primary management of acute promyelocytic leukemia. J Clin Oncol. 2010;28(6):1047–53.
56. Hu J, Liu YF, Wu CF, Xu F, Shen ZX, Zhu YM, et al. Long-term efficacy and safety of all-trans retinoic acid/arsenic trioxide-based therapy in newly diagnosed acute promyelocytic leukemia. Proc Natl Acad Sci U S A. 2009;106(9):3342–7.

57. Ohnishi K, Yoshida H, Shigeno K, Nakamura S, Fujisawa S, Naito K, et al. Prolongation of the QT interval and ventricular tachycardia in patients treated with arsenic trioxide for acute promyelocytic leukemia. Ann Intern Med. 2000;133(11):881–5.
58. Westervelt P, Brown RA, Adkins DR, Khoury H, Curtin P, Hurd D, et al. Sudden death among patients with acute promyelocytic leukemia treated with arsenic trioxide. Blood. 2001;98(2):266–71.
59. Unnikrishnan D, Dutcher JP, Varshneya N, Lucariello R, Api M, Garl S, et al. Torsades de pointes in 3 patients with leukemia treated with arsenic trioxide. Blood. 2001;97(5):1514–6.
60. Niu C, Yan H, Yu T, Sun HP, Liu JX, Li XS, et al. Studies on treatment of acute promyelocytic leukemia with arsenic trioxide: remission induction, follow-up, and molecular monitoring in 11 newly diagnosed and 47 relapsed acute promyelocytic leukemia patients. Blood. 1999;94(10):3315–24.
61. Douer D, Tallman MS. Arsenic trioxide: new clinical experience with an old medication in hematologic malignancies. J Clin Oncol. 2005;23(10):2396–410.
62. Hei TK, Liu SX, Waldren C. Mutagenicity of arsenic in mammalian cells: role of reactive oxygen species. Proc Natl Acad Sci U S A. 1998;95(14):8103–7.
63. Cuzick J, Evans S, Gillman M, Price Evans DA. Medicinal arsenic and internal malignancies. Br J Cancer. 1982;45(6):904–11.
64. Sanz MA, Grimwade D, Tallman MS, Lowenberg B, Fenaux P, Estey EH, et al. Management of acute promyelocytic leukemia: recommendations from an expert panel on behalf of the European LeukemiaNet. Blood. 2009;113(9):1875–91.
65. Mathews V, Chandy M, Srivastava A. Arsenic trioxide in the management of acute promyelocytic leukaemia. Natl Med J India. 2001;14(4):215–22.
66. Mrozek K, Heinonen K, de la Chapelle A, Bloomfield CD. Clinical significance of cytogenetics in acute myeloid leukemia. Semin Oncol. 1997;24(1):17–31.
67. Slack JL, Arthur DC, Lawrence D, Mrozek K, Mayer RJ, Davey FR, et al. Secondary cytogenetic changes in acute promyelocytic leukemia—prognostic importance in patients treated with chemotherapy alone and association with the intron 3 breakpoint of the PML gene: a Cancer and Leukemia Group B study. J Clin Oncol. 1997;15(5):1786–95.
68. De Botton S, Chevret S, Sanz M, Dombret H, Thomas X, Guerci A, et al. Additional chromosomal abnormalities in patients with acute promyelocytic leukaemia (APL) do not confer poor prognosis: results of APL 93 trial. Br J Haematol. 2000;111(3):801–6.
69. Mathews V, Thomas M, Srivastava VM, George B, Srivastava A, Chandy M. Impact of FLT3 mutations and secondary cytogenetic changes on the outcome of patients with newly diagnosed acute promyelocytic leukemia treated with a single agent arsenic trioxide regimen. Haematologica. 2007;92(7):994–5.
70. Gilliland DG. FLT3-activating mutations in acute promyelocytic leukaemia: a rationale for risk-adapted therapy with FLT3 inhibitors. Best Pract Res Clin Haematol. 2003;16(3):409–17.
71. Gilliland DG, Griffin JD. The roles of FLT3 in hematopoiesis and leukemia. Blood. 2002;100(5):1532–42.
72. Marasca R, Maffei R, Zucchini P, Castelli I, Saviola A, Martinelli S, et al. Gene expression profiling of acute promyelocytic leukaemia identifies two subtypes mainly associated with Flt3 mutational status. Leukemia. 2006;20(1):103–14.
73. Gale RE, Hills R, Pizzey AR, Kottaridis PD, Swirsky D, Gilkes AF, et al. Relationship between FLT3 mutation status, biologic characteristics, and response to targeted therapy in acute promyelocytic leukemia. Blood. 2005;106(12):3768–76.
74. Callens C, Chevret S, Cayuela JM, Cassinat B, Raffoux E, de Botton S, et al. Prognostic implication of FLT3 and Ras gene mutations in patients with acute promyelocytic leukemia (APL): a retrospective study from the European APL Group. Leukemia. 2005;19(7):1153–60.
75. Chillon MC, Santamaria C, Garcia-Sanz R, Balanzategui A, Maria Eugenia S, Alcoceba M, et al. Long FLT3 internal tandem duplications and reduced PML-RARalpha expression at diagnosis characterize a high-risk subgroup of acute promyelocytic leukemia patients. Haematologica. 2010;95(5):745–51.
76. Thirugnanam R, George B, Chendamarai E, Lakshmi KM, Balasubramanian P, Viswabandya A, et al. Comparison of clinical outcomes of patients with relapsed acute promyelocytic leukemia induced with arsenic trioxide and consolidated with either an autologous stem cell transplant or an arsenic trioxide-based regimen. Biol Blood Marrow Transplant. 2009;15(11):1479–84.
77. Ganesan S, Alex AA, Chendamarai E, Balasundaram N, Palani HK, David S, et al. Rationale and efficacy of proteasome inhibitor combined with arsenic trioxide in the treatment of acute promyelocytic leukemia. Leukemia. 2016;30(11):2169–78.
78. Mathews V, Korula A, Kulkarni U, Ganesan S, David S, Alex AA, Nisham PN, Abraham A, Srivastava A, Lakshmi KM, Balasubramanian P, George B. Management of relapsed acute promyelocytic leukemia post ATO upfront therapy: open-labeled phase II study evaluating role of proteasome inhibition. Blood. 2016;128(22):446.
79. Mathews V. De-escalation of treatment for acute promyelocytic leukaemia? Lancet Haematol. 2015;2(9):e348–9.
80. Powell BL, Moser B, Stock W, Gallagher RE, Willman CL, Stone RM, et al. Arsenic trioxide improves event-free and overall survival for adults with acute promyelocytic leukemia: North American Leukemia Intergroup Study C9710. Blood. 2010;116(19):3751–7.

19 Therapy-Related Acute Promyelocytic Leukemia

Kristen Pettit and Richard A. Larson

Abbreviations

AML	Acute myeloid leukemia
APL	Acute promyelocytic leukemia
ATO	Arsenic trioxide
ATRA	All-trans retinoic acid (tretinoin)
CR	Complete remission
DNMT3A	DNA methyltransferase 3A
FLT3	FMS-like tyrosine kinase-3 receptor
GIMEMA	Gruppo Italiano Malattie EMatologiche dell'Adulto
IDH1/2	Isocitrate dehydrogenase 1 and 2
LCH	Langerhans cell histiocytosis
MDS	Myelodysplastic syndrome
MS	Multiple sclerosis
OS	Overall survival
PML	Promyelocytic leukemia
RARA	Retinoic acid receptor alpha
RT	Radiation therapy
t-APL	Therapy-related acute promyelocytic leukemia
TET2	Tet oncogene family member 2 isocitrate
t-MN	Therapy-related myeloid neoplasm

K. Pettit, M.D. • R.A. Larson, M.D. (✉)
Department of Medicine and the Comprehensive Cancer Center, University of Chicago, 5841 S. Maryland Ave, MC2115, Chicago, IL 60637, USA
e-mail: kpettit@medicine.bsd.uchicago.edu; rlarson@medicine.bsd.uchicago.edu

Introduction

Exposure to DNA-damaging agents, either by certain cytotoxic drugs or by radiation therapy, has been shown to predispose to later development of myeloid malignancies including myelodysplastic syndrome (MDS), myeloproliferative neoplasms (MPN), and acute myeloid leukemia (AML), which together constitute the World Health Organization category of therapy-related myeloid neoplasms (t-MN) [1]. t-MN currently accounts for about 10–20% of AML and MDS cases and exhibits characteristic chromosomal abnormalities and latency periods as well as poor prognoses in most cases [2]. t-MN after exposure to alkylating agents or radiation typically develops 5–7 years after initial therapy and is most often associated with a complex karyotype or abnormalities of chromosomes 5 or 7. There is often an antecedent myelodysplastic phase [3, 4]. t-MN after exposure to topoisomerase II inhibitors develops more quickly, generally within 1–3 years, and often involves rearrangements at chromosome bands11q23 or 21q22 [5, 6].

Less commonly, t-MN will present with a t(15;17)(q22;q21) and clinical features of acute promyelocytic leukemia (APL). These cases of therapy-related acute promyelocytic leukemia (t-APL) most commonly arise after exposure to topoisomerase II inhibitors but have also been observed after alkylating agents, antimitotic agents, and radiation therapy. t-APL represents a

O. Abla et al. (eds.), *Acute Promyelocytic Leukemia*, https://doi.org/10.1007/978-3-319-64257-4_19

distinct subset of t-MN with clinical features, treatment options, and prognosis similar to those now seen in de novo APL.

Several rich sources of clinical information on t-APL are available in the literature and will be discussed throughout this chapter (see Table 19.1). In the largest series of t-APL cases to date, Beaumont et al. examined in detail 106 cases of t-APL diagnosed at 45 medical centers in three European countries between 1982 and 2001 [7]. In the same article, that group reviewed 77 pooled case reports from the literature up to that point [8]. In 2000, the International Workshop on the relationship of prior therapy to balanced chromosome aberrations in therapy-related myelodysplastic syndromes and acute leukemia was held in Chicago and described 511 cases of t-MNs, including 41 cases of t-APL [9]. In addition, Pulsoni et al. reported on the Italian cooperative group Gruppo Italiano Malattie EMatologiche dell'Adulto (GIMEMA) experience between 1984 and 1998 comparing 51 cases of t-APL to 641 cases of de novo APL [10]. Together, these reports help form the basis of clinical knowledge of t-APL.

Epidemiology

t-APL is an uncommon disease that accounts for a small proportion of all APL and t-MN cases. Earlier studies in particular highlighted the infrequency of t-APL diagnoses. Detourmignies et al. examined 284 cases of APL that were diagnosed between 1982 and 1991 at 7 European medical centers and found that only 16 cases (5.6%) were related to prior cytotoxic therapy [8]. Among the GIMEMA APL cohort, t-APL accounted for 4.8% of the 51 cases studied [10]. Kantarjian et al. reported on 112 patients with t-MNs seen at the MD Anderson Cancer Center between 1973 and1985 and found that only two cases (1.8%) had a t(15;17) [11]. Among 63 patients with t-MNs seen at the University of Chicago prior to 1985, 2 (3%) had a t(15;17) and clinical characteristics of

Table 19.1 Key t-APL case series

Series	Number of patients	Primary diagnosis	Exposure	Latency, months	Outcomes
French, Spanish, and Belgian report [7]	106	Breast cancer 60% Non-Hodgkin lymphoma 15% Hodgkin lymphoma 2% Other solid tumors 23% Nonmalignant disorders 2%	Combined chemotherapy and RT 46% Chemotherapy alone 28% RT alone 26%	25 (range, 4–276)	Those in pre-ATRA era (*n* = 14), CR 87% In ATRA era, CR 80% 8-year OS 59%
Literature review [7, 8]	77	Breast cancer 17% Non-Hodgkin lymphoma 5% Hodgkin lymphoma 16% Other solid tumors 31% Nonmalignant disorders 29%	Not reported	25	Not reported
International Workshop [9]	41	Breast cancer 44% Non-Hodgkin lymphoma 17% Hodgkin lymphoma 10% Other solid tumors 27% Nonmalignant conditions 2%	Combined chemotherapy and RT 54% Chemotherapy alone 17% RT alone 21%	29 (range, 9–175)	CR 74% Number in continuous CR at 5 years 57%
GIMEMA [10]	51	Breast cancer 29% Non-Hodgkin lymphoma 18% Hodgkin lymphoma 6% Other solid tumors 47%	Combined chemotherapy and RT 20% Chemotherapy alone 20% RT alone 33% Surgery alone 27%	36 (range, 8–366)	CR 97% 4-year OS 84%

APL [12]. The 2000 International Workshop in Chicago identified 8% of t-MN with balanced chromosome aberrations as t-APL [9].

While still rare, the incidence of t-APL appears to be on the rise although this may be the result of greater recognition for this striking disease. Beaumont et al. reported on 106 patients with t-APL diagnosed between 1982 and 2001 in France, Spain, and Belgium and found that 26 of those patients were diagnosed with t-APL in the first 10-year period, compared to 80 who were diagnosed in the second 10-year period [7]. Other centers have noted an apparent increase in the number of cases of t-APL as well, even after retrospectively examining all prior APL diagnoses to determine whether prior cytotoxic exposure had been overlooked and the therapy-related cases had been misclassified in earlier years. At the University Hospital of Lille, France, the proportion of APL cases that occurred after prior cytotoxic therapy rose considerably from 5% in the 1984–1993 period to 22% between 1994 and 2000 [7, 13]. A similar trend was noted at the MD Anderson Cancer Center, where 2% of all APL cases were therapy-related in 1986, compared to 12% in 1996 [11, 14]. Therefore, there may be a true increase in the incidence of t-APL as opposed to increased recognition of t-APL as an entity. This rise largely parallels the rising incidence of t-MN overall over the past few decades and may reflect increased use of specific leukemogenic therapies as well as improved survivorship from primary malignancies [15, 16].

Disease Presentation

Clinical Features

In general, clinical characteristics seen in t-APL parallel those of de novo APL. t-APL is seen across all adult age groups, with median age at diagnosis between 49 and 57 years [7–10]. Hematologic parameters are comparable between therapy-related and de novo groups [7, 9, 10]. Female predominance of t-APL has been demonstrated in multiple studies, most likely reflecting the frequency of topoisomerase II inhibitor use and radiation therapy for the treatment of breast and gynecologic malignancies [7, 9, 10, 14]. This differs from de novo APL, which exhibits no predisposition by sex. The GIMEMA group noted several other differences in those with t-APL compared to de novo disease in their study [10]. They found that those with t-APL presented with a worse performance status ($P < 0.005$) and older age ($P < 0.05$). Those with therapy-related disease also had higher fibrinogen levels and few hemorrhagic complications than their de novo counterparts. Elliott et al. found a slightly lower BMI in patients with therapy-related disease, but other clinical features were similar [17]. Overall, these few small differences in clinical features do not translate to differences in clinical outcome, as will be discussed below.

Pathologic Features

Pathologic features of t-APL, including cytologic, cytogenetic, and molecular abnormalities, have been shown to be similar to those seen in de novo APL. Duffield et al. compared bone marrow specimen from nine patients with t-APL to those with de novo disease and found no differences in morphology or immunophenotype between the two groups [18]. In contrast to non-promyelocytic t-MN where an antecedent myelodysplastic phase is common, cases of t-APL lack such a phase and present with overt leukemia [7, 19].

In addition to t(15;17), other chromosomal abnormalities occasionally occur in APL. The incidence and types of additional abnormalities found in t-APL are similar to those also seen in de novo APL. While the prognostic impact of additional chromosomal abnormalities in APL has been a matter of debate in the past, in the current era of therapy, they do not seem to confer adverse risk [20–23]. Overall in APL, 26–33% of cases harbor additional chromosomal abnormalities, the most common being trisomy 8 (12%), followed by abnormalities in chromosomes 9 (2%), 7 (2%), 21 (2%), and 17 (1%) [20]. Beaumont et al. reported a similar incidence of additional chromosomal abnormalities in t-APL, with a slightly different distribution. Within this group, trisomy 8 was seen in only 5% of cases, and the remaining abnormalities predominantly involved chromosomes 5, 7, or 17 [7]. Among the 41 cases analyzed through the International Workshop, 41% of cases included additional abnormalities, most frequently trisomy 8 in 12%. There was no association between additional chromosomal abnormalities and either age or type of previous therapy in this series. While occasional variant translocations involving RARA that confer resistance to standard therapy have been reported in de novo APL, they are rare, and such cytogenetic variants have not been reported in t-APL.

Molecular profiling has been reported for a small number of patients with t-APL. FMS-like tyrosine kinase-3 receptor (*FLT3*) gene mutations are commonly seen in de novo APL. However, they do not appear to connote the same negative prognosis that is seen in non-promyelocytic AML. Several groups have compared the frequency of *FLT3* mutations between therapy-related and de novo APL cases and reported somewhat discordant results. Yin et al. found a high incidence of *FLT3* mutations (42% of 12 t-APL cases studied) [24]. Ottone et al. found a similar incidence, 30% in t-APL compared to 44% in de novo APL ($P = 0.50$) [25]. Duffield et al. found that all five t-APL cases studied had a *FLT3* mutation compared to 59% of de novo cases ($P = 0.41$) [18]. This variation may be due to the small numbers in each series and to differences in the patient population studied. One study focused on patients with prior malignancies, while another focused on patients with multiple sclerosis (MS). Ottone et al. also tested for mutations in several other genes associated with myeloid malignancies, including tet oncogene family member 2 (*TET2*), isocitrate dehydrogenases 1 and 2 (*IDH1* and *IDH2*), and DNA methyltransferase 3A (*DNMT3A*) [25]. They found a *DNMT3A* pathogenic mutation in one t-APL case but none in the de novo APL group. They reported one *IDH1* mutation in a de novo case. *TET2* polymorphisms were common in both groups. Further evaluation with larger cohort sizes and more extensive mutation panels will clarify the mutational profiles of these two disorders.

Prior Diagnosis and Exposures

t-APL has been reported following a variety of therapies used for several different malignant and nonmalignant disorders (see Table 19.2). The most commonly implicated antecedent therapies are topoisomerase II-targeting agents such as mitoxantrone, etoposide, and anthracyclines (particularly epirubicin) [7, 9, 10]. The mechanism by which topoisomerase II inhibitors initiate development of t-APL has been described in detail by Grimwade and colleagues and will be discussed below (see Pathogenesis). However, t-APL has also been described after treatment with other DNA-damaging therapies such as alkylating agents, antimetabolites, external beam radiation, and radioactive iodine. The leukemogenic risk may be dose-dependent for some agents such as etoposide, but not for others such as mitoxantrone [26–28]. While t-APL typically develops rapidly with a median latency of 25–32 months, cases have been reported as early as 4 months after first exposure and as late as 276 months after therapy [7, 9, 28, 29]. Thus, the latency period, both at

Table 19.2 Risk factors for the development of t-APL

t-APL risk factors
Primary diagnosis
Malignant
Breast cancer
Non-Hodgkin lymphoma
Hodgkin lymphoma
Uterine cancer
Testicular cancer
Other solid tumors
Nonmalignant
Multiple sclerosis
Psoriasis
Langerhans cell histiocytosis
Exposures
Topoisomerase II inhibitors
Mitoxantrone
Etoposide
Anthracyclines
Bimolane
Radiation therapy
External beam radiation
Radioactive iodine

median and the range, is similar to what is observed in cases of non-promyelocytic t-MN that develops after topoisomerase II inhibitors.

The majority of t-APL cases have arisen after treatment for solid malignancies. In the Beaumont series of 106 t-APL cases, the most common primary disorder was breast cancer (60%) followed by non-Hodgkin lymphoma (15%), Hodgkin lymphoma (2%), uterine cancer (4%), lung cancer (1%), other solid tumors (19%), and, rarely, nonmalignant disorders (2%). Treatments for these primary tumors included chemotherapy alone (28%), radiation alone (26%), or both (46%). Most patients received an alkylating agent or a topoisomerase II inhibitor, in 64% and 57%, respectively [7]. Findings were similar in the 41 patients included in the International Workshop, where breast cancer was again the most common primary diagnosis (44%), followed by non-Hodgkin lymphoma (17%), Hodgkin lymphoma (10%), other solid tumors (27%), and nonmalignant conditions (2%). Most had received both chemotherapy and radiation (54%), though in this series, fewer received chemotherapy alone (17%) and more received radiation alone (29%) [9].

While the largest series of t-APL cases have primarily identified those that develop after treatment of primary cancers, the literature is ripe with smaller series and case reports describing t-APL after treatment for nonmalignant disorders. Multiple reports describe an association between APL and psoriasis, particularly after treatment with the antimitotic drugs, bimolane and razoxane. Both of these drugs function through inhibition of topoisomerase II and were previously used in China to treat both neoplastic disorders and psoriasis [30, 31]. Ge et al. reported on 17 cases of APL in patients with psoriasis diagnosed over 10 years at the First Affiliated Hospital at Harbin Medical University, China [32]. These cases represented 8.3% of all APL diagnoses at that center during that time period. Only four patients had received prior therapy with bimolane, suggesting that there could be additional risk conferred by the underlying psoriasis itself. Another report by Wang et al. examined 100 cases of acute leukemia that developed in patients with psoriasis [33]. In their series, APL was by far the most common leukemia subtype, present in 53 of the cases. Of those, 40% had been treated with bimolane or related analogues, 42% had been treated with agents other than bimolane, and 18% had not been treated. Various theories have been proposed to explain the increased leukemia susceptibility among patients with psoriasis even in the absence of treatment, including antigenic stimulation, and the presence of chromosomal fragile sites [34, 35]. Interestingly, downregulation of the retinoic acid receptor alpha (RARA) in the epidermis leads to abnormal keratinocyte proliferation that is responsive to retinoic acid therapy, suggesting some biologic similarity between APL and psoriasis. These authors speculate that additional predisposition to APL may exist in these psoriasis patients even prior to DNA-damaging agents [36, 37].

Children treated for Langerhans cell histiocytosis (LCH) with etoposide have also been found to have increased risk for t-APL. In an analysis of 77 case reports of t-APL, 12 of those cases were found to have occurred in children with LCH. All 12 had been treated with etoposide, and 9 of the 12 had received cumulative doses >4500 mg/m^2 [7, 26, 27]. However, in another series of 348 patients with LCH treated at several European medical centers with etoposide, no cases of t-APL were reported. In this series, all patients received total etoposide doses of <2000 mg/m^2, suggesting a dose-dependent leukemogenic effect of this agent [26].

Similarly, patients with multiple sclerosis (MS) treated with the topoisomerase II inhibitor mitoxantrone have developed t-APL. Ammatuna et al. reported on 33 patients at various European medical centers who had MS and were subsequently diagnosed with t-APL [28]. Among those patients, 30/33 had received mitoxantrone. Their median cumulative dose of mitoxantrone was 112 mg and ranged from only 14 mg in one patient up to 242 mg, suggesting an idiosyncratic relationship and the lack of a dose-response risk in this situation. The three patients who had not received mitoxantrone had been treated with steroids alone, interferon beta with sequential steroids, and interferon beta plus azathioprine. Many additional case reports of t-APL after mitoxantrone for MS can be found in the literature [38–46]. Other leukemogenic risk factors may be present in some patients with MS, such as genetic variants involving DNA repair (*BRCA2* and *XRCC5*) that could predispose to translocation events or variants affecting the metabolism of chemotherapeutics (such as *CYP3A4*) that could result in increased cellular exposure to drugs such as mitoxantrone [47].

Several cases of APL after immunosuppressive treatment alone for nonmalignant conditions have been reported, but it is controversial whether these cases should be considered therapy-related. In Japanese centers, two children developed APL after receiving living donor partial orthotopic liver transplantation. The first was 12 years old and received a liver transplant for ornithine transcarbamylase deficiency, followed by tacrolimus and azathioprine immunosuppression posttransplant. Azathioprine has been associated with t-MN after solid organ transplantation [48]. The second, a 4-year-old girl, received a liver transplant for congenital biliary atresia and received tacrolimus after transplant. APL developed after latencies of 21 months and 46 months, respectively. Both were treated with all-trans retinoic acid (ATRA, tretinoin) and chemotherapy, and both attained complete remissions (CR), which were ongoing at the time of publication [49]. One case of APL in a patient with Crohn's disease treated with the anti-TNF alpha monoclonal antibody infliximab has been reported in the literature [50]. It would be difficult to infer causality from this single case report alone. Treatment with TNF antagonists and the presence of inflammatory bowel disease have both been associated with increased risk of developing lymphoid neoplasms, but a causal link to myeloid neoplasms remains unclear [51–54].

Pathogenesis

In virtually all cases of APL, a balanced translocation between the long arms of chromosomes 15 and 17 results in juxtaposition of the promyelocytic leukemia (*PML*) gene with the retinoic acid receptor alpha (*RARA*) gene [55, 56]. The resulting *PML-RARA* fusion protein functions as an aberrant retinoid receptor that resists physiologic retinoid-induced differentiation of myeloid cells [57]. In cases of de novo APL, the inciting factors that lead to this translocation event are largely unknown. In contrast, in t-APL, the molecular mechanisms underlying the cleavage of DNA strands and subsequent translocation are well described. This is particularly true after treatment with topoisomerase II inhibitors, which represents the most common setting for development of t-APL.

Topoisomerases are enzymes that regulate the DNA topology through the introduction of single- or double-stranded DNA breaks at specific breakpoints. In the case of topoisomerase II, the enzyme generates transient double-stranded breaks through the formation of a covalent cleavage complex, thus allowing for modulation of DNA supercoiling and release of knots or tangles. DNA repair mechanisms subsequently religate the cleaved DNA strands. Modern pharmacology has been successful in exploiting these mechanisms for therapeutic purposes, and today topoisomerase II is a crucial target for a number of chemotherapeutic agents. Chemotherapeutics that affect topoisomerase II can be divided into two categories. The first includes compounds that decrease the overall activity of the enzyme, such as anthracyclines (i.e., epirubicin, daunorubicin, and doxorubicin). The second group increases transition levels of the topoisomerase II-DNA cleavage complexes, leading to inhibition of cell replication and transcription. Drugs in this category are referred to as topoisomerase II poisons and include etoposide and mitoxantrone [58, 59].

The association between myeloid neoplasms and topoisomerase II-damaging agents has been recognized for quite some time, but only more recently have the molecular mechanisms underlying this relationship come to light. Mistry et al. examined differences in the genomic breakpoint regions between three groups of patients: those with t-APL that developed after exposure to mitoxantrone, those with t-APL that developed after other exposures (e.g., radiation therapy or epirubicin), and those with de novo APL [60]. They found that the breakpoints in cases of t-APL arising after mitoxantrone treatment were clustered in an eight base pair region in intron 6 within the *PML* gene. This breakpoint region corresponded to a site that was preferentially cleaved by mitoxantrone at nine times the frequency that was seen in the absence of the drug. While breakpoints in *RARA* were more dispersed, they similarly corresponded to preferential sites of DNA cleavage by mitoxantrone. Short, homologous sequences in *PML* and *RARA* were observed, suggesting that DNA repair occurred by nonhomologous end joining. One of their patients had only received 15 mg of mitoxantrone, supporting previous observations for an absence of dose-response effect with mitoxantrone. A subsequent series of 12 patients with t-APL that developed after treatment with mitoxantrone for MS demonstrated that the *PML* breakpoint fell within the previously identified breakage "hotspot" in 42% of cases [41]. An extension of this study included 23 patients with t-APL and demonstrated DNA breakpoints within the *PML* "hotspot" in 39% of t-APL cases overall, compared to none of the de novo cases ($P = 0.007$) [61]. In addition, breakpoints in *RARA* were found to cluster in a region of intron 2 in 65% of t-APL cases compared to 28% of de novo cases.

Patients who developed t-APL after treatment with epirubicin have also been found to share breakpoints that cluster within specific hotspots. Mays et al. examined genomic features in six patients who developed t-APL after treatment with epirubicin for breast cancer and observed specific breakpoint clustering within both *PML* and *RARA* loci [62]. Within *PML*, three of the six patients were found to have breakpoints in intron 6 that occurred at close approximation to one another, which was unlikely to occur by chance ($P = 0.014$). These intron 6 breakpoints occurred outside of the hotspot region that had previously been identified for mitoxantrone-induced APL cases. Other *PML* breakpoints were found in intron 3 and exon 7. The *RARA* breakpoints occurred within intron 2 in all six cases. In two of those cases, the breakpoints occurred within four nucleotides of each other, which was unlikely to occur by chance ($P = 0.017$). In all cases, the breakpoints in both chromosomes were found to occur at preferential sites for epirubicin-induced DNA cleavage by topoisomerase II.

From these observations, models have been generated by Grimwade and coworkers to depict the formation of the leukemogenic balanced translocation of chromosomes 15 and 17 after exposure to a topoisomerase II inhibitor (see Fig. 19.1) [62]. In this model, topoisomerase II

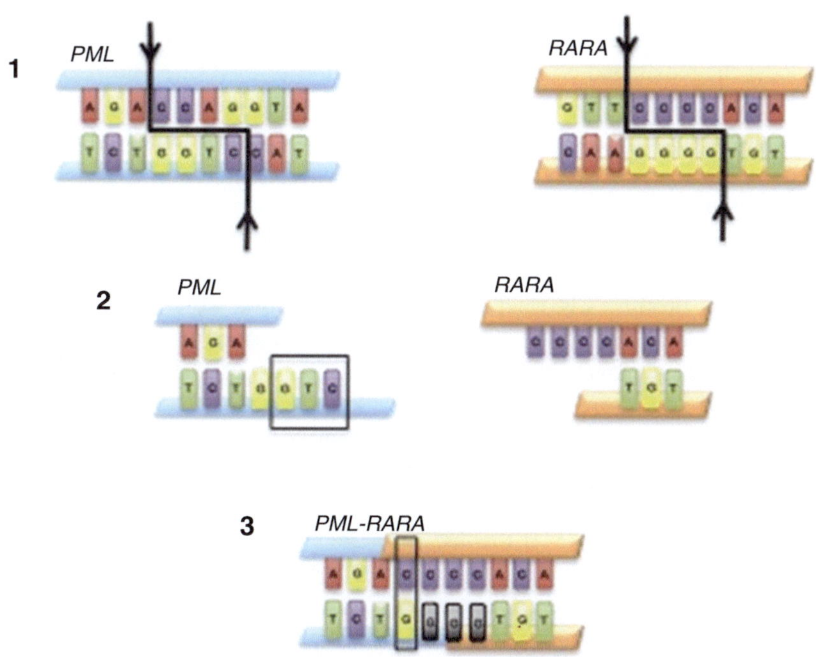

Fig. 19.1 Model for the mechanism of *PML-RARA* translocation in topoisomerase II inhibitor-induced t-APL. (*1*) Topoisomerase II induces 4-bp nicks in double-stranded DNA at preferential sites within *PML* and *RARA* genes. (*2*) Exonucleases digest bases from 5′ overhang (indicated by *black box*). (*3*) Nonhomologous end joining occurs (indicated by *black box*), followed by template-directed DNA polymerization (indicated by *gray text*) and strand ligation, resulting in the formation of a *PML-RARA* fusion gene (Reproduced with permission) [62]

induces 4 base pair nicks in double-stranded DNA at preferential sites within *PML* and *RARA* genes on chromosomes 15 and 17, respectively, and on other genes. Exonucleolytic processing occurs, followed by nonhomologous end joining. Gaps are filled by template-directed DNA polymerization and mismatch repair mechanisms, and strands are ligated. If this results in translocation between chromosomes 15 and 17, the *PML-RARA* fusion gene may be generated. The discovery of susceptible breakage sites and creation of this model for translocation formation have illuminated the likely molecular mechanisms for t-APL development and perhaps represent a step toward discovering mechanisms for the pathogenesis of de novo APL.

Treatment Approaches

While most t-MN confer a significantly worse prognosis compared to their cytogenetically matched de novo counterparts, those with APL seem to do similarly well regardless of whether the disease is related to prior cytotoxic therapy [2, 7, 10, 63, 64]. A report from the GIMEMA retrospectively identified 51 patients with APL after a prior cancer diagnosis and compared the outcomes of these patients to those with de novo APL [10]. The majority of t-APL patients (31 out of 51) were treated with a standard regimen of ATRA plus idarubicin. Despite older age and worse performance status among the t-APL patients in this series, outcomes were equally good between the two groups. CR rates were 97% and 93% in the t-APL group and de novo APL group, respectively, and 4-year overall survival (OS) was 85% and 78%, respectively. Other case series similarly show encouraging long-term survival for patients with t-APL treated with ATRA plus chemotherapy [7, 9, 65].

In the era of arsenic trioxide (ATO) therapy, these favorable and comparable outcomes between de novo and t-APL have held up. Dayyani et al. conducted a retrospective analysis of 29 patients with t-APL treated at the MD Anderson Cancer Center and compared outcomes of patients treated with ATRA/ATO ($n = 19$) to those treated with ATRA/anthracycline-based chemotherapy ($n = 10$) [66]. Remission rates were similar between the two groups, with CRs in 89% and 70%, respectively ($P = 0.35$). Median OS was not reached at last follow-up for the ATRA/ATO group, compared to 161 weeks for the ATRA/chemotherapy group ($P = 0.79$). Similarly, Ge et al. examined 17 patients with psoriasis-associated t-APL treated with ATO-based induction and post-remission therapy and reported an 88% CR rate and estimated a 3-year OS rate of 77% ± 12% [32]. Given this overall favorable response profile, patients with t-APL should be treated according to conventional APL treatment algorithms, and one can expect favorable outcomes quite similar to those with de novo disease. In contrast to other t-MN, intensification of therapy based on therapy-related status, such as inclusion of allogeneic stem cell transplantation, is typically not necessary in t-APL to achieve cure.

Although primary chemotherapy resistance is common in other t-MN subtypes, drug resistance is rare in t-APL. In de novo APL, acquired mutations in *PML* or *RARA* have been shown to confer resistance to ATRA or ATO infrequently [67–71]. One such case of ATO resistance in a patient with t-APL has been analyzed and reported on by Iaccarino et al. [72]. The patient was found to have a point mutation in *PML* in both the rearranged and unrearranged alleles, as well as two mutations in the rearranged *RARA* gene, none of which were present prior to ATO treatment. Madan et al. characterized the molecular signature of relapsed APL and found that mutations in *PML* or *RARA* were commonly acquired at the time of relapse [73]. Further study is needed to determine whether patients with APL may benefit from screening for these or similar mutations to identify those at risk for developing relapse or resistance.

Future Directions

While much has been learned about t-APL over the past 15 years, additional questions remain. Further clarification is needed regarding the apparent rise in incidence of t-APL in recent years.

Preventive strategies such as minimizing exposure to topoisomerase II inhibitors and radiation therapy whenever possible may be helpful in mitigating this upturn. Whether adjunctive therapy with hematopoietic growth factors such as filgrastim facilitates the leukemogenic effects of intensive chemotherapy remains to be determined. Further evaluation of screening strategies for early detection of t-APL in the most high-risk situations, prior to the development of complications such as bleeding, is also warranted. A genetic predisposition to t-APL may exist in a proportion of patients, as is the case in other t-MNs; however, this requires further investigation [74]. In addition, molecular characterization of t-APL by high-throughput methods may identify those at higher risk for drug resistance or relapse. Lastly, models for the pathogenesis of t-APL may help elucidate mechanisms of de novo disease development.

Conclusions

Treatment with certain agents, particularly topoisomerase II inhibitors, can result in DNA damage within specific hotspots that predispose to development of balanced translocations in chromosomes 15 and 17. Radiation therapy is also implicated in these chromosomal rearrangements. t-APL is associated with a short latency period and typically develops within 2–3 years after the causative exposure. While the breakpoints in t-APL differ from those found in de novo APL, the phenotype that results is largely identical. Clinical and pathologic features of t-APL closely reflect those of de novo disease. Outcomes are similar to de novo APL, and same treatment algorithms should be employed.

References

1. Arber DA, Orazi A, Hasserjian R, Thiele J, Borowitz MJ, Le Beau MM, et al. The 2016 revision to the World Health Organization classification of myeloid neoplasms and acute leukemia. Blood. 2016;127(20):2391–405. PubMed PMID: 27069254.
2. Granfeldt Ostgard LS, Medeiros BC, Sengelov H, Norgaard M, Andersen MK, Dufva IH, et al. Epidemiology and clinical significance of secondary and therapy-related acute myeloid leukemia: a National Population-Based Cohort Study. J Clin Oncol. 2015;33(31):3641–9. PubMed PMID: 26304885.
3. Rowley JD, Golomb HM, Vardiman JW. Nonrandom chromosome abnormalities in acute leukemia and dysmyelopoietic syndromes in patients with previously treated malignant disease. Blood. 1981;58(4):759–67. PubMed PMID: 7272506.
4. Traweek ST, Slovak ML, Nademanee AP, Brynes RK, Niland JC, Forman SJ. Clonal karyotypic hematopoietic cell abnormalities occurring after autologous bone marrow transplantation for Hodgkin's disease and non-Hodgkin's lymphoma. Blood. 1994;84(3):957–63. PubMed PMID: 8043877.
5. Pedersen-Bjergaard J, Rowley JD. The balanced and the unbalanced chromosome aberrations of acute myeloid leukemia may develop in different ways and may contribute differently to malignant transformation. Blood. 1994;83(10):2780–6. PubMed PMID: 8180374.
6. Ratain MJ, Rowley JD. Therapy-related acute myeloid leukemia secondary to inhibitors of topoisomerase II: from the bedside to the target genes. Ann Oncol. 1992;3(2):107–11. PubMed PMID: 1318741.
7. Beaumont M, Sanz M, Carli PM, Maloisel F, Thomas X, Detourmignies L, et al. Therapy-related acute promyelocytic leukemia. J Clin Oncol. 2003;21(11):2123–37. PubMed PMID: 12775738.
8. Detourmignies L, Castaigne S, Stoppa AM, Harousseau JL, Sadoun A, Janvier M, et al. Therapy-related acute promyelocytic leukemia: a report on 16 cases. J Clin Oncol. 1992;10(9):1430–5. PubMed PMID: 1517786.
9. Andersen MK, Larson RA, Mauritzson N, Schnittger S, Jhanwar SC, Pedersen-Bjergaard J. Balanced chromosome abnormalities inv(16) and t(15;17) in therapy-related myelodysplastic syndromes and acute leukemia: report from an international workshop. Genes Chromosomes Cancer. 2002;33(4):395–400. PubMed PMID: 11921273.
10. Pulsoni A, Pagano L, Lo Coco F, Avvisati G, Mele L, Di Bona E, et al. Clinicobiological features and outcome of acute promyelocytic leukemia occurring as a second tumor: the GIMEMA experience. Blood. 2002;100(6):1972–6. PubMed PMID: 12200354.
11. Kantarjian HM, Keating MJ, Walters RS, Beran M, McLaughlin P, McCredie KB, et al. The association of specific "favorable" cytogenetic abnormalities with secondary leukemia. Cancer. 1986;58(4):924–7. PubMed PMID: 3719557.
12. Le Beau MM, Albain KS, Larson RA, Vardiman JW, Davis EM, Blough RR, et al. Clinical and cytogenetic correlations in 63 patients with therapy-related myelodysplastic syndromes and acute nonlymphocytic leukemia: further evidence for characteristic abnormalities of chromosomes no. 5 and 7. J Clin Oncol. 1986;4(3):325–45. PubMed PMID: 3950675.
13. Beaumont, M, JL Lai, E Simonnet, C Preudhomme, I Plantier, B Quesnel, F Bauters, and P Fenaux. Therapy related acute promyelocytic leukemia (tAPL): increasing incidence, especially after nonHodgkin's lymphoma (NHL) treated intensively? Blood. 2000;96(11):321a.

14. Pollicardo N, O'Brien S, Estey EH, al-Bitar M, Pierce S, Keating M, et al. Secondary acute promyelocytic leukemia. Characteristics and prognosis of 14 patients from a single institution. Leukemia. 1996;10(1):27–31. PubMed PMID: 8558933.
15. Allan JM, Travis LB. Mechanisms of therapy-related carcinogenesis. Nat Rev Cancer. 2005;5(12):943–55. PubMed PMID: 16294218.
16. Seedhouse C, Russell N. Advances in the understanding of susceptibility to treatment-related acute myeloid leukaemia. Br J Haematol. 2007;137(6):513–29. PubMed PMID: 17539774.
17. Elliott MA, Letendre L, Tefferi A, Hogan WJ, Hook C, Kaufmann SH, et al. Therapy-related acute promyelocytic leukemia: observations relating to APL pathogenesis and therapy. Eur J Haematol. 2012;88(3):237–43. PubMed PMID: 22023492.
18. Duffield AS, Aoki J, Levis M, Cowan K, Gocke CD, Burns KH, et al. Clinical and pathologic features of secondary acute promyelocytic leukemia. Am J Clin Pathol. 2012;137(3):395–402. PubMed PMID: 22338051. Pubmed Central PMCID: 3578661.
19. Pedersen-Bjergaard J, Christiansen DH, Desta F, Andersen MK. Alternative genetic pathways and cooperating genetic abnormalities in the pathogenesis of therapy-related myelodysplasia and acute myeloid leukemia. Leukemia. 2006;20(11):1943–9. PubMed PMID: 16990778.
20. De Botton S, Chevret S, Sanz M, Dombret H, Thomas X, Guerci A, et al. Additional chromosomal abnormalities in patients with acute promyelocytic leukaemia (APL) do not confer poor prognosis: results of APL 93 trial. Br J Haematol. 2000;111(3):801–6. PubMed PMID: 11122141.
21. Cervera J, Montesinos P, Hernandez-Rivas JM, Calasanz MJ, Aventin A, Ferro MT, et al. Additional chromosome abnormalities in patients with acute promyelocytic leukemia treated with all-trans retinoic acid and chemotherapy. Haematologica. 2010;95(3):424–31. PubMed PMID: 19903674. Pubmed Central PMCID: 2833072.
22. Ono T, Takeshita A, Iwanaga M, Asou N, Naoe T, Ohno R, et al. Impact of additional chromosomal abnormalities in patients with acute promyelocytic leukemia: 10-year results of the Japan Adult Leukemia Study Group APL97 study. Haematologica. 2011;96(1):174–6. PubMed PMID: 20884714. Pubmed Central PMCID: 3012784.
23. Hernandez JM, Martin G, Gutierrez NC, Cervera J, Ferro MT, Calasanz MJ, et al. Additional cytogenetic changes do not influence the outcome of patients with newly diagnosed acute promyelocytic leukemia treated with an ATRA plus anthracyclin based protocol. A report of the Spanish group PETHEMA. Haematologica. 2001;86(8):807–13. PubMed PMID: 11522536.
24. Yin CC, Glassman AB, Lin P, Valbuena JR, Jones D, Luthra R, et al. Morphologic, cytogenetic, and molecular abnormalities in therapy-related acute promyelocytic leukemia. Am J Clin Pathol. 2005;123(6):840–8. PubMed PMID: 15899774.
25. Ottone T, Cicconi L, Hasan SK, Lavorgna S, Divona M, Voso MT, et al. Comparative molecular analysis of therapy-related and de novo acute promyelocytic leukemia. Leuk Res. 2012;36(4):474–8. PubMed PMID: 22071137.
26. Haupt R, Fears TR, Heise A, Gadner H, Loiacono G, De Terlizzi M, et al. Risk of secondary leukemia after treatment with etoposide (VP-16) for Langerhans' cell histiocytosis in Italian and Austrian-German populations. Int J Cancer. 1997;71(1):9–13. PubMed PMID: 9096658.
27. Group TFLCHS. A multicentre retrospective survey of Langerhans' cell histiocytosis: 348 cases observed between 1983 and 1993. The French Langerhans' Cell Histiocytosis Study Group. Arch Dis Child. 1996;75(1):17–24. PubMed PMID: 8813865. Pubmed Central PMCID: 1511663.
28. Ammatuna E, Montesinos P, Hasan SK, Ramadan SM, Esteve J, Hubmann M, et al. Presenting features and treatment outcome of acute promyelocytic leukemia arising after multiple sclerosis. Haematologica. 2011;96(4):621–5. PubMed PMID: 21193421. Pubmed Central PMCID: 3069242.
29. Rowley JD, Olney HJ. International workshop on the relationship of prior therapy to balanced chromosome aberrations in therapy-related myelodysplastic syndromes and acute leukemia: overview report. Genes Chromosomes Cancer. 2002;33(4):331–45. PubMed PMID: 11921269.
30. Frantz CE, Smith H, Eades DM, Grosovsky AJ, Eastmond DA. Bimolane: in vitro inhibitor of human topoisomerase II. Cancer Lett. 1997;120(2):135–40. PubMed PMID: 9461029.
31. Xue Y, Lu D, Guo Y, Lin B. Specific chromosomal translocations and therapy-related leukemia induced by bimolane therapy for psoriasis. Leuk Res. 1992;16(11):1113–23. PubMed PMID: 1434747.
32. Ge F, Zhang Y, Cao F, Li J, Hou J, Wang P, et al. Arsenic trioxide-based therapy is suitable for patients with psoriasis-associated acute promyelocytic leukemia—a retrospective clinical study. Hematology. 2016;21(5):287–94. PubMed PMID: 26871996.
33. Wang Y, Mi Y, Li D, Xue Y, Bian S, Wang J. Acute leukemia association with psoriasis: a report on 100 patients from a single center in China. Am J Hematol. 2010;85(5):378–9. PubMed PMID: 20425800.
34. Soderberg KC, Jonsson F, Winqvist O, Hagmar L, Feychting M. Autoimmune diseases, asthma and risk of haematological malignancies: a nationwide case-control study in Sweden. Eur J Cancer. 2006;42(17):3028–33. PubMed PMID: 16945522.
35. Lu HL, Li WD, Wen HQ, et al. Chromosome aberration rate of lymphocytes in peripheral blood and fragile site of psoriasis patients. Chin J Dermatol. 1998;11:112.
36. van de Kerkhof PC. Update on retinoid therapy of psoriasis in: an update on the use of retinoids in dermatology. Dermatol Ther. 2006;19(5):252–63. PubMed PMID: 17014480.
37. Feng S, Lin L, Wu Q, Zhou W, Shao C. Study on the expression of RXRalpha in patients with psoriasis

vulgaris. Eur J Dermatol. 2006;16(1):33–8. PubMed PMID: 16436339.

38. Ellis R, Boggild M. Therapy-related acute leukaemia with mitoxantrone: what is the risk and can we minimise it? Mult Scler. 2009;15(4):505–8. PubMed PMID: 19251838.
39. Colovic N, Suvajdzic N, Kraguljac Kurtovic N, Djordjevic V, Dencic Fekete M, Drulovic J, et al. Therapy-related acute leukemia in two patients with multiple sclerosis treated with Mitoxantrone. Biomed Pharmacother. 2012;66(3):173–4. PubMed PMID: 22440894.
40. Bosca I, Pascual AM, Casanova B, Coret F, Sanz MA. Four new cases of therapy-related acute promyelocytic leukemia after mitoxantrone. Neurology. 2008;71(6):457–8. PubMed PMID: 18678830.
41. Hasan SK, Mays AN, Ottone T, Ledda A, La Nasa G, Cattaneo C, et al. Molecular analysis of t(15;17) genomic breakpoints in secondary acute promyelocytic leukemia arising after treatment of multiple sclerosis. Blood. 2008;112(8):3383–90. PubMed PMID: 18650449. Pubmed Central PMCID: 2954750.
42. Ramkumar B, Chadha MK, Barcos M, Sait SN, Heyman MR, Baer MR. Acute promyelocytic leukemia after mitoxantrone therapy for multiple sclerosis. Cancer Genet Cytogenet. 2008;182(2):126–9. PubMed PMID: 18406875.
43. Ledda A, Caocci G, Spinicci G, Cocco E, Mamusa E, La Nasa G. Two new cases of acute promyelocytic leukemia following mitoxantrone treatment in patients with multiple sclerosis. Leukemia. 2006;20(12):2217–8. PubMed PMID: 17051242.
44. Nollet S, Berger E, Deconinck E, Baldauf E, Rumbach L. Acute leukaemia in two multiple sclerosis patients treated with mitoxantrone. Rev Neurol. 2006;162(2):195–9. PubMed PMID: 16518259. Leucemies aigues chez deux patients atteints de sclerose en plaques et traites par mitoxantrone.
45. Ghalie RG, Mauch E, Edan G, Hartung HP, Gonsette RE, Eisenmann S, et al. A study of therapy-related acute leukaemia after mitoxantrone therapy for multiple sclerosis. Mult Scler. 2002;8(5):441–5. PubMed PMID: 12356214.
46. Vicari AM, Ciceri F, Folli F, Lanzi R, Colombo B, Comi G, et al. Acute promyelocytic leukemia following mitoxantrone as single agent for the treatment of multiple sclerosis. Leukemia. 1998;12(3):441–2. PubMed PMID: 9529141.
47. Hasan SK, Buttari F, Ottone T, Voso MT, Hohaus S, Marasco E, et al. Risk of acute promyelocytic leukemia in multiple sclerosis: coding variants of DNA repair genes. Neurology. 2011;76(12):1059–65. PubMed PMID: 21346221.
48. Offman J, Opelz G, Doehler B, Cummins D, Halil O, Banner NR, et al. Defective DNA mismatch repair in acute myeloid leukemia/myelodysplastic syndrome after organ transplantation. Blood. 2004;104(3):822–8. PubMed PMID: 15090454.
49. Sato T, Kobayashi R, Iguchi A, Nakajima M, Koizumi S, Furukawa H, et al. Acute promyelocytic leukemia after living donor partial orthotopic liver transplantation in two Japanese girls. Leuk Lymphoma. 2005;46(7):1057–60. PubMed PMID: 16019558.
50. Mohammad F, Vivekanandarajah A, Haddad H, Shutty CM, Hurford MT, Dai Q. Acute promyelocytic leukaemia (APL) in a patient with Crohn's disease and exposure to infliximab: a rare clinical presentation and review of the literature. BMJ Case Rep. 2014;2014. PubMed PMID: 24842356. Pubmed Central PMCID: 4039892.
51. Mir Madjlessi SH, Farmer RG, Weick JK. Inflammatory bowel disease and leukemia. A report of seven cases of leukemia in ulcerative colitis and Crohn's disease and review of the literature. Dig Dis Sci. 1986;31(10):1025–31. PubMed PMID: 3463495.
52. Anderson LA, Pfeiffer RM, Landgren O, Gadalla S, Berndt SI, Engels EA. Risks of myeloid malignancies in patients with autoimmune conditions. Br J Cancer. 2009;100(5):822–8. PubMed PMID: 19259097. Pubmed Central PMCID: 2653768.
53. Askling J, Brandt L, Lapidus A, Karlen P, Bjorkholm M, Lofberg R, et al. Risk of haematopoietic cancer in patients with inflammatory bowel disease. Gut. 2005;54(5):617–22. PubMed PMID: 15831904. Pubmed Central PMCID: 1774486.
54. Brown SL, Greene MH, Gershon SK, Edwards ET, Braun MM. Tumor necrosis factor antagonist therapy and lymphoma development: twenty-six cases reported to the Food and Drug Administration. Arthritis Rheum. 2002;46(12):3151–8. PubMed PMID: 12483718.
55. de The H, Lavau C, Marchio A, Chomienne C, Degos L, Dejean A. The PML-RAR alpha fusion mRNA generated by the t(15;17) translocation in acute promyelocytic leukemia encodes a functionally altered RAR. Cell. 1991;66(4):675–84. PubMed PMID: 1652369.
56. Kakizuka A, Miller WH Jr, Umesono K, Warrell RP Jr, Frankel SR, Murty VV, et al. Chromosomal translocation t(15;17) in human acute promyelocytic leukemia fuses RAR alpha with a novel putative transcription factor, PML. Cell. 1991;66(4):663–74. PubMed PMID: 1652368.
57. Grignani F, Ferrucci PF, Testa U, Talamo G, Fagioli M, Alcalay M, et al. The acute promyelocytic leukemia-specific PML-RAR alpha fusion protein inhibits differentiation and promotes survival of myeloid precursor cells. Cell. 1993;74(3):423–31. PubMed PMID: 8394219.
58. Deweese JE, Osheroff N. The DNA cleavage reaction of topoisomerase II: wolf in sheep's clothing. Nucleic Acids Res. 2009;37(3):738–48. PubMed PMID: 19042970. Pubmed Central PMCID: 2647315.
59. Lo-Coco F, Hasan SK. Understanding the molecular pathogenesis of acute promyelocytic leukemia. Best Pract Res Clin Haematol. 2014;27(1):3–9. PubMed PMID: 24907012.
60. Mistry AR, Felix CA, Whitmarsh RJ, Mason A, Reiter A, Cassinat B, et al. DNA topoisomerase II

in therapy-related acute promyelocytic leukemia. N Engl J Med. 2005;352(15):1529–38. PubMed PMID: 15829534.
61. Hasan SK, Ottone T, Schlenk RF, Xiao Y, Wiemels JL, Mitra ME, et al. Analysis of t(15;17) chromosomal breakpoint sequences in therapy-related versus de novo acute promyelocytic leukemia: association of DNA breaks with specific DNA motifs at PML and RARA loci. Genes Chromosomes Cancer. 2010;49(8):726–32. PubMed PMID: 20544846.
62. Mays AN, Osheroff N, Xiao Y, Wiemels JL, Felix CA, Byl JA, et al. Evidence for direct involvement of epirubicin in the formation of chromosomal translocations in t(15;17) therapy-related acute promyelocytic leukemia. Blood. 2010;115(2):326–30. PubMed PMID: 19884644. Pubmed Central PMCID: 2808156.
63. Borthakur G, Lin E, Jain N, Estey EE, Cortes JE, O'Brien S, et al. Survival is poorer in patients with secondary core-binding factor acute myelogenous leukemia compared with de novo core-binding factor leukemia. Cancer. 2009;115(14):3217–21. PubMed PMID: 19441109. Pubmed Central PMCID: 4184418.
64. Larson RA, Le Beau MM. Prognosis and therapy when acute promyelocytic leukemia and other "good risk" acute myeloid leukemias occur as a therapy-related myeloid neoplasm. Mediterr J Hematol Infect Dis. 2011;3(1):e2011032. PubMed PMID: 21869918. Pubmed Central PMCID: 3152454.
65. Jantunen E, Heinonen K, Mahlamaki E, Penttila K, Kuittinen T, Lehtonen P, et al. Secondary acute promyelocytic leukemia: an increasingly common entity. Leuk Lymphoma. 2007;48(1):190–1. PubMed PMID: 17325866.
66. Dayyani F, Kantarjian H, O'Brien S, Pierce S, Jones D, Faderl S, et al. Outcome of therapy-related acute promyelocytic leukemia with or without arsenic trioxide as a component of frontline therapy. Cancer. 2011;117(1):110–5. PubMed PMID: 20803607. Pubmed Central PMCID: 4287232.
67. Schachter-Tokarz E, Kelaidi C, Cassinat B, Chomienne C, Gardin C, Raffoux E, et al. PML-RARalpha ligand-binding domain deletion mutations associated with reduced disease control and outcome after first relapse of APL. Leukemia. 2010;24(2):473–6. PubMed PMID: 19865110.
68. Gallagher RE, Moser BK, Racevskis J, Poire X, Bloomfield CD, Carroll AJ, et al. Treatment-influenced associations of PML-RARalpha mutations, FLT3 mutations, and additional chromosome abnormalities in relapsed acute promyelocytic leukemia. Blood. 2012;120(10):2098–108. PubMed PMID: 22734072. Pubmed Central PMCID: 3437597.
69. Tomita A, Kiyoi H, Naoe T. Mechanisms of action and resistance to all-trans retinoic acid (ATRA) and arsenic trioxide (As2O 3) in acute promyelocytic leukemia. Int J Hematol. 2013;97(6):717–25. PubMed PMID: 23670176.
70. Zhu HH, Qin YZ, Huang XJ. Resistance to arsenic therapy in acute promyelocytic leukemia. N Engl J Med. 2014;370(19):1864–6. PubMed PMID: 24806185.
71. Lehmann-Che J, Bally C, de The H. Resistance to therapy in acute promyelocytic leukemia. N Engl J Med. 2014;371(12):1170–2. PubMed PMID: 25229938.
72. Iaccarino L, Ottone T, Divona M, Cicconi L, Cairoli R, Voso MT, et al. Mutations affecting both the rearranged and the unrearranged PML alleles in refractory acute promyelocytic leukaemia. Br J Haematol. 2016;172(6):909–13. PubMed PMID: 26728337.
73. Madan V, Shyamsunder P, Han L, Mayakonda A, Nagata Y, Sundaresan J, et al. Comprehensive mutational analysis of primary and relapse acute promyelocytic leukemia. Leukemia. 2016;30(8):1672–81. PubMed PMID: 27063598. Pubmed Central PMCID: 4972641.
74. Churpek JE, Marquez R, Neistadt B, Claussen K, Lee MK, Churpek MM, et al. Inherited mutations in cancer susceptibility genes are common among breast cancer survivors who develop therapy-related leukemia. Cancer. 2016;122(2):304–11. https://doi.org/10.1002/cncr.29615. Epub 7 Dec 2015. PMID: 26641009.

20 Rare Acute Leukemia Variants Involving Retinoic Acid Receptor Genes

Laura Cicconi and Oussama Abla

Introduction

Acute promyelocytic leukemia (APL) is typically characterized by the balanced reciprocal translocation t(15;17)(q24.1;q21.2) which fuses the promyelocytic leukemia (*PML*) and retinoic acid receptor-α (*RARA*) gene. *PML-RARA* oncoprotein is the key pathogenetic player in APL pathogenesis and acts through the transcriptional repression on multiple RARA target genes, causing the inhibition of cellular differentiation and uncontrolled proliferation of undifferentiated elements [1]. Rarely, patients presenting with clinical and morphological features suggestive of APL lack either cytogenetic evidence of t(15;17) or molecular evidence of PML-RARA and are subsequently recognized to harbor instead variant translocations involving *RARA* gene fused to partner genes other than PML [1–3]. Another member of the retinoic acid receptor family (i.e., RAR gamma) has been recently reported to be rearranged to *PML* and to another gene *NUP98* in single-case report of suspected APL lacking PML-RARA transcript, again highlighting the contribution of RA receptors in this form of leukemia [4, 5]. To date, at least 12 variant translocations involving *RARA* have been identified, including *ZBTB16/RARA* (formerly named *PLZF-RARA*) [6], *NPM-RARA*, *NuMA-RARA* [7], *STAT5B/RARA* [8], *PRKAR1A/RARA* [9], *BCOR/RARA* [10], *FIP1L1/RARA* [11], *OBFC2A/RARA* [12], *GTF2I/RARA* [13], and the most recent *IRF2BP2/RARA* [14] *and FNDC3B/RARA* [15].

In this chapter, we will discuss the clinical, morphological, cytogenetic, and molecular features, as well as the treatment outcome of these rare APL variants.

L. Cicconi, M.D. (✉)
Department of Biomedicine and Prevention, University Tor Vergata, via Montpellier 1, Rome, Italy
e-mail: cicconi.laura@yahoo.it

O. Abla, M.D.
Division of Hematology/Oncology, Department of Pediatrics, Hospital for Sick Children, Toronto, ON, Canada

Genetic *RARA* Variants

The first case of an alternative translocation involving *RARA* but not *PML* gene was described in 1993 by Chen and colleagues at the Shanghai Institute of Hematology, where a patient with evident morphologic features of APL was found to harbor the balanced translocation t(11;17)(q23;q21) instead of the classical t(15;17) [6]. In this case, molecular studies revealed that *RARA* gene was fused to a gene located on chromosome 11, termed at the time *PLZF*, encoding for a transcriptional factor. Few years later in 1997, a European Working Group was formed to study cases with morphologic and cytochemical features of APL lacking the typical t(15;17) studied by conventional karyotype [2, 16]. Of the initial 60 cases, the majority (42/60)

O. Abla et al. (eds.), *Acute Promyelocytic Leukemia*, https://doi.org/10.1007/978-3-319-64257-4_20

harbored cryptic *PML-RARA* gene rearrangements demonstrated by FISH and RT-PCR that were not previously identified through conventional karyotype due to insertions or complex translocations. However, in 12/60 cases (20%), a variant translocation involving *RARA* locus on chromosome 17q21 was identified. In particular, 11 cases were characterized by t(11;17)(q23;q21) with ZTBTB16/RARA and one case by t(5;17) (q35;q21) with *NPM-RARA* rearrangement.

In the last two decades, a number of variant gene partners rearranged with *RARA* have been identified, and those cases are estimated to account for 1–2% of all APL cases. Interestingly, all these variants contain the exact same *RARA* gene sequence as the translocation breakpoints always map in the second intron of the *RARA* gene. At the protein level, all the oncoproteins harbor the C-terminal *RARA* B through F domains which mediate the functions of DNA binding, retinoid X receptor (RXR) heterodimerization, ligand binding (ATRA), corepressor binding, and coactivator interaction functions [17]. At the clinical level, despite the constant involvement of *RARA* gene, the sensitivity of these genetic variants to molecularly targeted therapies like all *trans*-retinoic acid (ATRA) and arsenic trioxide (ATO) employed in *PML-RARA*-positive APL is not the same, with the majority (i.e., ZTBTB16/RARA) being resistant to these agents. All the clinico-biological characteristics and treatment response data of RARA variants are reported in Table 20.1.

Table 20.1 Biological and clinical features of variant gene fusions involving *RAR* receptor genes.

Fusion gene	Cytogenetics	In vitro sensitivity to ATRA	In vitro sensitivity to ATO	Therapy and outcome
ZTBTB16-RARA	t(11;17)(q23;q21)	Resistant	Resistant	Major series reported insensitivity to ATRA [2, 21] and therapeutic strategies including intensive chemotherapy and stem cell transplant are generally adopted for young and/or fit patients. Case reports have described response to ATRA with differentiation effects [22, 23]
NPM1-RARA	t(5;17)(q35;q21)	Responsive	Not tested	Case reports have shown CR with ATRA + chemotherapy. Relapses have been reported in 4/8 cases [29]. ATO therapy has been used in only one relapsed case with success [33]
STAT5B-RARA	der(17)	Resistant	Not tested	The majority of patients with *STAT5B/RARA*-positive APL showed resistance to both ATO and ATRA as the majority (six out of seven) of them experienced single or multiple relapses [38, 40–42]
BCOR-RARA	t(X;17)(p11;q12)	Not tested	Not tested	The single patient reported achieved CR through leukemic cell differentiation with ATRA and Tamibarotene, but not with ATO. The patient relapsed several times and needed allo-HSCT to maintain remission [10]
FIP1L1-PDGFRα	t(4;17)(q12;q21)	Responsive	Not tested	The patient achieved CR with ATRA therapy alone [11]
IRF2BP2-RARA	t(1;17)(q14;q21)	Responsive	Not tested	The first case achieved CR by ATRA + GO and ATO but relapsed 10 months later [14]. Grimwade and colleagues described differentiation of blasts with hematologic response with ATRA alone [55]. In the last case, the patient was resistant to ATRA and chemotherapy [57]

Table 20.1 (continued)

Fusion gene	Cytogenetics	In vitro sensitivity to ATRA	In vitro sensitivity to ATO	Therapy and outcome
FNDC3B-RARA	t(3;17)(q26;q21)	Not tested	Not tested	The patient initially responded to ATRA + chemotherapy and developed differentiation syndrome. Relapse was documented +8 months after the beginning of maintenance [15]
NuMA-RARA	t(11;17)(q13;q21)	Responsive	Not tested	The only patient reported was sensitive to ATRA [7]
PRKAR1A/RARA	der(17)	Not tested	Not tested	Treatment of a single patient with ATRA, idarubicin, and arsenic trioxide induced cytogenetic complete remission [9]
OBFC2A/RARA	t(2;17)(q32;q21)	Responsive	Not tested	The patient achieved CR with ATRA + chemotherapy and remained disease-free [12]
GTF2I/RARA	t(7;17)(q11;q21)	Not tested	Not tested	The only described patient failed to achieve CR with ATRA and ATO therapy [13]
NUP98/RARG	t(11;12)(p15;q13)	Primary blast cells resulted responsive to ATRA [65]; transfected cells resulted resistant [64]	Not tested	The only patient described was treated with ATRA only for 1 day at diagnosis and with ATRA in combination with chemotherapy at relapse; it is therefore impossible to evaluate the clinical sensitivity to this agent [4]
PML-RARG	t(12;15)(q13;q22)	Not tested	Not tested	The patient resulted resistant to a short course of therapy with ATRA (18 days) [5]

Translocation t(11;17)(q23;q21) APL with the *ZBTB16/RARA* Fusion Gene

The most common APL variant is t(11;17)(q23;q21) which fuses *ZBTB16* (formerly PLZF or promyelocytic leukemia zinc finger) with *RARA* and results in the production of the *ZBTB16-RARA* fusion protein.

APL with the t(11;17)(q23;q21) was first described in 1993 by Chen and colleagues at the Shanghai Institute of Hematology [6]. Within a large series of APL cases, the authors identified a patient with a morphologic diagnosis of APL whose leukemic cells did not harbor the *PML-RARA* fusion gene and contained instead a t(11;17)(q23;q21) translocation [6]. This cytogenetic variant was fully characterized at the molecular level by the same investigators in collaboration with other researchers including S. Waxman in the USA and A. Zelent in the UK [6]. As a result of the t(11;17), the *RARA* gene was fused in-frame with the coding sequences of a new gene, termed *ZBTB16* (for promyelocytic leukemia zinc finger), which encoded a putative transcription factor containing nine zinc finger motifs related to the Drosophila gene Kruppel and was expressed in at least two isoforms differing for the N-terminal region of the protein. The location of the translocation breakpoints within the *RARA* and *ZBTB16* genes suggested that in addition to the *ZBTB16-RARA* hybrid gene, expressed by the *ZBTB16* gene promoter from the derivative 11q+ chromosome, the reciprocal *RARA-ZBTB16* fusion gene was expressed from the derivative 17q− chromosome. Interestingly, both *PML-RARA* and *ZBTB16-RARA* genes were shown to contain identical portions of the *RARA* gene, indicating the importance of RARA functional domains in the etiology of this disease.

Pathophysiology Studies on Cell Lines and Mouse Models

Pandolfi and colleagues from Harvard University in the USA demonstrated through mouse models the pathophysiology of the leukemogenesis driven by ZBTB16-RARA chimeric protein and discovered important implications related to the response to APL therapy, in particular to ATRA [18]. In fact, they demonstrated that *both ZBTB16-RARA* and *PML-RARA* have a critical leukemogenic role, but they retain important biologic differences due to the distinct PML and ZBTB16 moieties involved in the translocations with RARA. In order to understand the two models of leukemogenesis and their response to ATRA treatment, they generated transgenic mice expressing either ZBTB16-RARA or PML-RARA. Leukemias developing in *ZBTB16-RARA* mice were characterized by leucocytosis in the peripheral blood accompanied by infiltration of promyelocytes and myelocytes retaining their capacity to generate terminal maturing forms in all organs. These features were more similar to the phenotype observed in chronic myeloid leukemia phenotype and distinct from PML-RARA-driven leukemias, in which the most prominent feature consisted in the accumulation of immature myeloid blasts blocked at the promyelocytic stage. Importantly, PML-RARA- and ZBTB16-RARA-driven leukemias differed in terms of their sensitivity to ATRA: opposite to classical PML-RARA leukemia, ZBTB16-RARA leukemia generated in mice was resistant to this agent [18]. The biological basis underlying this therapy response difference was in part unraveled by Pandolfi and colleagues. In fact, similarly to PML-RARA, the ZBTB16-RARalpha fusion protein was shown to act as a transcriptional repressor, but its activity was more potent as compared to PML-RARA [18]. Previous studies had already shown that in the absence of the ligand (RA), RARA forms complexes with multiple corepressor proteins (SMRT, N-CoR, Sin3, and HDACs). The work of Pandolfi and colleagues demonstrated that the interaction of SMRT with ZBTB16-RARA via its ZBTB16 moiety is more stable than PML-RARA-SMRT interaction, and this might explain the lack of responsiveness to ATRA. Interestingly, experiments in ZBTB16-RARA transgenic mice showed that increased ATRA doses are effective in inducing complete clinical remission. Moreover, these investigators reported that the combination of histone deacetylase inhibitors such as Trichostatin A (TSA) and ATRA was able to overcome the transcriptional repression ZBTB16-RARalpha-expressing leukemia cells [18].

The advent of arsenic trioxide (ATO) therapy in APL at the end of the 1990s prompted investigators to test the sensitivity of t(11;17)(q23;q21) to ATO alone or in combination with ATRA. de Thé and colleagues from Hopital St. Louis in Paris showed that ATO failed to induce apoptosis in primary blasts of a t(11;17)(q23;q21) APL in vitro [19]. Similar results were obtained by Pandolfi and colleagues, who reported that neither in ZBTB16-RARA transgenic mice nor in nude mice transplanted with ZBTB16-RARA cells ATO or ATO + ATRA in combination showed any efficacy [20]. Arsenic trioxide, known to induce aggregation of PML nuclear bodies, left the microspeckled ZBTB16-RARA localization completely unaffected. However, de Thé and colleagues showed that ATRA treatment led to ZBTB16-RARA protein degradation, similar to what demonstrated in PML-RARA-positive APL [19]. However, ZBTB16-RARA degradation was not accompanied by differentiation or apoptosis, suggesting that therapeutic strategies aimed solely at degrading the ZBTB16-RARA oncoprotein may not be effective in t(11;17) APL and that other molecular events might be responsible for resistance to ATRA and ATO in this leukemic subset.

Clinical Characteristics and Therapeutic Approaches

ZBTB16-RARA-positive leukemias are very rare, and only case reports or small case series have been reported up to date. As to phenotypic features, t(11;17) leukemias fall into an unusual morphologic spectrum of APL. The cases with *ZBTB16-RARA* t(11;17) APL are characterized by a predominance of blasts with regular nuclei, coarse granules, or, less often, fine or no granules and a more condensed nuclear chromatin compared with classic APL; there is also an increased number of Pelger-like cells or hypogranular neutrophils [16].

In general, the t(11;17) APL variant seems to have morphologic features intermediate between FAB M2 and FAB M3 subtypes. These features have also been described in two cases that lacked t(11;17) but harbored cryptic *ZBTB16-RARA* rearrangements [16]. The *ZBTB16-RARA* APL variant is also immunophenotypically unique since it is more commonly associated with CD56 expression compared with classic APL.

At the clinical level, Licht and colleagues reported six patients who all failed to achieve complete remission with ATRA or chemotherapy +/− ATRA [21]. On the contrary, Grimwade and colleagues reported in their series that 10 out of 11 patients achieved complete remission, 6 of whom with ATRA employed for first-line therapy alone or in combination with chemotherapy [2]. Case reports have, however, questioned the absolute resistance of this rare variant to retinoids. Jansen and colleagues have reported complete remission (CR) through blast cell differentiation in a patient harboring ZBTB16-RARA rearrangement by using granulocyte colony-stimulating factor (G-CSF), combined with ATRA [22]. Similarly, Petti et al. have reported in one case the achievement of a CR with ATRA and hydroxyurea, documenting a differentiating effect produced by this therapy on leukemic blasts [23].

NPM-RARA Fusion Gene

The second APL variant is t(5;17)(q35;q21) which results in the fusion of *NPM* (nucleophosmin gene) to *RARA*, producing the *NPM-RARA* fusion gene [24]. NPM1 is a nucleolar phosphoprotein, ubiquitously expressed, that has an essential role in transporting components of the ribosome and other proteins between the cytoplasm and the nucleolus [25]. Rearrangement of *NPM1* gene has been previously reported in t(2;5) positive lymphomas where NPM1 is fused to the ALK tyrosine kinase, generating the *NPM-ALK* fusion in anaplastic large cell lymphoma [26]. *NPM1* is also fused to the *MLF1* gene in t(3;5)(q25.1;q34-35) leading to the *NPM-MLF1* fusion gene in myelodysplastic syndromes and AML [27]. In addition, it is now well known that *NPM1* gene is recurrently mutated in AML with normal karyotype and represents a separate genomic entity in the WHO classification of AML [28].

In 1994, Corey et al. reported the first case of t(5;17)(q35;q21) in a 4-year-old girl with APL, from whose leukemic blasts they isolated cDNA and identified the NPM-RARA fusion transcript [29]. The encoded NPM-RARA protein represented a fusion between the N-terminal 117 amino acids of NPM and the 503 C-terminal amino acids of RARA [24]. Interestingly, NPM-RARA protein contains the same 118 N-terminal nucleophosmin sequences of the NPM-ALK fusion protein found in anaplastic lymphomas [26]. NPM-RARA APL cases have a morphologic and phenotypic profile similar to PML-RARA-positive APL, but Auer rods tend to be absent in *NPM-RARA*-positive cases; in addition, these blasts may display small azurophilic granules, abundant cytoplasm, and regular nuclear outline [2, 29, 30].

At the biologic level, the expression of NPM-RARA inhibits myeloid differentiation and induces leukemia in mouse models [31]. Similar to transgenic PML-RARA models, the NPM-RARA mice had a prolonged latency in leukemia development, ranging between 18 and 24 months and presented with leukemic blasts with monocytoid features resembling acute myelomonocytic leukemia. Similarly to PML-RARA APL, NPM-RARA fusion protein interacts with the corepressor protein SMRT in a manner that is less sensitive than wild-type RARA to dissociation by retinoic acid. NPM-RARA-positive blasts were shown *in vitro* to retain the ability to achieve terminal differentiation in the presence of pharmacological concentration of ATRA [31]. In addition, already in the first reported case of NPM-RARA, the patient was able to achieve complete remission with ATRA treatment [29].

More recently, proteomic analysis identified tumor necrosis factor receptor type 1-associated DEATH domain protein (TRADD) as an important binding partner for NPM-RARA. Biological assessment showed that NPM-RARA expression impaired TNF-induced signaling through TRADD, blunting TNF-mediated activation of caspase 3 and caspase 8, and consequently blocking apoptosis [32].

Five of the eight APL patients with *NPM-RARA* fusion gene described up to now were children, aged 12 years or less [30]. Extramedullary presentation of leukemia was common in this subset, with four cases (50%) presenting with myeloid sarcoma [30].

ATO therapy has been employed only in one case of NPM-RARA leukemia, and the authors reported long-term response to this agent after multiple relapses. However, no clear conclusions can be drawn in this regard [33].

NuMA-RARA Fusion Gene

The APL variant, t(11;17)(q13;q21), leads to the fusion between *nuclear mitotic apparatus (NuMA)* and *RARA* genes and was identified by Wells et al. in 1996 in a 6-year-old boy [7]. NuMA protein plays a role in mitosis, specifically in the formation of spindle pores and spindle asters and in the reformation of daughter nuclei [34]. The *NuMA-RARA* fusion gene joins exons encoding the retinoic acid and DNA-binding domains of *RARA* to 5′ exons of *NuMA*. The NuMA-RARA fusion protein exists in sheet-like nuclear aggregates with which normal NuMA partly co-localizes [7].

The first reported case was a 6-month-old boy who presented with multiple cutaneous lesions and peripheral blood morphologic and immunophenotypic characteristics resembling typical APL [35]. Bone marrow karyotype revealed a clonal cytogenetic abnormality, t(11;17)(q13;q21) with molecular evidence of *RARA* rearrangement but without involvement of *PML* or *ZBTB16*. The patient was treated with ATRA and achieved complete remission; he remained in morphological remission at 38 months after autologous stem-cell transplant [35]. Transgenic mouse models harboring NuMA-RARA were generated and showed to rapidly develop a myeloproliferative disease-like myeloid leukemia at early age. This leukemia was indistinguishable from human APL, demonstrating that NuMA-RARA is sufficient for disease development in APL mouse models [36].

STAT5B/RARA Fusion Gene

In this variant form, the signal transducer and activator of transcription 5b (*STAT5B*) have been shown to rearrange with *RARA* with consequent *STAT5B-RARA* fusion due to a 3 Mb interstitial deletion event on the long arm of chromosome 17 (17q21). STAT proteins are a family of latent cytosolic transcription factors activated by Janus kinase (JAK) tyrosine kinases, with seven members: STAT 1, 2, 3, 4, 5a, 5b, and 6. STAT5B is widely expressed on a number of tissues including hematopoietic progenitors. The aberrant activation of this family of proteins has been implicated in cell transformation and oncogenesis [37]. The first case of APL with *STAT5B/RARA* fusion was reported in a male patient in 1999 [8], and since then a total of eight cases have been reported [38]. The pathogenetic role of *STAT5B-RARA* remains unclear. *STAT5B-RARA* can enhance STAT3 activity and may contribute to leukemogenesis by interaction with the STAT3 oncogene pathway [39]. A literature review by Strehl et al. in 2013 showed that patients with *STAT5B/RARA*-positive APL are resistant to both ATO and ATRA as the majority (6 out of 7) of them experienced single or multiple relapses [38]. The only patient who remained relapse-free for more than 2 years received ATRA, ATO, and chemotherapy followed by allogeneic hematopoietic stem-cell transplant (HSCT) in the first molecular CR. Additional three patients were reported [40–42], and all resulted to be resistant to differentiation therapy. Therefore, because of the very poor prognosis of patients with *STAT5B/RARA*-positive APL, these patients might benefit from allogeneic HSCT in the first remission.

PRKAR1A/RARA Fusion Gene

The *PRKAR1A* gene encodes the regulatory subunit type I-α (RI-α) of cyclic adenosine monophosphate (cAMP)-dependent protein kinase (PKA) [43]. *PRKAR1A* is involved in another gene rearrangement with the *RET* proto-oncogene in papillary thyroid carcinomas [44], and *PRKAR1A* inactivating mutations or downregulation has been found in some sporadic adrenocortical tumors [45]. The first and only case of *PRKAR1A/RARA* fusion gene reported to date was a 66-year-old man with APL, whose leukemic cell karyotype showed 47,XY,+22[5]/46,XY[30] without the classic t(15;17) translocation. FISH studies disclosed a del(17)(q21)(5′RARA−,RARA+)

plus a split *RARA* signal with *RARA* break-apart probe [9]. Nested RT-PCR confirmed the presence of the PRKAR1A/RARA fusion transcript. The patient was treated with ATRA, ATO, and chemotherapy which induced complete molecular remission; at the time of report, he had remained disease-free for 2 years from diagnosis. Because the patient received treatment with multiple agents including ATRA, ATO, and different types of chemotherapy, it is difficult to definitely assess the sensitivity to ATRA or ATO without *in vitro* experiments or mouse models [9].

FIP1L1/RARA Fusion Gene

This fusion gene was identified in 2008 in a 90-year-old woman, whose karyotype showed 47, XX, t(4;17)(q12;q21), and trisomy 8. FISH analysis showed that 94% of the bone marrow cells had the *RARA* split signal but no *PML-RARA* fusion signals. Sequence analysis of the identified fusion gene, from the reverse sequence of *RARA* exon 3, identified Fip1-like1 or *FIP1L1* as the partner gene of *RARA*. Cloning of the *FIP1L1/RARA* showed three in-frame isoforms of this fusion gene fusing *RARA* exon 3 to *FIP1L1* [11]. *FIP1L1* is known to form a fusion gene with *PDGFRA* that causes chronic eosinophilic leukemia [46]. Furthermore, *FIP1L1/RARA* was also isolated from a case of juvenile myelomonocytic leukemia (JMML) [47].

FIP1L1/RARA forms a homodimer, which represses retinoic acid-dependent transcriptional activity at the lowest concentration of ATRA, showing responsiveness similar to that of *PML-RARA*. Indeed, the patient achieved a CR with ATRA therapy alone [11].

BCOR/RARA Fusion Gene

The BCL6 corepressor, BCOR, is a ubiquitously expressed nuclear protein, which directly interfaces to proto-oncoprotein BCL6 through the BCOR-BCL6-binding domain [48]. BCOR also associates with histone deacetylases (HDACs) and polycomb repressive complex 1 components, which indicates that it might suppress gene transcription by epigenetic mechanisms [49]. BCOR was reported to be critical for early embryonic development, mesenchymal stem-cell function, and lymphoid cell differentiation, and mutations in the gene have been linked with human-inherited diseases such as the oculofaciocardiodental and lenz microphthalmia syndromes [50].

The *BCOR/RARA* fusion was first reported in 2010 in a 45-year-old man with APL whose blasts showed a unique morphology with round inclusions and rectangular cytoplasmic bodies [10]. Karyotype analysis detected a novel chromosomal translocation described as 45, -Y, t(X;17)(p11.2;q12)[19]/46, XY[1]. FISH analysis indicated one intact and two split signals of *RARA* and two intact signals of *PML*. RT-PCR revealed BCOR cDNA from exons 9 to 12 to be fused to *RARA* exon 3. The chimeric cDNA had an in-frame codon from *BCOR* through *RARA*, creating a 1931 amino acid fusion protein described as *BCOR/RARA* [10]. The patient clinical course showed that coagulopathy at diagnosis was relieved by ATRA and tamibarotene, but not by ATO. Leukemic cell differentiation was accomplished with ATRA and tamibarotene. Despite initial response, the patient relapsed several times and eventually needed allogeneic HSCT to prolong remission [10].

Other Very Rare Variants

Four novel fusion genes involving *RARA* were recently identified: the *OBFC2A/RARA* [12], *GTF2I/RARA* [13], *IRF2BP2-RARA* [14], and *FNDC3-RARA* [15].

The *OBFC2A*, oligonucleotide/oligosaccharide-binding fold containing 2A, gene is located at chromosome 2q32.3 and encodes human single-stranded DNA-binding protein 2, which plays a role in DNA damage response and genomic stability. The *OBFC2A/RARA* was identified in a 59-year-old man with APL whose bone marrow karyotype showed clonal der(2)t(2;17)(q32;q21), and FISH revealed an extra *RARA* signal with the *PML-RARA* probe and a 3′ *RARA* green signal with the

RARA break-apart probe on der(2) [12]. Array comparative genomic hybridization (CGH) showed a loss in 2q32.2 and a gain in 17q21.2. The breakpoints were located within the *OBFC2A* gene in 2q32.2 and the *RARA* gene in 17q21.2. RT-PCR with direct sequence analysis showed that the *RARA* portion of the transcript started in exon 3 and was fused in-frame to exon 5 of *OBFC2A*. This fusion appeared to be sensitive to ATRA both in vitro and clinically, since the patient achieved a CR with ATRA and chemotherapy and remained disease-free for 1 year after diagnosis [12].

The *GTF2I*, general transcription factor 2I, gene is located at 7q11.23 and is ubiquitously expressed; it encodes a phosphoprotein with broad roles in transcription and signal transduction involving growth signaling, cell cycle regulation, and transforming growth factor beta 1 (TGFB1) signaling [13]. The *GTF2I/RARA* was recently identified in a 35-year-old man with APL whose bone marrow karyotype showed 46, XY, and del(7q22), while FISH analysis revealed that a split *RARA* signal was inserted into the disrupted 7q region documenting the presence of submicroscopic t(7;17)(q?;q21) translocation [13]. RT-PCR showed that the *GTF2I/RARA* resulted from the fusion between exon 6 of *GTF2I* and exon 3 of *RARA*. This fusion was resistant to both ATRA and ATO, since the patient failed to achieve complete remission with these agents and died after 146 days from diagnosis due to intracranial bleeding [13].

The *IRF2BP2* gene, located on chromosome 1q42.3, encodes a nuclear protein that specifically interacts with the C-terminal transcriptional repression domain of IRF2. IRF2BP2 acts as a corepressor factor in the process of repression of nuclear factor of activated T cells (NFAT) transactivation, mediating the regulation of genes involved in cell cycle, differentiation, and apoptosis [51]. Interestingly, IRF2BP2 is directly regulated by TP53, and its overexpression can inhibit apoptosis by impeding TP53-mediated transactivation of the *TP21* and *BAX* genes [51]. *IRF2BP2* was described as a fusion partner of *CDX1* in the t(1;5)(q42;q32) in mesenchymal chondrosarcoma and was found mutated in chronic lymphocytic leukemia and primary central nervous system lymphoma [52–54].

In APL cases harboring the IRF2BP2-RARA fusion transcript, the *IRF2BP2* intron 1 infused to intron 2 of *RARA* gene located on chromosome [14, 55].

In vitro studies have shown that the IRF2BP2-RARA fusion has the capacity to transform primary hematopoietic stem cells and to induce an ATRA-responsive leukemia. In fact, similarly to PML-RARA, IRF2BP2-RARA induces repression at retinoid response elements, that is reversed by pharmacological doses of ATRA [56]. Two reported IRF2BP2-RARA patients received ATRA in combination with chemotherapy or ATO and achieved complete remission with evidence of differentiation, but one patient relapsed after 10 months. One additional patient was treated with ATRA and chemotherapy but was resistant [14, 55, 57].

Finally, *FNDC3B* is another fusion partner described to be rearranged with *RARA* gene [15]. FNDC3B was originally described as factor involved in adipocyte differentiation process, and it contains nine fibronectin type III (FN3) domains, which are known to mediate protein interactions. In the recently described case, a 36-year-old male presented with a clinical picture suggestive for APL, characterized by hypergranular blasts in bone marrow; CD13, CD15, CD33, and CD117 positivity; and CD34 and HLA-DR negativity by flow cytometry and coagulopathy. However, RT-PCR and FISH failed to identify *PML-RARA,* but still FISH showed that 72% of cells had a split RARA signal. Karyotype analysis showed 45,X,-Y,t(3;17)(q26;q21)[8]/46,XY[5], and through 5′-rapid amplification of cDNA ends, the authors identified *FNDC3B* as *RARA* partner. Authors showed that exon 24 of *FNDC3B* was fused to exon 3 of *RARA*, generating a 1461 amino acid protein, containing eight FN3 domains of *FNDC3B* and the DNA-binding and ligand-binding domains of *RARA*. The patient was treated with 7 + 3 regimen including ATRA and entered into remission: of note, the patient experienced ATRA differentiation syndrome on day 4 of therapy. After initial response, the patient relapsed 8 months after the start of maintenance therapy [15].

Treatment Strategies

It is well known that *RARA* plays a key role in the development of APL. Study of the variant translocations has provided strong support for the pathogenetic role of the interaction between X-RARA fusion proteins and corepressors in the myeloid maturational arrest that characterizes APL [17, 58]. In fact, under normal conditions, ATRA causes ligand-dependent conformational changes in wild-type RARA that induces the dissociation of nuclear corepressors, facilitating cellular differentiation. In case of *PML-RARA* fusion, cellular differentiation is blocked since the physiologic concentrations of ATRA are sufficient to induce the conformational change that is required for the corepressor release. Thus, high concentrations of ATRA are required to induce release of the corepressor complex from the APL chimeric fusion proteins so that coactivators can activate transcription, which results in the terminal differentiation of the APL blasts [59].

NPM-RARA, *NuMA-RARA*, *PRKAR1A/RARA*, *BCOR/RARA,* and *FIP1L1/RARA* have all been reported to have a high affinity for corepressor molecules, and similarly to *PML-RARA*, they need high levels of ATRA to induce the release of corepressor complex and allow transcription and differentiation to proceed [9, 10, 17, 24, 60]. Therefore, patients with these variants can potentially achieve remission with treatment regimens similar to those employed for classic APL. Although patients with *NPM-RARA* and *BCOR/RARA* usually respond to ATRA similarly to patients with classic APL, studies have reported a higher risk of relapse in these patients [10, 29]. Arsenic trioxide is currently regarded as the most effective agent in APL harboring *PML-RARA* fusion gene. Arsenic trioxide combined to ATRA has produced up to 100% of OS rates in lower-risk APL and is currently indicated for front-line and salvage therapy [61]. ATO induces differentiation and apoptosis of leukemic cells via multiple mechanisms, with the main ones being the activation of caspase proteins cascade and the direct degradation of PML-RARA oncoprotein [3]. The latter effect is mediated by direct ATO binding to PML moiety of PML-RARA and subsequent SUMOylation and polyubiquitination of PML-RARA which is finally degradated by the ubiquitin-proteasome pathway [3]. Disregarding ZBTB16-RARA-positive APL which has been demonstrated to be resistant to ATO both in vivo and in vitro, the sensitivity of other rare APL variants to ATO has not been well documented yet, and only single-case reports are available. Chen et al. reported a long-term survival in an APL patient with variant *NPM-RARA* who relapsed four times and each time responded well to ATO or ATO-based re-induction therapies [33]. Also, *PRKAR1A/RARA* variant appears to be sensitive to ATO [9], while *BCOR/RARA*-positive leukemia seems resistant to this agent [10]. STAT5B-RARA variant has been almost consistently reported not to be sensitive to both ATRA and ATO [10].

APL Variants Involving RARG Gene

The retinoic acid receptor genes (RARA, RARB, RARG) share a high sequence homology with conserved DNA-binding and ligand-binding domains [62]. Despite their high structural homology, until recently genetic variants of APL reported in the literature exclusively involved the nuclear receptor alpha of the RAR family. In 2011, investigators from La Fè Hospital in Valencia first described the involvement of *RARG* gene as fusion partner with NUP98 in an AML case with morphological features of APL [4]. More recently, in 2017, investigators from South Korea have reported an even more peculiar case with morphologic and immunophenotypic features of classical hypergranular APL harboring *RARG* gene fused to *PML*. The latter is the first case to be reported involving *PML* in combination with an alternative *RAR* gene receptors [5].

NUP98-RARG Fusion Gene

Investigators from Hospital La Fé in Valencia (Spain) reported in 2011 a unique case of acute promyelocytic leukemia involving another subtype of the RAR family, i.e., RARgamma (RARG) receptor [4]. The patient presented with acute myeloid leukemia showing morphologic and immunophenotypic features consistent with the classical hypergranular subtype of APL. However, FISH and RT-PCR were both negative for PML-RARA, and G-banding karyotype analysis revealed a translocation t(11;12)(p15;q13). Through CGH array and RT-PCR, investigators demonstrated a novel rearrangement fusing together exon 12 of *NUP98* gene and exon 4 of *RARG* genes [4]. The NUP98 gene has been described to be involved in recurrent AML translocations and encodes for a protein component of the nuclear pore complex that regulates the nucleocytoplasmic transport of proteins and mRNAs [63]. Subsequent studies conducted in murine models have shown that NUP98-RARG homodimers were able to transform primary hematopoietic stem/progenitors [64]. Cells harboring this fusion protein disclose a specific nuclear localization pattern of NUP98-RARG homodimers together with the ability to recruit both RXRA and wild-type NUP98 but also exhibited transcriptional properties similar to other *RARA* fusions found in APL [64]. Regarding sensitivity to target therapies, contrasting results are present in available studies. The patient described in the single-case report was treated with a standard 7 + 3 schedule including cytarabine and idarubicin as induction therapy and subsequently underwent consolidation chemotherapy followed by autologous peripheral blood stem-cell transplant. After 2 years the patient relapsed and was treated with ATRA + chemotherapy obtaining CR; unfortunately he died from infectious complications during umbilical cord transplantation. The patient was treated with ATRA only for one day and with ATRA in combination with chemotherapy at relapse; it is therefore difficult to analyze the clinical sensitivity to this agent [4, 65]. Resistance to ATRA was demonstrated in an i*n vitro* study by the same Spanish investigators in the patient's leukemic cells harboring *NUP98-RARG* fusion [65]; an opposite result was suggested by a subsequent *in vitro* study using a *NUP98-RARG* construct, where cells were sensitive to this compound [64].

PML-RARG Fusion Gene

Investigators from South Korea very recently described the case of a 64-year-old woman presenting with a clinical picture of cytopenia and laboratory coagulopathy, whose bone marrow showed infiltration by atypical hypergranular promyelocytes with Auer rods characterized by immunophenotypic positivity for CD13, CD33, CD45, CD117, and cMPO and negativity for HLA-DR [5]. The t(15;17)(q22;q21) translocation was not detected by karyotyping; instead, a clonal translocation t(12;15)(q13;q22) was identified in 13 of 20 metaphases analyzed. FISH analysis for *PML-RARA* fusion showed *PML* split signals that were identified to be located on der(12)t(12;15)(q13;q22) and der(15)t(12;15)(q13;q22) from metaphase FISH and corresponding G-banded chromosomes. With whole-genome sequencing techniques, *PML* partner gene was identified as *RARG* on 12q13, and the results were validated by nested RT-PCR and Sanger sequencing. Two different PML-RARG transcripts were identified, with the longer transcript fusing PML exon 3 to exon 1 of RARG and the shorter fusing PML exon 3 and exon 2 of RARG. At the DNA level, the genomic breakpoint was located in *PML* intron 3 (as in bcr3 PML-RARA isoform) and at the protein level, the original RARG amino acid sequence was conserved, and DBD and LBD RARG domains remained functional after fusion. Concerning ATRA sensitivity, the patient was treated for 18 days with ATRA and showed no response [5]. However, no clinical conclusions can be drawn in light of the early discontinuation of ATRA.

Conclusions

Rare acute leukemia variants involving retinoic acid receptor genes represent very rare cases that share the involvement of *RAR* genes, either *RARA* of *RARG* isoforms, but retain heterogeneity in laboratory features and response to targeted therapy. Thus, the identification of some of these variants is important both for prognostic implications and for their sensitivity to targeted drugs.

References

1. de Thé H, Lavau C, Marchio A, Chomienne C, Degos L, Dejean A. The PML-RARα fusion mRNA generated by the t(15;17) translocation in acute promyelocytic leukemia encodes a functionally altered RAR. Cell. 1991;66(4):675–84.
2. Grimwade D, Biondi A, Mozziconacci MJ, Hagemeijer A, Berger R, Neat M, et al. Characterization of acute promyelocytic leukemia cases lacking the classic t(15;17): results of the European Working Party. Groupe Francais de Cytogenetique Hematologique, Groupe de Francais d'Hematologie Cellulaire, UK Cancer Cytogenetics Group and BIOME. Blood. 2000;96(4):1297–308.
3. Wang ZY, Chen Z. Acute promyelocytic leukemia: from highly fatal to highly curable. Blood. 2008;111:2505–15.
4. Such E, Cervera J, Valencia A, Barragan E, Ibanez M, Luna I, et al. A novel NUP98/RARG gene fusion in acute myeloid leukemia resembling acute promyelocytic leukemia. Blood. 2011;117(1):242–5.
5. Ha J-S, Do YR, Ki C-S, Lee C, Kim D-H, Lee W, et al. Identification of a novel PML-RARG fusion in acute promyelocytic leukemia. Leukemia. 2017;31(9):1992–1995.
6. Chen SJ, Zelent A, Tong JH, Yu HQ, Wang ZY, Derre J, et al. Rearrangements of the retinoic acid receptor alpha and promyelocytic leukemia zinc finger genes resulting from t(11;17)(q23;q21) in a patient with acute promyelocytic leukemia. J Clin Invest. 1993;91(5):2260–7.
7. Wells RA, Catzavelos C, Kamel-Reid S. Fusion of retinoic acid receptor α to NuMA, the nuclear mitotic apparatus protein, by a variant translocation in acute promyelocytic leukaemia. Nat Genet [Internet]. 1997;17(1):109–13. http://www.nature.com/doifinder/10.1038/ng0997-109
8. Arnould C, Philippe C, Bourdon V, Grégoire MJ, Berger R, Jonveaux P. The signal transducer and activator of transcription STAT5b gene is a new partner of retinoic acid receptor α in acute promyelocytic-like leukaemia. Hum Mol Genet. 1999;8(9):1741–9.
9. Catalano A, Dawson MA, Somana K, Opat S, Schwarer A, Campbell LJ, et al. Brief report: the PRKAR1A gene is fused to RARA in a new variant acute promyelocytic leukemia. Blood. 2007;110(12):4073–6.
10. Yamamoto Y, Tsuzuki S, Tsuzuki M, Handa K, Inaguma Y, Emi N. BCOR as a novel fusion partner of retinoic acid receptor alpha in a t(X;17)(p11;q12) variant of acute promyelocytic leukemia. Blood. 2010;116(20):4274–83.
11. Kondo T, Mori A, Darmanin S, Hashino S, Tanaka J, Asaka M. The seventh pathogenic fusion gene FIP1L1-RARA was isolated from a t(4;17)-positive acute promyelocytic leukemia. Haematologica. 2008;93:1414–6. Italy.
12. Won D, Shin SY, Park CJ, Jang S, Chi HS, Lee KH, et al. OBFC2A/RARA: a novel fusion gene in variant acute promyelocytic leukemia. Blood [Internet]. 2013;121(8):1432–5. http://www.ncbi.nlm.nih.gov/pubmed/23287866
13. Li J, Zhong H-Y, Zhang Y, Xiao L, Bai L-H, Liu S-F, et al. GTF2I-RARA is a novel fusion transcript in a t(7;17) variant of acute promyelocytic leukaemia with clinical resistance to retinoic acid. Br J Haematol. 2015;168:904–8. England.
14. Yin CC, Jain N, Mehrotra M, Zhang J, Protopopov A, Zuo Z, et al. Identification of a novel fusion gene, IRF2BP2-RARA, in acute promyelocytic leukemia. J Natl Compr Canc Netw. 2015;13(1):19–22.
15. Cheng CK, Wang AZ, Wong THY, Wan TSK, Cheung JS, Raghupathy R, et al. FNDC3B is another novel partner fused to RARA in the t(3;17)(q26;q21) variant of acute promyelocytic leukemia. Blood. 2017;129:2705–9.
16. Sainty D, Liso V, Cantù-Rajnoldi A, Head D, Mozziconacci MJ, Arnoulet C, et al. A new morphologic classification system for acute promyelocytic leukemia distinguishes cases with underlying PLZF/RARA gene rearrangements. Blood [Internet]. 2000;96(4):1287–96. http://www.ncbi.nlm.nih.gov/pubmed/10942370
17. Redner RL. Variations on a theme: the alternate translocations in APL. Leuk Off J Leuk Soc Am Leuk Res Fund UK. 2002;16(10):1927–32.
18. He LZ, Guidez F, Tribioli C, Peruzzi D, Ruthardt M, Zelent A, et al. Distinct interactions of PML-RARalpha and PLZF-RARalpha with co-repressors determine differential responses to RA in APL. Nat Genet. 1998;18(2):126–35.
19. Koken MH, Daniel MT, Gianni M, Zelent A, Licht J, Buzyn A, et al. Retinoic acid, but not arsenic trioxide, degrades the PLZF/RARalpha fusion protein, without inducing terminal differentiation or apoptosis, in a RA-therapy resistant t(11;17)(q23;q21) APL patient. Oncogene [Internet]. 1999;18(4):1113–8. http://www.ncbi.nlm.nih.gov/pubmed/10023688
20. Rego EM, He LZ, Warrell RPJ, Wang ZG, Pandolfi PP. Retinoic acid (RA) and As2O3 treatment in transgenic models of acute promyelocytic leukemia (APL) unravel the distinct nature of the leukemogenic process induced by the PML-RARalpha and PLZF-RARalpha oncoproteins. Proc Natl Acad Sci U S A. 2000;97(18):10173–8.
21. Licht JD, Chomienne C, Goy A, Chen A, Scott AA, Head DR, et al. Clinical and molecular characterization of a rare syndrome of acute promyelocytic leukemia associated with translocation (11;17). Blood [Internet]. 1995;85(4):1083–94. http://www.bloodjournal.org/content/85/4/1083.abstract

22. Jansen JH, de Ridder MC, Geertsma WM, Erpelinck CA, van Lom K, Smit EM, et al. Complete remission of t(11;17) positive acute promyelocytic leukemia induced by all-trans retinoic acid and granulocyte colony-stimulating factor. Blood [Internet]. 1999;94(1):39–45. m:%5CProject Team Management%5CPreclinical Programs%5CScientific Information%5CPDF Articles%5CBLD94(1)39.pdf
23. Petti MC, Fazi F, Gentile M, Diverio D, De Fabritiis P, De Propris MS, et al. Complete remission through blast cell differentiation in PLZF/RARalpha-positive acute promyelocytic leukemia: in vitro and in vivo studies. Blood. 2002;100(3):1065–7.
24. Redner RL, Rush EA, Faas S, Rudert WA, Corey SJ. The t(5;17) variant of acute promyelocytic leukemia expresses a nucleophosmin-retinoic acid receptor fusion. Blood [Internet]. 1996;87(3):882–6. http://www.ncbi.nlm.nih.gov/pubmed/8562957
25. Yung BYM. Oncogenic role of nucleophosmin/B23. Chang Gung Med J. 2007;30(4):285–93.
26. Morris S, Kirstein M, Valentine M, Dittmer K, Shapiro D, Saltman D, et al. Fusion of a kinase gene, ALK, to a nucleolar protein gene, NPM, in non-Hodgkin's lymphoma. Science [Internet]. 1994;263(5151):1281–4. http://www.sciencemag.org/cgi/doi/10.1126/science.8122112
27. Yoneda-Kato N, Look AT, Kirstein MN, Valentine MB, Raimondi SC, Cohen KJ, et al. The t(3;5)(q25.1;q34) of myelodysplastic syndrome and acute myeloid leukemia produces a novel fusion gene, NPM-MLF1. Oncogene [Internet]. 1996;12(2):265–75. http://www.ncbi.nlm.nih.gov/pubmed/8570204
28. Falini B, Nicoletti I, Martelli MF, Mecucci C. Acute myeloid leukemia carrying cytoplasmic/mutated nucleophosmin (NPMc+ AML): biologic and clinical features. Blood. 2007;109:874–85.
29. Corey SJ, Locker J, Oliveri DR, Shekhter-Levin S, Redner RL, Penchansky L, et al. A non-classical translocation involving 17q12 (retinoic acid receptor alpha) in acute promyelocytic leukemia (APML) with atypical features. Leukemia [Internet]. 1994;8(8):1350–3. http://www.ncbi.nlm.nih.gov/pubmed/8057672
30. Kikuma T, Nakamachi Y, Noguchi Y, Okazaki Y, Shimomura D, Yakushijin K, et al. A new transcriptional variant and small azurophilic granules in an acute promyelocytic leukemia case with NPM1/RARA fusion gene. Int J Hematol. 2015;102(6):713–8.
31. Redner RL, Corey SJ, Rush EA. Differentiation of t(5;17) variant acute promyelocytic leukemic blasts by all-trans retinoic acid. Leukemia [Internet]. 1997;11(7):1014–6. http://www.ncbi.nlm.nih.gov/pubmed/9204984
32. Chattopadhyay A, Hood BL, Conrads TP, Redner RL. Extrinsic apoptosis is impeded by direct binding of the APL fusion protein NPM-RAR to TRADD. Mol Cancer Res [Internet]. 2014;12(9):1283–91. http://www.ncbi.nlm.nih.gov/pubmed/25033841
33. Chen Y, Gu L, Zhou C, Wu X, Gao J, Li Q, et al. Relapsed APL patient with variant NPM-RARalpha fusion responded to arsenic trioxide-based therapy and achieved long-term survival. Int J Hematol. 2010;91(4):708–10.
34. Saredi A, Howard L, Compton DA. NuMA assembles into an extensive filamentous structure when expressed in the cell cytoplasm. J Cell Sci [Internet]. 1996;109(Pt 3):619–30. http://www.ncbi.nlm.nih.gov/pubmed/8907707
35. Wells RA, Hummel JL, De Koven A, Zipursky A, Kirby M, Dubé I, et al. A new variant translocation in acute promyelocytic leukaemia: molecular characterization and clinical correlation. Leuk Off J Leuk Soc Am Leuk Res Fund, UK [Internet]. 1996;10(4):735–40. http://www.ncbi.nlm.nih.gov/pubmed/8618456
36. Sukhai MA, Wu X, Xuan Y, Zhang T, Reis PP, Dubé K, et al. Myeloid leukemia with promyelocytic features in transgenic mice expressing hCG-NuMA-RARalpha. Oncogene [Internet]. 2004;23(3):665–78. http://www.ncbi.nlm.nih.gov/pubmed/14737102
37. Bromberg J. Stat proteins and oncogenesis. J Clin Investig. 2002;109:1139–42.
38. Strehl S, Konig M, Boztug H, Cooper BW, Suzukawa K, Zhang S-J, et al. All-trans retinoic acid and arsenic trioxide resistance of acute promyelocytic leukemia with the variant STAT5B-RARA fusion gene. Leukemia. 2013;27:1606–10. England.
39. Dong S, Tweardy DJ. Interactions of STAT5b-RARalpha, a novel acute promyelocytic leukemia fusion protein, with retinoic acid receptor and STAT3 signaling pathways. Blood. 2002;99(8):2637–46.
40. Pessina C, Basilico C, Genoni A, Meroni E, Elli L, Granata P, et al. A new acute myeloid leukemia case with STAT5B-RARA gene fusion due to 17q21.2 interstitial deletion. Leuk Lymphoma. 2017;58(8):1977–80.
41. Wang Y-Y, Hao J, Liu Z-Y, Weng X-Q, Sheng Y, Jiang C-L, et al. Novel STAT5B-RARA fusion transcript in acute promyelocytic leukemia: identification and treatment response. Leuk Lymphoma. 2015;56:2731–4. England.
42. Kluk MJ, Abo RP, Brown RD, Kuo FC, Dal Cin P, Pozdnyakova O, et al. Myeloid neoplasm demonstrating a STAT5B-RARA rearrangement and genetic alterations associated with all-trans retinoic acid resistance identified by a custom next-generation sequencing assay. Cold Spring Harb Mol case Stud. 2015;1(1):a000307.
43. Bossis I, Stratakis CA. Minireview: PRKAR1A: normal and abnormal functions. Endocrinology. 2004;145:5452–8.
44. Bongarzone I, Monzini N, Borrello MG, Carcano C, Ferraresi G, Arighi E, et al. Molecular characterization of a thyroid tumor-specific transforming sequence formed by the fusion of ret tyrosine kinase and the regulatory subunit RI alpha of cyclic AMP-dependent protein kinase A. Mol Cell Biol. 1993;13(1):358–66.
45. Bertherat J, Groussin L, Sandrini F, Matyakhina L, Bei T, Stergiopoulos S, et al. Molecular and functional analysis of PRKAR1A and its locus (17q22-24)

in sporadic adrenocortical tumors: 17q losses, somatic mutations, and protein kinase a expression and activity. Cancer Res. 2003;63(17):5308–19.

46. Cools J, Stover EH, Gilliland DG. Detection of the FIP1L1-PDGFRA fusion in idiopathic hypereosinophilic syndrome and chronic eosinophilic leukemia. Methods Mol Med. 2006;125(4):177–87.
47. Buijs A. Bruin M. Fusion of FIP1L1 and RARA as a result of a novel t(4;17)(q12;q21) in a case of juvenile myelomonocytic leukemia. Leukemia. 2007;21:1104–8. England.
48. Ghetu AF, Corcoran CM, Cerchietti L, Bardwell VJ, Melnick A, Privé GG. Structure of a BCOR corepressor peptide in complex with the BCL6 BTB domain dimer. Mol Cell. 2008;29(3):384–91.
49. Fan Z, Yamaza T, Lee JS, Yu J, Wang S, Fan G, et al. BCOR regulates mesenchymal stem cell function by epigenetic mechanisms. Nat Cell Biol [Internet]. 2009;11(8):1002–9.
50. Ng D, Thakker N, Corcoran CM, Donnai D, Perveen R, Schneider A, et al. Oculofaciocardiodental and Lenz microphthalmia syndromes result from distinct classes of mutations in BCOR. Nat Genet [Internet]. 2004;36(4):411–6.
51. Roy AL. Biochemistry and biology of the inducible multifunctional transcription factor TFII-I: 10 years later. Gene. 2012;492:32–41.
52. Nyquist KB, Panagopoulos I, Thorsen J, Haugom L, Gorunova L, Bjerkehagen B, et al. Whole-transcriptome sequencing identifies novel IRF2BP2-CDX1 fusion gene brought about by translocation t(1;5)(q42;q32) in mesenchymal chondrosarcoma. PLoS One. 2012;7(11):e49705.
53. Schuh A, Becq J, Humphray S, Alexa A, Burns A, Clifford R, et al. Monitoring chronic lymphocytic leukemia progression by whole genome sequencing reveals heterogeneous clonal evolution patterns. Blood. 2012;120(20):4191–6.
54. Bruno A, Boisselier B, Labreche K, Marie Y, Polivka M, Jouvet A, et al. Mutational analysis of primary central nervous system lymphoma. Oncotarget. 2014;5(13):5065–75.
55. Jovanovic JV, Carmen Chillón M, Vincent-Fabert C, Dillon R, Voisset E, Gutiérrez NC, et al. The IRF2BP2-RARα fusion generated by a cryptic rearrangement transforms hematopoietic stem/progenitor cells and induces retinoid sensitive acute promyelocytic leukemia (APL). Blood [Internet]. 2014;124(21):2325.
56. Jovanovic JV, Chillon MC, Vincent-Fabert C, Dillon R, Voisset E, Gutierrez NC, et al. The cryptic IRF2BP2-RARA fusion transforms hematopoietic stem/progenitor cells and induces retinoid-sensitive acute promyelocytic leukemia. Leukemia. 2017;31(3):747–51.
57. Yin CC, Jain N, Mehrotra M, Zhagn J, Protopopov A, Zuo Z, et al. Identification of a novel fusion gene, IRF2BP2-RARA, in acute promyelocytic leukemia. J Natl Compr Canc Netw [Internet]. 2015;13(1):19–22.
58. Adams J, Nassiri M. Acute promyelocytic leukemia a review and discussion of variant translocations. Arch Pathol Lab Med. 2015;139:1308–13.
59. Guidez F, Ivins S, Zhu J, Söderström M, Waxman S, Zelent A. Reduced retinoic acid-sensitivities of nuclear receptor corepressor binding to PML- and PLZF-RARα underlie molecular pathogenesis and treatment of acute Promyelocytic Leukemia. Blood [Internet]. 1998;91(8):2634–42.
60. Iwasaki J, Kondo T, Darmanin S, Ibata M, Onozawa M, Hashimoto D, et al. FIP1L1 presence in FIP1L1-RARA or FIP1L1-PDGFRA differentially contributes to the pathogenesis of distinct types of leukemia. Ann Hematol. 2014;93(9):1473–81.
61. Lo-Coco F, Avvisati G, Vignetti M, Thiede C, Orlando SM, Iacobelli S, et al. Retinoic acid and arsenic trioxide for acute promyelocytic leukemia. N Engl J Med. 2013;369(2):111–21.
62. Di Masi A, Leboffe L, De Marinis E, Pagano F, Cicconi L, Rochette-Egly C, et al. Retinoic acid receptors: from molecular mechanisms to cancer therapy. Mol Asp Med. 2015;41:1–115.
63. Moore MAS, Chung KY, Plasilova M, Schuringa JJ, Shieh JH, Zhou P, et al. NUP98 dysregulation in myeloid leukemogenesis. Ann N Y Acad Sci. 2007;1106:114–42.
64. Qiu JJ, Zeisig BB, Li S, Liu W, Chu H, Song Y, et al. Critical role of retinoid/rexinoid signaling in mediating transformation and therapeutic response of NUP98-RARG leukemia. Leukemia [Internet]. 2015;29(5):1153–62.
65. Such E, Cordon L, Sempere A, Villamon E, Ibanez M, Luna I, et al. In vitro all-trans retinoic acid sensitivity of acute myeloid leukemia blasts with NUP98/RARG fusion gene. Ann Hematol. 2014;93:1931–3. Germany.

Management of Treatment-Related Complications in Acute Promyelocytic Leukemia

21

Ombretta Annibali and Giuseppe Avvisati

Introduction

Since the first use, by Chinese investigators, of all-*trans* retinoic acid (ATRA) [1] and of arsenic trioxide (ATO) [2] in the treatment of acute promyelocytic leukemia (APL), the survival rates of this type of leukemia have significantly improved reaching 80–90% of all the patients receiving therapeutic regimens including one or both these drugs [3]. Despite that, severe hemorrhagic and to a less extent thrombotic complications can still occur and cause early death (see Chap. 5). Further, new toxicities related to the use of ATRA and ATO have emerged which may complicate the course of this disease. Herein, we describe the management of complications, other than thrombohemorrhagic, observed in APL patients related to the use of ATRA and/or ATO.

Common Complications Shared by ATRA and ATO in APL

Differentiation Syndrome

The first identified complication of ATRA treatment was the differentiation syndrome (DS), previously referred to as retinoic acid syndrome (RAS) [4]. This syndrome is a relatively common and potentially severe complication seen in patients with APL treated with ATRA [4] and/or ATO [5] characterized in its first description by fever, dyspnea, hypotension, and pleural and pericardial effusions. It occurs in about 10–25% of APL patients during the first days or weeks after the start of ATRA and/or ATO [6–8]. So far, no reliable factors can predict which patients are more or less likely to develop DS after treatment with ATRA or ATO. Nevertheless, an increased incidence has been reported in patients with an elevated white blood cell (WBC) count at diagnosis or a rapidly increasing WBC count [9]. It is important, however, to recognize that the syndrome can also occur in the absence of an elevated WBC count. Another factor which has been proposed as predictive of DS is an elevated body mass index (BMI) [10].

The etiology of DS is not fully understood, but it is thought to be due to the release of inflammatory vasoactive cytokines causing capillary leak syndrome with fever, edema, rash, and hypotension [11–13]. It has also been suggested that the maturation of promyelocytes induced by ATRA or ATO may induce changes in the adhesive properties of APL cells that promote the aggregation of promyelocytes, with subsequent leukostasis, vessel occlusion, and tissue infiltration by the maturing cells [14].

DS has been defined by the GIMEMA group as *definitely present* in the presence of the

O. Annibali, M.D., Ph.D. • G. Avvisati, M.D., Ph.D. (✉)
UOC Hematology, Stem Cell Transplantation, University Hospital Campus Bio Medico, Via Alvaro del Portillo 21, Rome 00128, Italy
e-mail: g.avvisati@unicampus.it

O. Abla et al. (eds.), *Acute Promyelocytic Leukemia*, https://doi.org/10.1007/978-3-319-64257-4_21

following five signs and symptoms: fever, dyspnea, pleural and/or pericardial effusion, pulmonary infiltrates on chest radiograph, and weight gain >5 kg; DS is defined as "indeterminate" in the presence of two to four of the above signs and symptoms, associated or not with lower extremity edema and/or hypotension [15]. More recently, the PETHEMA group revised the DS grading system and classified patients into those with severe DS (presence of four or more of the following signs and symptoms: dyspnea, unexplained fever, weight gain greater than 5 kg, unexplained hypotension, acute renal failure, and, particularly, a chest radiograph demonstrating pulmonary infiltrates or pleuropericardial effusion) or moderate DS (presence of 2–3 of the previous signs or symptoms) [16].

Until now, no single sign or symptom has been identified to be sufficient to diagnose DS, since these symptoms may be associated with other conditions such as infections, septic shock, or hemorrhage. Considering that the diagnosis can be subtle and elusive, a high index of suspicion is required for the early recognition of DS. In case of suspected DS, it is recommended to discontinue the administration of ATRA and/or ATO and to administer dexamethasone (10 mg total dose, intravenous every 12 h for a minimum of 3 days) associated with a diuretic (furosemide) if needed; however, some investigators suggest that ATRA and/or ATO treatment should be discontinued only in case of severe DS [16]. In order to reduce the incidence and severity of DS, some clinical trials have included the administration of prophylactic steroids to all patients with APL during induction therapy [15, 17, 18]. However, a prospective randomized trial is required to determine whether this approach decreases the incidence and mortality of DS. In patients with respiratory distress, temporary cessation of ATRA and/or ATO is recommended. Both drugs may be restarted once the syndrome has resolved.

In some patients, DS may also cause a significant decline in the left ventricular ejection fraction (LVEF) [19], and there are reports of coronary vasospasm and myocardial stunning in the setting of this syndrome [20, 21].

Hyperleukocytosis

Hyperleukocytosis is a well-known and frequent side effect of both ATRA [22, 23] and ATO [24, 25]. The marked increase in the WBC count is due to the rapid maturation induced by ATRA and/or ATO of a large mass of leukemic cells, which may result in leukostasis. Hyperleukocytosis can be successfully managed using hydroxyurea.

Complications Related to the Use of ATRA in APL

Pseudotumor Cerebri

Idiopathic intracranial hypertension (IIH), commonly called pseudotumor cerebri (PTC), is the second most common complication of ATRA, initially described by Mahmoud et al. in children with APL [26]. Children and adolescents with APL treated with ATRA have higher rates of PTC (9%, especially in children <10 years of age) [7] compared to adults (3% in large adult trials) [27]; PTC may or may not be associated with DS. The incidence in children decreased with the use of lower doses of ATRA (25 mg/m^2/day) in the most recent pediatric clinical trials [28]. In fact, a lower dose of ATRA had proven to be effective in a previously reported dose reduction trial for adult APL [29]. However, despite such reduction, both headaches and PTC are still observed. The risk of PTC may increase with the concurrent use of azole antifungal agents, which can increase ATRA plasma levels by inhibiting cytochrome P450-mediated ATRA catabolism [30]. PTC has also been anecdotally reported with the use of ATO [31].

The diagnosis of PTC during APL treatment is routinely suspected in patients with severe headache, nausea and vomiting, papilledema, retinal hemorrhage, ocular pain, and visual changes and/or vision loss. The risk of vision loss increases if PTC is prolonged. Patient evaluation should include neurologic and ophthalmologic examination (ocular fundi and visual fields assessment), cerebrospinal fluid (CSF) opening pressure and cell count, and neuroimaging studies such as a computed tomography (CT) or magnetic resonance imaging (MRI). The diagnosis of PTC is confirmed in the presence of elevated CSF opening pressure, normal CSF cell count, and negative neuroimaging studies. If symptoms persist, therapeutic options include the temporary discontinuation or dose reduction of ATRA, major analgesic drugs (codeine or morphine sulfate), and/or the administration of steroids and acetazolamide [27]. In the majority of reported cases, PTC tends to be transient and reversible and can be resolved with medical intervention.

The mechanism of ATRA-related PTC is similar to that of vitamin A toxicity, which is a known cause of PTC, since high doses of ATRA can enhance the production of the CSF. In a study comparing CSF retinol levels in patients with idiopathic PTC to those without PTC, a higher level of vitamin A was noted in the CSF of affected patients, none of whom had known vitamin A toxicity [32]. In addition, ATRA may alter the lipid constituents of the arachnoid villi, which disturbs the normal transport system thus preventing the absorption of CSF [33].

In 2013, the diagnostic criteria for PTC syndrome were modified and currently include papilledema, normal neurologic exam except for cranial nerve abnormalities, normal neuroimaging without evidence of hydrocephalus, mass or structural lesion, and no abnormal meningeal enhancement on MRI or contrast-enhanced CT, normal CSF composition, and elevated CSF opening pressure (250 mm CSF in adults or 280 mm CSF in children). Further, the diagnosis can be made in the absence of papilledema if all of the above criteria are satisfied and the patient has unilateral or bilateral abducens nerve palsy. If there is neither papilledema nor a sixth cranial nerve palsy, the diagnosis can be suggested, but not confirmed with additional neuroimaging characteristics [34]. Although headache is the most common presenting symptom of PTC [35], it is not part of the 2013 diagnostic criteria.

Mucocutaneous Complications

The toxicity of ATRA, other than DS, is dose related [36] and mostly involves the skin and mucous membranes. Dermatologic complications consist of skin/mucous membrane dryness (77%), rash (54%), pruritus (20%), alopecia (14%), and skin changes (14%). The mucocutaneous complications of ATRA treatment include dryness of the skin, cheilitis, erythema, pruritus, alopecia, skin changes, Sweet's syndrome, and, very rarely, scrotal ulcerations.

Skin Dryness

Most APL patients on ATRA treatment may develop this complication, which is generally associated with erythema of the skin, mouth, eyes, and lips (cheilitis). In its severe form, this complication may mimic exfoliative dermatitis, a rare and potentially serious skin disorder, in which the skin is diffusely red and inflamed with varying degrees and types of scaling [37].

Cheilitis

Cheilitis is an acute or chronic inflammation of the lips which may be caused by systemic or topical retinoids. It usually involves the lip vermilion and the vermilion border, although the surrounding skin and oral mucosa may also be affected. Common symptoms include erythema, dryness, scaling, fissuring, edema, itching, and burning. It is a frequently observed side effect during ATRA treatment, but most cases are mild to moderate. Patients should be advised to avoid lip balms containing flavors, preservatives, propolis, lanolin, and other potential allergens. Simple emollients can be liberally used in combination with topical corticosteroids, which can help in reducing inflammation and pruritus [37].

Erythema Nodosum

Erythema nodosum is a very rare complication of ATRA treatment. Kuo et al. have described four patients with classic APL who developed erythema nodosum during ATRA therapy [38]. Fever and subsequent multiple painful erythematous nodules over the extremities developed between days 12 and 19, respectively, after ATRA therapy. Skin biopsy was consistent with erythema nodosum. All patients received a short course of steroids, with rapid resolution of the fever and skin lesions. All patients achieved complete remission without withdrawal of ATRA [38].

Sweet's Syndrome

Sweet's syndrome is an acute febrile neutrophilic dermatosis characterized by nonpruritic skin lesions on the face, neck, chest, and extremities associated with fever [39, 40]. Skin biopsy shows a predominantly neutrophilic infiltration in the dermis without leukocytoclastic vasculitis. The cutaneous lesions and the clinical symptoms improve rapidly after starting treatment with systemic corticosteroids. The etiology can be idiopathic (72%), parainflammatory to infections, autoimmune disorders, vaccination (16%), paraneoplastic to hemoproliferative disorders or solid malignant tumors (11%), or pregnancy related (2%) [40]. Few cases of Sweet's syndrome have been described in the medical literature following the initiation of ATRA therapy in APL [41–44]. The recognition of Sweet's syndrome induced by ATRA therapy is of clinical importance because it requires management different from that for cutaneous infection (herpes virus, fungi) or drug-induced vasculitis. Corticosteroids rapidly improve the cutaneous and systemic signs, allowing ATRA therapy to be continued without interruption in some cases [42].

Sweet's syndrome has been also associated with DS [44], since these two syndromes share several features such as fever, infiltration of neutrophils, and dramatic improvement with steroid therapy. However, in addition to the previous case, in the literature there is only another case of Sweet's syndrome preceding DS [7].

Scrotal Ulcerations

Another adverse effect of ATRA treatment in APL is represented by scrotal ulcerations [45–48]. It remains unclear why the ulcers occur on the scrotum, but it may be that the thin skin of this area may be more susceptible to retinoic acid and thus more prone to develop lesions. However, its pathogenesis remains unknown. In almost all patients, genital ulcers with concomitant fever appeared after 17–32 days from the start of ATRA. Intravenous dexamethasone was able to control the progression of scrotal ulcers in some patients; however ATRA should be discontinued in case of failure of steroid therapy. Therefore, it is important to recognize genital ulcers associated with ATRA in order to take the appropriate measures.

Lipid Profile

In most patients treated with doses >50 mg/m^2/day of ATRA, mild to moderate increase in triglyceride level has been observed. However, discontinuation of ATRA and the use of drugs against hypertriglyceridemia are not usually recommended [49].

Rare Adverse Effects of ATRA in APL

Other very rare complications of ATRA treatment in APL have been reported and include endocrine and metabolic adverse effects, such as hypercalcemia, male infertility, bone marrow necrosis, fibrosis, and acute pancreatitis [50]. Investigators dealing with the treatment of APL should keep in mind the possibility that signs and symptoms indicating these rare complications may appear acutely during ATRA induction or during follow-up as late complications. Discontinuation of ATRA is mandatory in case of acute onset of hypercalcemia, pancreatitis, or bone marrow fibrosis. ATRA may be restarted once the patient has recovered from the complication and definitely discontinued in case of recurrence.

Complications Related to the Use of ATO in APL

Arsenic trioxide (ATO) treatment is associated with several toxicities including prolongation of QTc interval, hepatotoxicity, neurotoxicity, mucocutaneous toxicities, fluid retention, and nephrotoxicity. Usually, none of these complications is known to compromise the successful control of APL by ATO. However, during the consolidation phase, occurrence of these complications is very rare, so it is possible that complications are due to toxic effects of the drug together with toxic products released by leukemic cells. The side effects of ATO are dose related, and in the presence of severe complications, the dose of this drug should be reduced or discontinued. In this regard, it is interesting to note that a lower ATO dosage of 0.8 mg/Kg has been reported to be equally effective for patients with APL [51].

Prolongation of QTc Interval

Electrocardiographic (ECG) prolongation of the QTc interval is a common and well-documented side effect of ATO, while it is not observed with ATRA treatment. The GIMEMA-SAL-AMLSG APL0406 trial reported prolonged QTc interval in 15 patients in the ATRA-ATO group (16%) [24]. QTc prolongation can lead to torsade de pointes-type ventricular arrhythmia, which can be potentially fatal. In this context, possible interaction with other drugs that prolong the QTc interval must be taken into account because several drugs are responsible to prolong QT interval and/or induce torsade de pointes [52]. For this reason, close ECG and electrolytes monitoring is necessary during treatment with ATO. In particular, the Mg^{++} and K^{+} levels should always be kept in the high normal range, taking into account possible concomitant treatments that may deplete electrolytes (e.g., amphotericin B, furosemide, etc.).

QT interval is represented by the QRS complex, the ST segment, and the T wave. Its measurement starts from the deepest point of Q wave to the end of T wave. This interval greatly depends on the heart rate, and several formulas have been proposed to adjust the QT interval for heart rate in order to obtain the corrected QT interval (QTc); however, none of these proposed formulas is entirely satisfactory [53–55]. Despite that, data from the medical literature indicate that one of the most simple methods for adjusting the QT interval for heart rate is the Framingham formula [55]. Applying this formula, a QTc (corrected QT) interval > 450 milliseconds (ms) for men and >460 ms for women must be considered prolonged. Despite the relatively high frequency of QT prolongation during ATO treatment, clinically significant arrhythmias are very rare and none were reported in the most recent trials employing ATO as first-line therapy. International guidelines recommend maintaining potassium and magnesium concentrations above 4.0 mEq/L and 1.8 mg/dL, respectively, in order to reduce the risk of QTc prolongation and to discontinue other concurrent drugs that may cause QTc prolongation during ATO therapy [27]. In patients with a prolonged QTc interval above 500 msec, ATO should be withheld, electrolytes repleted, and other drugs that may prolong QTc interval discontinued until normalization of the QTc [27].

Hepatotoxicity

Hepatotoxicity during ATO treatment is defined as an increase in serum bilirubin and/or ALT and/or alkaline phosphatase >5 times the normal upper level. This toxicity has frequently been reported in studies employing ATO with or without ATRA, especially in terms of increase in liver enzymes (mostly ALT and AST, less frequently alkaline phosphatase and bilirubin). This complication may occur in up to 60% of cases [24]; however it is generally reversible and successfully managed with a decrease or temporary discontinuation of ATO and/or ATRA. No cases of hepatic failure have been reported in recent trials [24, 25].

In general, hepatotoxicity develops about 5–10 days after initiation of ATO. The peak transaminase levels rarely exceed five times the upper reference value [56]. Increases in bilirubin and ductal enzymes including alkaline phosphatase and γ-glutamyl transpeptidase (γ-GT) are uncommon and if present should prompt investigation for other causes of cholestasis. A few cases of fulminant hepatic failure have been reported when ATO was used in patients with newly diagnosed APL [57]; however, this phenomenon has not been confirmed subsequently. When the transaminases are less than three times normal, our experience shows that ATO therapy can be continued at half the original dose. The liver function usually normalizes within a week, and resumption of full dose treatment or at the reduced dose is subsequently well tolerated [57]. This transient hepatotoxicity may or may not recur during subsequent ATO treatment. However, when the transaminases exceed three times normal, temporary cessation of ATO treatment may be needed. The hepatotoxicity usually resolves within a week, and treatment at half the original dose, with gradual escalation to full dose, can be restarted.

Distinct from intravenous (IV) ATO, the full dose of oral ATO enters first the portal circulation and subsequently the liver; despite that, oral ATO does not cause more liver toxicity than IV ATO.

Data from chronic arsenic poisoning studies suggest that liver fibrosis, cirrhosis, and hepatocellular carcinoma may occur [58–60]. Therefore, a prolonged therapeutic use of ATO may require close monitoring. So far, cirrhosis and hepatocellular carcinoma during the follow-up of APL treated with therapeutic doses of ATO have not been reported. In chronic carriers of hepatitis B virus (HBV), lamivudine prophylaxis to prevent viral reactivation has been advocated [61] although such a strategy has not been validated in control trials. Since both HBV and chronic arsenic exposure predispose to cirrhosis and hepatocellular carcinoma [62], it may be prudent to prescribe prophylactic antiviral treatment to avoid potential synergistic ATO and HBV hepatic damage. Finally, other hepatotoxic drugs used in the clinical course of leukemia, including antibiotics and the azole antifungal drugs, should also be used with caution during ATO therapy.

Neurotoxicity

Peripheral neuropathy is reported in up to 10% of ATO-treated patients [63, 64]. The incidence may be even higher when other predisposing conditions are present, including old age, diabetes mellitus, multiple myeloma, and the concurrent administration of neurotoxic drugs. A glove and stocking sensory neuropathy is typical, with electrophysiological studies showing reduced sensory action potentials with delayed conduction. Muscle atrophy has been occasionally reported after prolonged exposure [65]. Gradual improvement occurs when ATO is reduced in dosage or discontinued. Sural nerve biopsies performed in a few severe cases have not shown specific histopathological features. Severe functional deficits are unusual, and the presence of serious neuropathies during ATO treatment should prompt investigations for other causes. The blood-brain barrier (BBB) prevents heavy metals, including arsenic, from penetrating the CNS. Therefore, CNS side effects and encephalopathies during ATO therapy have not been reported. Hence, mental confusion in a patient on ATO should lead to investigations for other causes, such as CNS leukemia, viral encephalitis, alcoholism, or metabolic derangements. For similar reasons, the CNS may be a sanctuary site for leukemic cells, and isolated CNS relapse in patients who responded to front-line ATO treatment has been described [66]. Suspected Wernicke's encephalopathy associated with ATO treatment has been reported [67]. However, abnormalities in thiamine pyrophosphate and erythrocyte transketolase levels in consecutive patients on prolonged ATO treatment have not been observed, so that routine vitamin B_1 supplements do not seem to be warranted. Long-term follow-up has not shown unusual CNS manifestations in patients after chronic treatment with ATO, although behavioral abnormalities have been reported in animals with chronic arsenic exposure since birth [68].

Entry of arsenic into the CNS, however, may occur when the BBB is compromised. In a case of meningeal relapse of APL treated with oral ATO, penetration of arsenic into the cerebrospinal fluid to therapeutically meaningful levels has been demonstrated [69].

A prominent but innocuous side effect when ATO is combined with ATRA is severe headache [70]. Brain CT scan and fundoscopic examination have occasionally shown signs of PTC [31]. Although this side effect is stressful and alarming, the headache usually responds well to analgesic treatment and dose splitting of ATRA or ATO, and no long-term sequelae have been reported.

Dermatologic Toxicity

Chronic arsenic exposure results in various skin manifestations, including hyperpigmentation, keratosis, and squamous cell carcinoma (SCC). The therapeutic use of ATO results in cumulative doses well below that reported environmental or occupational arsenic exposure that leads to these skin manifestations [58]. The commonest dermatologic problem during ATO treatment is increased skin pigmentation [60]. So far, squamous cell carcinoma has not been reported. Abnormal pigmentation is reversible after cessation of ATO treatment. If severe or persistent pigmentation occurs, then other causes, including porphyria and hemosiderosis, must be excluded [71].

Skin rash is the second most common problem. A late-onset painful and erythematous rash can be observed after prolonged arsenic treatment, which could be related partly to the vasoconstrictive effects of the drug [72]. The concomitant use of ATRA may also worsen the skin rash. In severe cases, temporary dose reduction or even cessation of ATO may be required. An allergic type, measles-like, pruritic rash has also been observed [64]. Skin rashes usually respond well to corticosteroid treatment, and ATO treatment can be continued without interruption.

Fluid Retention

Edema of the hands, legs, and face after ATO treatment has also been described [65], which may be related to fluid retention as part of the APL-related DS.

Viral Reactivation

In addition to HBV reactivation, another intriguing side effect of ATO treatment is reactivation of latent herpes virus (HSV) infections [73]. Both herpes simplex and herpes zoster (VZV) reactivation may occur. During ATO treatment, VZV reactivation occurs in up to 25% of patients within the first year of treatment [74]. Recognition of this association is important, since the timely treatment of VZV may shorten the duration of symptoms and decrease post-herpetic complications.

Nephrotoxicity

Since ATO has a predominant renal excretion, its dose should be reduced in patients with renal dysfunction. With appropriate dose adjustment and monitoring of arsenic levels, a patient with relapsed APL, on continuous peritoneal dialysis, has been successfully treated with oral ATO [75].

Miscellaneous Toxicities

Gastrointestinal symptoms have been frequently reported with IV ATO [64]. For patients receiving oral ATO, mild nausea and dyspepsia are common [76]. Most patients respond to symptomatic treatment, and cessation or dose reduction of arsenic compounds is usually not required. Carcinogenicity and mutagenicity are common concerns for antineoplastic agents. In populations exposed to chronic environmental arsenic, a higher incidence of skin and liver cancer has been observed, together with chromosomal instability [77]. An increased incidence of cancer of the skin, lung, and liver has also been reported after industrial and agricultural arsenic exposure [78, 79]. The risk of secondary cancers after ATO treatment is not well defined.

Conclusions

The introduction of ATRA and ATO as targeted therapy for APL has significantly improved the long-term outcome of this disease, which was once considered one of the most fatal malignancies. With the combined use of these agents, patients are now able to achieve a cure rate of 85–90%. However, it is important to recognize that both of these agents have toxicities different from those observed with anthracyclines or other chemotherapeutic agents. Table 21.1 summarizes recommendations for the management of DS and other serious complications observed with the use of ATRA and ATO in APL.

Table 21.1 Management of the most common complications associated with the use of ATRA and/or ATO in APL

Drug	Complication	Signs and symptoms	Management
ATRA and/or ATO	Differentiation syndrome	**GIMEMA definition**: • *Definitely present* 1. Fever 2. Dyspnea 3. Hypotension 4. Pleural and pericardial effusions 5. Weight gain >5 kg • *Indetermined* 2 or 4 of the above **PETHEMA definition**: • *Severe DS* 1. Fever 2. Weight gain >5 kg 3. Hypotension 4. Acute renal failure 5. Pulmonary infiltrates or pleuropericardial effusions • *Moderate DS* 2 or 3 of the above	• IV dexamethasone 10 mg BID until complete resolution of signs and symptoms • Temporary discontinuation of ATRA and/or ATO is mandatory in case of a definitely present or severe DS
	Hyperleukocytosis	• *Rapid WBC increase ($WBC > 10 \times 10^9/L$)*	• Hydroxyurea, gemtuzumab ozogamycin, or anthracyclines (idarubicin or daunorubicin) may be used
	Hepatotoxicity	• *Increase in serum bilirubin and/or ALT and/or alkaline phosphatase > 5 times the upper normal level*	• ATRA and/or ATO should be temporarily discontinued until normalization of hepatic function tests
ATRA	Pseudotumor cerebri	• ***DIAGNOSIS before*** 2013: • *Suspected* 1. Severe headache 2. Nausea and/or vomiting 3. Papilledema 4. Retinal hemorrhages 5. Visual changes and/or vision loss • *Confirmed* 1. Increased CSF pressure 2. Normal CSF composition 3. Normal neuroimaging • ***DEFINITION after*** 2013: • Papilledema • Cranial nerve abnormalities • Normal neuroimaging • Normal CSF composition • Elevated CSF opening pressure	• Temporary discontinuation of ATRA is recommended • Use of analgesics (opiates) to control headaches • Steroids and diuretics (acetazolamide or furosemide) • Close ophthalmological monitoring • Repeated lumbar punctures with CSF removal
ATO	QTc interval prolongation	• *Prolongation of corrected QT (QTc) interval > 500 ms*	• Withhold ATO until normalization of QTc interval • Patient must be monitored with daily ECG until normalization of QTc interval

References

1. Huang ME, Ye YC, Chen SR, Chai J, Lu JX, Zhoa L, et al. Use of all trans-retinoic acid in the treatment of acute promyelocytic leukemia. Blood. 1988;72:567–72.
2. Shen ZX, Chen GQ, Ni JH, Li XS, Xiong SM, Qiu QY, et al. Use of arsenic trioxide (As2O3) in the treatment of acute promyelocytic leukemia (APL): II. Clinical efficacy and pharmacokinetics in relapsed patients. Blood. 1997;89:3354–60.
3. Wang ZY, Chen Z. Acute promyelocytic leukemia: from highly fatal to highly curable. Blood. 2008;111:505–15.
4. Frankel SR, Eardley A, Lauwers G, Weiss M, Warrell RP Jr. The "retinoic acid syndrome" in acute promyelocytic leukemia. Ann Intern Med. 1992;117:292–6.
5. Camacho LH, Soignet SL, Chanel S, Ho R, Heller G, Scheinberg DA, et al. Leukocytosis and the retinoic acid syndrome in patients with acute promyelocytic leukemia treated with arsenic trioxide. J Clin Oncol. 2000;18:2620–5.
6. Tallman MS, Andersen JW, Schiffer CA, Appelbaum FR, Feusner JH, Ogden A, et al. All-trans-retinoic acid in acute promyelocytic leukemia. N Engl J Med. 1997;337:1021–8.
7. De Botton S, Dombret H, Sanz M, Miguel JS, Caillot D, Zittoun R, et al. Incidence, clinical features, and outcome of all trans-retinoic acid syndrome in 413 cases of newly diagnosed acute promyelocytic leukemia: the European APL Group. Blood. 1998;92:2712–8.
8. Soignet SL, Frankel SR, Douer D, Tallman MS, Kantarjian H, Calleja E, et al. United States multicenter study of arsenic trioxide in relapsed acute promyelocytic leukemia. J Clin Oncol. 2001;19:3852–60.
9. Vahdat L, Maslak P, Miller WH Jr, Eardley A, Heller G, Scheinberg DA, et al. Early mortality and the retinoic acid syndrome in acute promyelocytic leukemia: impact of leukocytosis, low-dose chemotherapy, PML/RAR-alpha isoform, and CD13 expression in patients treated with all-trans retinoic acid. Blood. 1994;84:3843–9.
10. Breccia M, Mazzarella L, Bagnardi V, Disalvatore D, Loglisci G, Cimino G, et al. Increased BMI correlates with higher risk of disease relapse and differentiation syndrome in patients with acute promyelocytic leukemia treated with the AIDA protocols. Blood. 2012;119:49–54.
11. Luesink M, Pennings JL, Wissink WM, Linssen PC, Muus P, Pfundt R, et al. Chemokine induction by all-trans retinoic acid and arsenic trioxide in acute promyelocytic leukemia: triggering the differentiation syndrome. Blood. 2009;114:5512–21.
12. Luesink M, Jansen JH. Advances in understanding the pulmonary infiltration in acute promyelocytic leukaemia. Br J Haematol. 2010;151:209 20.
13. Larson RS, Tallman MS. Retinoic acid syndrome: manifestations, pathogenesis, and treatment. Best Pract Res Clin Haematol. 2003;16:453–61.
14. Lin C-P, Huang MJ, Chang IY, Lin WY, Sheu YT. Retinoic acid syndrome induced by arsenic trioxide in treating recurrent all-trans retinoic acid resistant acute promyelocytic leukemia. Leuk Lymphoma. 2000;38:195–8.
15. Avvisati G, Lo-Coco F, Paoloni FP, Petti MC, Diverio D, Vignetti M, et al. AIDA0493 protocol for newly diagnosed acute promyelocytic leukemia: very long-term results and role of maintenance. Blood. 2011;117:4716–25.
16. Sanz MA, Montesinos P. How we prevent and treat differentiation syndrome in patients with acute promyelocytic leukemia. Blood. 2014;123:2777–82.
17. Sanz MA, Martin G, Gonzalez M, et al. Risk-adapted treatment of acute promyelocytic leukemia with all-trans-retinoic acid and anthracycline monochemotherapy: a multicenter study by the PETHEMA group. Blood. 2004;103:1237–43.
18. Wiley JS, Firkin FC. Reduction of pulmonary toxicity by prednisolone prophylaxis during all-trans retinoic acid treatment of acute promyelocytic leukemia. Australian Leukaemia Study Group. Leukemia. 1995;9:774–8.
19. Tallman MS, Andersen JW, Schiffer CA, Appelbaum FR, Feusner JH, Ogden A, et al. Clinical description of 44 patients with acute promyelocytic leukemia who developed the retinoic acid syndrome. Blood. 2000;95:90–5.
20. De Santis GC, Madeira MIA, de Oliveira LCO, Falcao RP, Rego EM. Cardiac stunning as a manifestation of ATRA differentiation syndrome in acute promyelocytic leukemia. Med Oncol. 2012;29:248–50.
21. Maqsood K, Mirrani G, Sarwar N, Burke JF. Coronary vasospasm mimicking ST-elevation myocardial infarction in a patient with ATRA-induced differentiation syndrome: a case report and review of literature. J Hematol. 2013;2:27–30.
22. Montesinos P, Bergua JM, Vellenga E, Rayón C, Parody R, de la Serna J, et al. Differentiation syndrome in patients with acute promyelocytic leukemia treated with all-trans retinoic acid and anthracycline chemotherapy: characteristics, outcome, and prognostic factors. Blood. 2009;113:775–83.
23. Kelaidi C, Chevret S, De Botton S, Raffoux E, Guerci A, Thomas X, et al. Improved outcome of acute promyelocytic leukemia with high WBC counts over the last 15 years: the European APL Group experience. J Clin Oncol. 2009;27:2668–76.
24. Lo-Coco F, Avvisati G, Vignetti M, Thiede C, Orlando SM, Iacobelli S, et al. Retinoic acid and arsenic trioxide for acute promyelocytic leukemia. N Engl J Med. 2013;369:111–21.
25. Burnett A, Russell NH, Hills RK, Bowen D, Kell J, Knapper S, et al. Arsenic trioxide and all-trans retinoic acid treatment for acute promyelocytic leukemia in all risk groups (AML17): results of a randomised, controlled, phase 3 trial. Lancet Oncol. 2015;16:1295–305.
26. Mahmoud HH, Hurwitz CA, Roberts WM, Santana VM, Ribeiro RC, Krance RA, et al. Tretinoin toxicity in children with acute promyelocytic leukemia. Lancet. 1993;342:1394–5.

27. Sanz MA, Grimwade D, Tallman MS, Lowenberg B, Fenaux P, Estey EH, et al. Management of acute promyelocytic leukemia recommendations from an panel on behalf of the European Leukemia Net. Blood. 2009;113:1875–91.
28. Testi AM, Biondi A, Lo Coco F, Moleti ML, Giona F, Vignetti M, et al. GIMEMA-AIEOP AIDA protocol for the treatment of newly diagnosed acute promyelocytic leukemia (APL) in children. Blood. 2005;106:447–53.
29. Castaigne S, Lefebvre P, Chomienne C, Suc E, Rigal-Huguet F, Gardiin C, et al. Effectiveness and pharmacokinetics of low-dose all-trans retinoic acid (25 mg/m2) in acute promyelocytic leukemia. Blood. 1993;82:3560–3.
30. Yarali N, Tavil B, Kara A, Ozkasap S, Tunç B. Acute renal failure during ATRA treatment. Pediatr Hematol Oncol. 2008;25:115–8.
31. Galm O, Fabry U, Osieka R. Pseudotumor cerebri after treatment of relapsed acute promyelocytic leukemia with arsenic trioxide. Leukemia. 2000;14:343–4.
32. Warner JE, Bernstein PS, Yemelyanov A, Alder SC, Farnsworth ST, Digre KB. Vitamin A in the cerebrospinal fluid of patients with and without idiopathic intracranial hypertension. Ann Neurol. 2002;52:647–50.
33. Anoop TM, Jain N, Nair SG, Narayanan G. All-trans-retinoic acid-induced pseudotumor cerebri in acute promyelocytic leukemia. J Neurosci Rural Pract. 2014;5:273–5.
34. Friedman DI, Liu GT, Digre KB. Revised diagnostic criteria for the pseudotumor cerebri syndrome in adults and children. Neurology. 2013;81:1159–65.
35. Mallery RM, Friedman DI, Liu GT. Headache and the pseudotumor cerebri syndrome. Curr Pain Headache Rep. 2014;18:1–8.
36. Sanz MA, Montesinos P, Vellenga E, Rayón C, de la Serna J, Parody R, et al. Risk-adapted treatment of acute promyelocytic leukemia with all-trans retinoic acid and anthracycline monochemotherapy: long-term outcome of the LPA 99 multicenter study by the PETHEMA Group. Blood. 2008;112:3130–4.
37. Yacoub MR, Berti A, Campochiaro C, Tombetti E, Ramirez GA, Nico A, Di Leo E, Fantini P, Sabbadini MG, Nettis E, Colombo G. Drug induced exfoliative dermatitis: state of the art. Clin Mol Allergy. 2016;14:9.
38. Kuo MC, Dunn P, Wu JH, Shih LY. All- trans-retinoic acid-induced erythema nodosum in patients with acute promyelocytic leukemia. Ann Hematol. 2004;83:376–80.
39. Sweet RD. An acute febrile neutrophilic dermatosis. Br J Dermatol. 1964;76:349–56.
40. Von den Driesch P. Sweet's syndrome (acute febrile neutrophilic dermatosis). J Am Acad Dermatol. 1994;31:535–56.
41. Arun B, Berberian B, Azumi N, Frankel SR, Luksenburg H, Freter C. Sweet's syndrome during treatment with all trans retinoic acid in a patient with acute promyelocytic leukemia. Leuk Lymphoma. 1998;31:613–5.
42. Christ E, Linka A, Jacky E, Speich R, Marincek B, Schaffner A. Sweet's syndrome involving the musculoskeletal system during treatment of promyelocytic leukemia with all trans retinoic acid. Leukemia. 1996;10:731–4.
43. Shirono K, Kiyofuji C, Tsuda H. Sweet's syndrome in a patient with acute promyelocytic leukemia during treatment with all-trans retinoic acid. Int J Hematol. 1995;62:183–7.
44. Takada S, Matumoto K, Sakura T, Shiozaki H, Miyawaki S. Sweet's syndrome followed by retinoic acid syndrome during the treatment of acute promyelocytic leukemia with all-trans retinoic acid. Int J Hematol. 1999;70:26–9.
45. Pavithran K, Arjun R, Aruna R, Thomas M. Scrotal ulceration during induction therapy of acute promyelocytic leukemia with ATRA. Am J Hematol. 2004;75:260–1.
46. Mori A, Tamura S, Katsuno T, et al. Scrotal ulcer occurring in patients with acute promyelocytic leukemia during treatment with all-trans-retinoic acid. Oncol Rep. 1999;6:55–8.
47. Charles KS, Kanaa M, Winfield DA, Reilly JT. Scrotal ulceration during ATRA therapy for acute promyelocytic leukemia. Clin Lab Haematol. 2000;22:171–4.
48. Esser AC, Nossa R, Shoji T, Sapadin AN. All-trans-retinoic acid induced scrotal ulceration in a patient with acute promyelocytic leukemia. J Am Acad Dermatol. 2000;43:316–7.
49. Kanamaru A, Takemoto Y, Tanimoto M, Murakami H, Asou N, Kobayashi T, et al. All-trans retinoic acid for the treatment of newly diagnosed acute promyelocytic leukemia. Blood. 2015;85:1202–6.
50. Hatake K, Uwai M, Ohtsuki T, Tomizuka H, Izumi T, Yoshida M, et al. Rare but important adverse effects of all-trans retinoic acid in acute promyelocytic leukemia and their management. Int J Hematol. 1997;66:13–9.
51. Shen Y, Shen ZX, Yan H, Chen J, Zeng XY, Li JM, et al. Studies on the clinical efficacy and pharmacokinetics of low-dose arsenic trioxide in the treatment of relapsed acute promyelocytic leukemia: a comparison with conventional dosage. Leukemia. 2001;15:735–41.
52. Gowda RM, Khan IA, Wilbur SL, Vasavada BC, Sacchi TJ. Torsade de pointes: the clinical considerations. Int J Cardiol. 2004;96:1–6.
53. Luo S, Michler K, Johnston P, Peter W, Macfarlane PW. A comparison of commonly used QT correction formulae: The effect of heart rate on the QTc of normal ECGs. J Electrocardiol. 2004;37(Suppl):81–90.
54. Indik JH, Pearson EC, Fried K, Woosley RL. Bazett and Fridericia QT correction formulas interfere with measurement of drug-induced changes in QT interval. Heart Rhythm. 2006;3:1003–7.
55. Sagie A, Larson ML, Goldberg RJ, Bengtson JR, Levy D. An improved method for adjusting the QT interval for heart rate (the Framingham Heart Study). Am J Cardiol. 1992;70:797–1.
56. Au WY, Kumana CR, Kou M, Mak R, Chan GC, Lam CW, et al. Oral arsenic trioxide in the treatment of relapsed acute promyelocytic leukemia. Blood. 2003;102:407–8.
57. Niu C, Yan H, Yu T, Sun HP, Liu JX, Li XS, et al. Studies on treatment of acute promyelocytic leukemia with arsenic trioxide: remission induction, follow-up, and molecular monitoring in 11 newly diagnosed and 47 relapsed acute promyelocytic leukemia patients. Blood. 1999;94:3315–24.

58. Mazumder DN, Das Gupta J, Santra A, Pal A, Ghose A, Sarkar S. Chronic arsenic toxicity in west Bengal—the worst calamity in the world. J Indian Med Assoc. 1998;96:4–7.
59. Guha Mazumder DN. Arsenic and liver disease. J Indian Med Assoc. 2001;99:318–20.
60. Liu J, Zheng B, Aposhian HV, Zhou Y, Chen ML, Zhang A, et al. Chronic arsenic poisoning from burning high-arsenic-containing coal in Guizhou, China. Environ Health Perspect. 2002;110:119–22.
61. Lau GK, Yiu HH, Fong DY, Cheng HC, Au WY, Lai LS, et al. Early is superior to deferred preemptive lamivudine therapy for hepatitis B patients undergoing chemotherapy. Gastroenterology. 2003;125:1742–9.
62. Lu JN, Chen CJ. Prevalence of hepatitis B surface antigen carrier status among residents in the endemic area of chronic arsenicism in Taiwan. Anticancer Res. 1991;11:229–33.
63. Lazo G, Kantarjian H, Estey E, Thomas D, O'Brien S, Cortes J. Use of arsenic trioxide (As2O3) in the treatment of patients with acute promyelocytic leukemia: the M. D. Anderson experience. Cancer. 2003;97:2218–24.
64. Ohnishi K, Yoshida H, Shigeno K, Nakamura S, Fujisawa S, Naito K, et al. Arsenic trioxide therapy for relapsed or refractory Japanese patients with acute promyelocytic leukemia: need for careful electrocardiogram monitoring. Leukemia. 2002;16:617–22.
65. Huang SY, Chang CS, Tang JL, Tien HF, Kuo TL, Huang SF, et al. Acute and chronic arsenic poisoning associated with treatment of acute promyelocytic leukaemia. Br J Haematol. 1998;103:1092–5.
66. Au WY, Ma SK, Ooi C, Liang R, Kwong YL. Unusual manifestations of acute leukemia. Case 1. CNS extramedullary relapse of acute promyelocytic leukemia after arsenic trioxide-induced remission. J Clin Oncol. 2000;18:3435–7.
67. Yip SF, Yeung YM, Tsui EY. Severe neurotoxicity following arsenic therapy for acute promyelocytic leukemia: potentiation by thiamine deficiency. Blood. 2002;99:3481–2.
68. Rodriguez VM, Carrizales L, Mendoza MS, Fajardo OR, Giordano M. Effects of sodium arsenite exposure on development and behavior in the rat. Neurotoxicol Teratol. 2002;24:743–50.
69. Au WY, Tam S, Kwong YL. Entry of elemental arsenic into the central nervous system in patients with acute promyelocytic leukemia during arsenic trioxide treatment. Leuk Res. 2008;32:357–8.
70. Au WY, Chim CS, Lie AK, Liang R, Kwong YL. Combined arsenic trioxide and all-trans retinoic acid treatment for acute promyelocytic leukaemia recurring from previous relapses successfully treated using arsenic trioxide. Br J Haematol. 2002;117:130–2.
71. Hughes GS Jr, Davis L. Variegate porphyria and heavy metal poisoning from ingestion of "moonshine". South Med J. 1983;76:1027–9.
72. Tsai SM, Wang TN, Ko YC. Mortality for certain diseases in areas with high levels of arsenic in drinking water. Arch Environ Health. 1999;54:186–93.
73. Tanvetyanon T, Nand S. Herpes zoster during treatment with arsenic trioxide. Ann Hematol. 2004;83:198–200.
74. Au WY, Kwong YL. Frequent varicella zoster reactivation associated with therapeutic use of arsenic trioxide: portents of an old scourge. J Am Acad Dermatol. 2005;53:890–2.
75. Au WY, Cheung GT, Yuen TW, Kumana CR, Kwong YL. Successful treatment of relapsed acute promyelocytic leukemia in a patient receiving continuous ambulatory peritoneal dialysis with oral arsenic trioxide. Arch Intern Med. 2005;165:1067–8.
76. Lu DP, Qiu JY, Jiang B, Wang Q, Liu KY, Liu YR, et al. Tetra-arsenic tetra-sulfide for the treatment of acute promyelocytic leukemia: a pilot report. Blood. 2002;99:3136–43.
77. Chou WC, Hawkins AL, Barrett JF, Griffin CA, Dang CV. Arsenic inhibition of telomerase transcription leads to genetic instability. J Clin Invest. 2001;108:1541–7.
78. Axelson O, Dahlgren E, Jansson CD, Rehnlund SO. Arsenic exposure and mortality: a case-referent study from a Swedish copper smelter. Br J Ind Med. 1978;35:8–15.
79. Luchtrath H. The consequences of chronic arsenic poisoning among Moselle wine growers. Pathoanatomical investigations of postmortem examinations performed between 1960 and 1977. J Cancer Res Clin Oncol. 1983;105:173–82.

Index

O. Abla et al. (eds.), *Acute Promyelocytic Leukemia*, https://doi.org/10.1007/978-3-319-64257-4

MIX
Papier aus verantwortungsvollen Quellen
Paper from responsible sources
FSC® C105338

If you have any concerns about our products,
you can contact us on
ProductSafety@springernature.com

In case Publisher is established outside the EU,
the EU authorized representative is:
Springer Nature Customer Service Center GmbH
Europaplatz 3, 69115 Heidelberg, Germany

Printed by Libri Plureos GmbH
in Hamburg, Germany